INTERNATIONAL HANDBOOK OF CROSS-CULTURAL NEUROPSYCHOLOGY

INTERNATIONAL HANDBOOK OF CROSS-CULTURAL NEUROPSYCHOLOGY

Edited by

Barbara P. Uzzell
Memorial Neurological Association

Marcel O. Pontón
Harbor-UCLA Medical Center

Alfredo Ardila
Florida International University

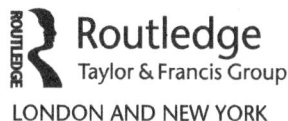

LONDON AND NEW YORK

First published 2007 by Lawrence Erlbaum Associates, Inc.

Published 2020 by Routledge
2 Park Square, Milton Park, Abingdon, Oxon OX14 4RN
52 Vanderbilt Avenue, New York, NY 10017

Routledge is an imprint of the Taylor & Francis Group, an informa business

Copyright © 2007 by Taylor & Francis

All rights reserved. No part of this book may be reprinted or reproduced or utilised in any form or by any electronic, mechanical, or other means, now known or hereafter invented, including photocopying and recording, or in any information storage or retrieval system, without permission in writing from the publishers.

Notice:
Product or corporate names may be trademarks or registered trademarks, and are used only for identification and explanation without intent to infringe.

ISBN 13: 978-0-8058-3586-1 (pbk)

Cover design by Kathryn Houghtaling Lacey

Library of Congress Cataloging-in-Publication Data

   p. cm.
   Includes bibliographical references and index.
ISBN 978-0-8058-3585-4 — 0-8058-3585-7 (cloth)
ISBN 978-0-8058-3586-1 — 0-8058-3586-5 (pbk.)

2004
—dc22   2004000000
                                                 CIP

Books published by Lawrence Erlbaum Associates are printed on acid-free paper, and their bindings are chosen for strength and durability.

Contents

Preface		ix
1	Grasping the Cross-Cultural Reality *B. P. Uzzell*	1
2	The Impact of Culture on Neuropsychological Test Performance *Alfredo Ardila*	23
3	The Art of Clinical Neuropsychology *Nathaniel William Nelson & Marcel Pontón*	45
4	Environmentalists and Nativists: The IQ Controversy in Cross-Cultural Perspective *Victor Nell*	63
5	Qualitative Assessment Within and Across Cultures *Carla Caetano*	93
6	Cognitive Abilities in Different Cultural Contexts *Alfredo Ardila & Kevin Keating*	109
7	Speech, Language, and Neuropsychological Testing: Implications for African Americans *Constance D. Qualls*	127

8 Developmental Perspectives: Culture and   145
    Neuropsychological Development During Childhood
    Lúcia W. Braga

 9 Executive Functions in Hispanics: Toward an Ecological   163
    Neuropsychology
    Carmen G. Armengol

10 Illiterates and Cognition: The Impact of Education   181
    Alfredo Ardila & Mónica Rosselli

11 Relationship Between Functional Brain Organization   199
    and Education
    Alexandre Castro-Caldas

12 Educational Effects on Cognitive Functions: 215
    Brain Reserve, Compensation, or Testing Bias?
    F. Ostrosky-Solís

13 Visuospatial Assessment in Cross-Cultural   227
    and Nonwestern Settings
    Roy Sugarman

14 Neural Circuit of Reading and Writing in the Japanese   253
    Language
    Makoto Iwata

15 Cross-Cultural Issues in Neuropsychology: Assessment   265
    of the Hispanic Patient
    Marcel Pontón & Marta E. Corona-LoMonaco

16 Clinical Neuropsychology of Spanish Speakers: 283
    The Challenge and Pitfalls of a Neuropsychology
    of a Heterogeneous Population
    Gabriel D. Salazar, Miguel Perez Garcia & Antonio E. Puente

17 Cultural Issues in Clinical Context With Asian Indian   303
    Patients: Guidelines for the Health Care Team
    Amee P. Shah

CONTENTS

18 Epidemiological, Social, and Cultural Aspects of Illness: 319
A Case Study of Brain Injuries, Stroke, and HIV/AIDS
in South Africa
Leah Gilbert & Stephen Tollman

19 Natural Recovery: An Ecological Approach 341
to Neuropsychological Recuperation
Tedd Judd & Roberta DeBoard

20 Emotions and Attitudes: Unbundling Sociocultural 371
Influences
Shirley G. Tollman

Author Index 383

Subject Index 389

Preface

Culture dictates what is and what is not relevant in a situation, and provides specific models for thinking, acting, and feeling. Cognitive abilities measured during neuropsychological assessments correlate with many factors including an individual's learning opportunities and contextual experiences within a culture. In cross-culture neuropsychology, cultural variations and similarities are evident.

Cultural diversity is an enormous, but frequently overlooked moderating variable. Theoretically, comparable cognitive disturbances can be found in every brain-damaged human regardless of cultural background, educational level, language, and ecological demands related to brain lesions. Although these may be identified, cultural influences are observable during assessment and rehabilitation of cognitive disturbances. Cultural differences reside clearer in contexts in which cognitive processes are viewed, than in noting the existence of a process in one culture group, and not in another. Culture dictates behavior, what is learned, and at what age. Consequently, different cultural environments lead to the development of different patterns of abilities, and may eventually influence organization of cognition abilities within the brain.

Clinical judgment can be biased by previous experiences from different cultures, by expectancy rates of pathology among certain groups, and by differences in socioeconomic levels. Development of a cross-cultural understanding can only occur through knowledge about the values of culture in which a brain-damaged individual lives. As clinical experiences increase with people from different cultures, the limitations of neuropsychological tools to make accurate assessments become evident. Neuropsychologists need to acknowledge the selected test instruments necessary for examining ethnic patients, the necessary language choices, the educational level influences, and the need for similar linguistically and culturally clinicians and patients. This handbook addresses cultural influences on cognitive processes as measured by neuropsychological instruments. It includes cross-culture aspects of 1) test-taking attitudes; 2) understanding health care systems; 3) understanding causality, disease, recovery, healing, rehabilitation, and caregiving; 4) behavioral and emotional attitudes and cultural norms; 5) communication pragmatics; and 6) epidemiological features in relation to cross-cultural neuropsychology.

Although it is impossible to address every single cultural group in the world, this handbook emphasizes major cultural distinctions to increase awareness of nuances, differences, and similarities between cultural groups on the continents of North and South America, Europe, Africa, Asia, and Australia where cultural diversity abounds and blends.

The contents of this handbook view assessments and rehabilitation from different perspectives, thereby offering opportunities for increasing knowledge and understanding, improving clinical skills and laying the groundwork for establishing international and cross-culture collaborations. The contributors feel the many professionals throughout the world, such as neuropsychologists, cross-cultural psychologists, social psychologists, cultural anthropologists, speech pathologists, sociologists, researchers, and international scientists, will find the material in this volume stimulating and a contribution to heightened awareness of cultural influences.

Publication of this handbook is long overdue in many ways. About 15 years ago, one of editors (BPU) approached several publishers about publishing a book addressing cultural influences on assessment and neurorehabilitation, and was informed there was no interest in such a topic in the neuropsychological community, and therefore no market for such a book. Time passage and ease of e-mail communication between neuropsychologists from different ethnic backgrounds has peaked interest. Most neuropsychologists now acknowledge cultural influences and want to increase their knowledge about the many ways culture influences assessment and rehabilitation across cultures. It is to those neuropsychologists who hunger for knowledge about cross-cultural factors that this book is dedicated. We, as editors, are grateful to the contributors who have steadfastly written informative and knowledge-filled chapters, and to Lawrence Erlbaum Associates Publishers who saw the importance of publishing this cross-culture book.

—B. P. Uzzell
—Marcel O. Pontón
—Alfredo Ardila

Chapter 1

Grasping the Cross-Cultural Reality

B. P. Uzzell
Memorial Neurological Association

Since their inception, countries around the world have been participants in a gigantic, ongoing multicultural experiment filled with cultural diversity found in both separate and overlapping geographic locations. The final outcome of the experiment is unknown, because it is ongoing. Types of coexistences, interactions, and isolations of cultures are not always predictable during this experiment. Culture edicts may induce peaceful, or not so peaceful coexistence between countries, but what role do cross-cultural edicts play in identifying commonalities and differences among cultures? The focus of this book is to provide knowledge about cross-cultural neuropsychology with is assessment and rehabilitation techniques within the context of multiculturalism.

Cultural diversity in the world has provided data not only about itself, but also about cross-cultural events and multiculturalism. These data are currently being influenced and modified by rapid air travel time and satellite communications, such as, the availability of electronic communication via e-mail, Internet, and worldwide television and radio broadcasts transmitted to many culturally diverse groups. Some say the distinctiveness among cultural groups may begin to fade as the worldwide communication accelerates.

CROSS-CULTURAL REALITY AND MULTICULTURALISM

Grasping the cross-cultural reality requires defining several terms in order to communicate with a consensual understanding. Multiculturalism within psychology has been called a social–intellectual movement promoting cultural diversity as a core principle while insisting on equality and respect of all cultural groups. At times, conflict occurs between the core principle of cultural diversity and equality in cultural groups. The apparent value and validity of psychological theories and practices (including neuropsychological theories and practices) depend on how well they fare during genuine intercultural dialogue (Fowers & Richardson, 1996). Understanding concepts of both multiculturalism and cross-cultural features require knowledge about the basic unit common to both, namely, "culture."

Cross-cultural considerations reflect a quest for universals across cultures that are common to several cultures. Determining suitable application of neuropsychological instruments developed within the United States or any other country requires recognition of cross-cultural findings. Whereas questions contained in a neuropsychological instrument may be understood and suitable in the culture in which it was developed, it may have a different meaning or no meaning in another culture. Principles of neuropsychology by necessity must include cross-cultural methods that defined and acknowledge diversity and universals between two or more different cultures or cultural areas.

A number of questions arise and require answers as cross-cultural principles in neuropsychology are derived. What happens when one cultural group crosses into the territory of another group? What is the effect of one culture on another? What are the opinions toward brain damage or brain injury within a given culture? How do different cultures assess and treat the brain damaged? Do neuropsychologists possess sufficient sensitivity and knowledge to assess and treat brain damaged outside of their own culture? If they do not, should neuropsychologists be trained to assess and treat brain-injured individuals outside their own culture? Assessment and treatment skills outside one's own culture require understanding and appreciating cultural diversity as the first step in developing cross-cultural principles of neuropsychology.

To assist in probing answers to these and many other questions, cross culturalists have identified three theoretical orientations; Absolutism, Relativism, and Universalism (Berry, Poortinga, Segall, & Dasen, 1992). Absolutism assumes human behaviors are basically the same in all cultures with cultural environment contributing little or nothing to the meaning of human behavior. This definition appears straightforward, but Absolutism can be a treacherous minefield for neuropsychologists. Assessments made with instruments in one culture, taken to another culture with a linguistic translation can lead to erroneous conclusions, if consequences of the culture on which the test instruments are based are not considered. Disastrous consequences of applying Absolutism are visible when tests of ability are taken cross-culturally without the same set of test assumptions being fulfilled across cultures.

1. GRASPING THE CROSS-CULTURAL REALITY

Relativism is the opposite of Absolutism, and initially was an attempt to guard against ethnocentric judgments. This position warns against making invalid cross-cultural comparisons. Relativists seem to have little or no interest in group similarities or differences, and consider context-free concepts and their measurements to be impossible. Relativism approach collects no data, and thus is useless for diagnosing and rehabilitating brain damage cross culturally.

Universalism assumes human characteristics common to all members of the species produce psychological givens with culture influencing their development and display. Universalism proceeds cautiously by applying a wide variety of methods and safeguards while making interpretations based on alternative culturally meanings. The approach armed with appropriate linguistic translation, administration by a "native" tester with familiar content enables ability tests to go cross culturally. Universalism has become more acceptable in psychological practice in the United States with strong preferences for quantification and universal metrics for comparison purposes. Because ability tests depend on applying the same set of cultural assumptions, reliability and validity of measurements are doubtful cross culturally. Ultimately the goal is to specify culturally sensitive strategies to apply appropriately to assess abilities in a wide range of cultural contexts (Greenfield, 1997). Cautious comparisons using methodological principles and safeguards within the purview of similarities and differences and the context of alternative culturally based meanings are required.

Questions neuropsychology no doubt must address now and in years to come, center around the universality of human underlying physiological phenomena that can be measured behaviorally across cultures. For example, after a human head sustains sufficient force to induce a loss of consciousness and brain damage, what universal behavioral sequelae can be observed and measured? What behavioral observations and measurements are tied to culture, and what ones are not? What behavioral observations and measurements are physiologically based? After brain damage to the primary language area, are there universal physiological changes behaviorally observed and measured regardless of the language spoken? And what are the culturally based behavioral observations and measurements after damage to the primary language area?

Another factor influencing neuropsychological assessment is the onset of the disease process. Recent evidence showing an earlier onset of dementia of the Alzheimer's type in Latinos than in Anglo individuals (Clark et al., 2005) may mean neuropsychological findings of such populations may be related to onset of disease process rather than cultural differences. Caution, however, advised further investigations of the disease processes of such cultural groups.

According to a published report (Berry & Dasen, 1974), the term, cross-cultural psychology, has been multicultural and inclusive. In contrast, another report (Segall, Lonner, & Berry, 1998) stated cross-cultural psychology was destined to become an unnecessary term when psychology finally takes into account the effects of culture on human behavior and vice versa. Although neuropsychology/psychology seems to be on the path of cultural awareness, it has not reached the point where all aspects of human behavior are clearly recognized within its culture milieu.

Culture, Acculturation, and Assimilation

Webster's dictionary defines culture as "the integrated pattern of human behavior that includes thought, speech, action and artifacts and depends upon man's capacity for learning and transmitting knowledge to succeeding generations." The initial phrase of this definition, "the integrated pattern of human behavior" is striking. These words state aspects of culture (thought, speech, action, and artifacts) that blend together to generate the integrated pattern of human behavior.

The second part of Webster's definition is concerned with the survival of a culture through a capacity of humans to learn an integrated pattern of human behavior and to transmit it to successive generations. The definition indicated culture exists not only in the present, but in the future as well. Perpetuation of culture requires absorption through learning and finding ways of transmitting knowledge to those yet to be born. Added to this mix is the influence of each successive generation with their ideas, concepts, and inventions on culture. The changing or fluid aspect of culture missing from Webster's definition needs to be addressed in applying neuropsychological measures. Although inability to learn a cultural pattern or to transmit the cultural pattern has been observed in neuropsychological measurements when brain abnormalities are detected, it is not necessarily associated with disruption of cultural learning, but may represent generational differences or isolation from the current or prevailing culture for various reasons.

The term, culture, implies sharing or agreeing with what is called social convention (Greenfield, 1997). Integration of unique components within a given culture sets one culture apart from another culture. Acculturation is the process of learning manners and style of the dominant, prevailing culture (Dashefsky & Shapiro, 1976) that begins during childhood and becomes the basis for adult behavior. Acculturation begins in childhood, after birth, with a set of cultural factors shaping behaviors during infancy. Reactions of parents and caregivers during periods of helplessness, or infancy, contribute to establishment of behaviors. Behaviors derived from Attachment Theory are based on three core hypotheses related to: (1) sensitivity of mothers or caregivers to infant behaviors (smiling, crying, and approaching); (2) later social competency based on security of attachment with the mother or caregiver; and (3) initiation of environmental explorations once a secure base has been established in infancy. Evidence suggests these tenets within core hypotheses; sensitivity, competency, and secure base are not universal, but biased by western thinking and viewed differently in the Far East. For example, Japanese parents prefer to anticipate the needs of infants by identification of situations that may stress infants and take anticipatory steps to minimize stress. In the West, parents wait until infants communicate their needs before addressing those needs.

Cultural differences later observed suggest that emotional openness, viewed as desirable in the United States, is not viewed similarly in Japan. Assertive, autonomous characteristics preferred by westerners are reportedly viewed by Japanese as immature and uncultivated. The secure base–exploration link viewed as necessary for social independence and self-reliance in the United States, is not preferred in Japan where more dependent/group behaviors are preferred (Rothbaum, Weisz, Pott, Miyake, & Morelli, 2000).

Aside from acculturation during development periods within a given culture, the term, acculturation, occurs in the context of continuous contact for extended periods of time of two or more groups from different cultures. Levels of acculturation are defined by the degree to which cultural values, beliefs, and practices are incorporated by members from another culture. It is most often applied to members of ethnic minority adopting the cultural values, beliefs, and practices of a dominant culture. Generally, the younger one is during emigration from the country of origin, and the longer one remains in a new culture, the more one becomes acculturated. This fact is recognized in some cultures. Japanese language contains a different word for first, second, third, fourth, and fifth generations of families living in an alternative culture specifying the degree of acculturation (Wong, 2000).

Methods of measuring acculturation are appearing and being applied to determine the effects of acculturation on neuropsychological measures. Such is the case with the application of a rating scale developed specifically for a study of Mexican Americans (Cuellar, Arnold, & Maldonado, 1995). Findings show higher levels of acculturation improved performances on a neuropsychological measure of interest, namely, the Wisconsin Card Sorting Test (Coffey, Marmol, Schock, & Adams, 2005). In another study, the degree of acculturation has determined neuropsychological outcomes following traumatic brain injury (TBI; Kennepohl, Shore, Nabors & Hanks, 2004).

Assimilation involves understanding and participating in institutions of a society-at-large. Through the process of participating, the society-at-large values are acquired. Both assimilation and acculturation have implications for selections and application of neuropsychological instruments and treatment techniques. Individuals from minority cultures not assimilated and not acculturated into a majority culture are more likely to hold on to the cultural norms of their minority cultures exclusively. As a result, it would be inappropriate to apply neuropsychological instruments of the majority culture to such groups. Neuropsychological instruments are suitable for individuals from minority cultures who have become fully assimilated and acculturated into a majority cultural group. Most difficult is selection of neuropsychological instruments for the in-between minority culture group who are partly acculturated and assimilated into the majority culture. How much of these measurements reflect the culture of origin, and how much of these measurements reflect the culture of the majority is difficult to dissect. With greater worldwide electronic communication, the numbers of this in-between group are increasing as individuals acquire some, but not all, aspects of another culture other than their own. A link between primary and secondary cultures has been language. Higher levels of assimilation and acculturation have been linked to greater language proficiency in another language than the primary one (Llorente, Taussig, Satz, & Perez, 2000). A need is always present to develop and assess language proficiency with better methods in order to gain knowledge about acculturation and assimilation in clinical settings. A call has been made for more culturally sensitive neuropsychological tests and normative data (Ferraro & McDonald, 2005).

Culture concepts and language proficiency studied by many social scientists for centuries have been mainly overlooked in conscious body of neuropsychological knowledge in the past. Behavioral measurements, stemming from culture, have a potential to influence test-taking behaviors of children and adults during neuropsychological assessment. Certainly more time needs to be spent on measuring and understanding the influences of cultural tenets on human behavior that influence neuropsychological assessments and rehabilitation treatments.

As human beings, we have the same basic needs, but how we meet those needs is generally culturally determined. Some populations or groups feel their cultures meet human, as well as spiritual needs, the best and want the rest of the world to follow their cultural decrees. Other world residents enjoy cultural diversity found in the world inhabitants, and think diversity should flourish. Although the history of the multicultural world experiment has been chronicled for centuries, its meaningfulness is not readily perceived nor similarly perceived by many of the current world inhabitants.

The distinctiveness of a multicultural experiment is apparent in the early history of North America. Europeans seem to believe culture was not present within North America until their arrival brought European cultures to North America. Yet Native North Americans greeted and assisted many European immigrant groups in adapting to the new environment. Both Native North Americans and European immigrants initially assimilated and acculturated aspects of each other's culture.

Interestingly, Native North Americans carry origins of another culture because they were not indigenous to the United States, but had Asiatic origins about 30,000 years ago. Nuclear DNA determined this origin. Mitochondria DNA techniques have gone further in localizing Asian origins of the Native North Americans to northern China, southeast Siberia or Mongolia (Schurr, 2000). Although the findings are based on physical distinctions, not cultural ones, they suggest the Native North American left an Asiatic culture, and began a new culture within the environment of North America. Although unknown, it would be interesting to determine if Native North Americans today share any similar aspects of the current Asiatic cultures of origin. Although this example suggests viewing any cultural group in the world as "Native," may be questionable.

Ethnicity

Ethnicity refers to the national origins of an individual that give rise to cultural expressions of norms, values, language, and customs passed down from generation to generation (Uswatte & Elliot, 1997). Although controversial for some time, race, has been considered a biological marker, and has become more accepted as a social construct when based on geohistorical locations. (Neville, 2000). Multicultural psychology prefers the term sociorace to underscore the role of sociohistorical realities of groups in examining racial identity (Helms, 1994).

Multiculturalism itself has sometimes been conceptualized as a moral movement intended to enhance dignity, rights, and recognized worth of marginalized groups. It has strived to conceptualize an individual or group with respect to culture and history, but generally has failed to be self-reflective about the contextual sources of its own ethical ideals. Indeed, more understanding of the contextual sources is needed (Dashefsky & Shapiro, 1976). Although multiculturalism does not necessarily represent the final truth in understanding cultural differences, its ideals and aspirations constitute a compelling claim to truth that can be projected (Fowers & Richardson, 1996). Neuropsychology has somewhat of a *laissez-faire* attitude of multiculturalism for years, recognizing many sociohistorical realities, but not recognizing ethnicity with the true consciousness necessary to systematically address assessment and rehabilitation issues.

Some efforts have been made to understand multiculturalism and cross-cultural neuropsychological through biculturalism. Cultural icons and language have been shown to be effective means of activating cultural constructs of bicultural individuals and enabling frame switching. During frame switching, a bicultural individual shifts between interpretive frames rooted in different cultures in response to cues in the social environment (Hong, Morris, Chiu, & Benet-Martinez, 2000). For example, bicultural children at school in the United States may speak English and are exposed to United States cultural constructs, but once home in the afternoon, they return to cultural constructs and language of their parents, whether they be Spanish, Mexican, Italian, German, French, Chinese, Polish, or some other culture.

Human behavior reportedly is meaningful only when viewed in the sociocultural context in which it occurs (Segall, 1979). Because clinical neuropsychologists assess and rehabilitate human behavior, knowledge of the sociocultural context becomes important. Sensitivity to cultural and ethnic differences has generally been ignored in neuropsychology until near the end of the 20th century. Fortunately, the situation is now changing as many neuropsychologists are beginning to acknowledge cultural diversity scientifically. Others are acknowledging cultural diversity politically. Nevertheless, challenges for creating a truly multicultural neuropsychology that understands cross-cultural neuropsychology are destined not only to unfold during the 21st century, but to be refined.

CROSS-CULTURAL ASSESSMENTS

For many years, anthropology and cross-cultural psychology have been sifting through a maze of concepts to establish understandings about the appropriate application of tests and interpretations. Quite advisable for cross-cultural neuropsychology as it develops is to note the findings from anthropology and cross-cultural psychology.

Language Factors During Assessment

At the heart of cross-cultural knowledge, investigation, and practice is symbolism and communication. If the examiner and the examinee do not share the same symbolic culture and communicate effectively, then conclusions drawn from cross-cultural assessment will most likely be erroneous. Valid cross-cultural test interpretations in neuropsychology are based on the human capacity to share symbolic representations. Often, both verbal and nonverbal symbols are not shared cross culturally. The same symbols may have the same, different, or no meanings cross culturally. Communication between examiner and examinee must be clearly understood. This is most obvious when examiner and examinee speak and understand different languages. Without shared symbolism during communication, neuropsychological assessment may not be possible, or if attempted, may be invalid. For measurements of neuropsychology to be valid cross culturally, both examiner and examinee should speak and understand the same symbolism or language. The question remains how comparable are measurements made with one set of symbols or language to measurements made with another set of symbols or language?

One solution for cross-cultural examination has been to translate items from tests based on values in one culture to that of another language and culture. Such a solution often creates more problems than it solves. Personal observations made 16 years ago showed that responses of a head-injured Guatemalan patient were not similar to the those usually made by Mexicans on a translated California Verbal Learning Test. Post assessment interviews with the Guatemalan revealed differences were not due to the presence of a head injury, but due to differences in language. Names of spices on the California Verbal Learning Test translated into Mexican language were different from those of Guatemalan speech, even though both languages are considered to be Spanish. The variation in words or symbols in the Spanish language was later documented in the literature (Ponton & Ardila, 1999).

More investigations into the effects of language on neuropsychological assessment are needed. Findings showing that demographics (age, education, gender) and to a lesser extent, language of test administration were determinants of semantic verbal fluency in a group of Latinos over the age of 60 living in California who were examined in their preferred language (English or Spanish) with the Spanish English Animal Test (Gonzalez, Mungas, & Haan, 2005) require further study and examination. Is animal naming a culture-free test if conducted in a preferred language, or findings attributable to some variable not examined in this study, such as acculturation? Furthermore, not only education but influences on the quality of education need to be considered (Shuttleworth et al., 2004).

Little thought has been given to the differences found in other common languages, such as English as spoken by Americans, British, and Australians or Scandinavian languages, spoken by Swedish, Danish, or Norwegian. Who should examine each of these groups neuropsychologically? Final consensus about whether the examiner and the examinee should have the same cultural background and speak the same precise language during neuropsychological assessment has not been made, but the trend is for the examiner and the examinee to speak the same language and come from the same culture. For instance, if an American examines a person from Great Britain or Australia, is it the same as when a British or Australian person is examined by an examiner from his/her own culture, even though they speak the same language, namely English? Is it the same if a nonnative examiner who has learned the language examines a native-speaking examinee? In the United States, neuropsychologists come from diverse culture groups; is it appropriate for bilingual neuropsychologists who have English as a second language to examine an individual who is has English as a primary language? If so, what is the application of the bicultural framework in these situations? These and other questions about selecting appropriate language need further research.

Often translators are used during assessment. In these circumstances, problems appear when the translation is not given verbatim to the examinee or to the examiner. The translator may feel the need to assist the examinee in making a response. When this happens, the true response of the examinee remains unknown and assessment is invalid. Likewise, the translator may feel a need to simplify the examinee's response in making a translation to the examiner, resulting in eliminating critical information or missed information. Responses depend on translations following structural rules of the language, dialect diversity, as well as demographic variables for accurate communication with a designated examinee undergoing neuropsychological assessment.

The relationship of the translator to the examinee may make a difference. If the translator is a relative, the social situation is different than if the translator is an employee of a translation service. The preexisting dynamic relationship between the examinee and the relative may affect translations. If the translator is a child of the examinee, the examinee may feel that his or her parental authority has been eroded when the power of communication is granted to the child by the examiner who is perceived as an authority figure.

Translations have not always been a successful solution for cross-cultural examinations for another reason, lack of normative data. Applications of translated standardized test have been interpreted as violating the assumptions on which the test has been normed, adding an additional potential source of variability (Wong, Strickland, Fletcher-Janzen, Ardila, & Reynolds, 2000). Using a standardized test normed in a different culture can lead to drawing inferences and erroneous conclusions because of this variability (Wilde, 2005). Reports of specific culture norms have begun to appear (Pontón et al., 1996; Echemendia & Harris, 2004; Fillenbaum et al., 2005).

Questions remain unanswered including validity of norms from test instruments after being translated from one language to another language in clinical situations. Although age and education levels impact norms in all cultural groups, neuropsychological norms obtained within one culture cannot be appropriately applied to another cultural group because assumptions underlying those norms may not be the same in different cultures. When Spanish norms were applied to Mexican American performances on the Wisconsin Card Sorting Text, no clinically significant differences were present. In contrast, English norms yielded significant differences, suggesting the inappropriateness of English norms to this group (Coffey, Marmol, Schock, & Adams, 2005).

Reports of subculture norms have begun to appear for older African American adults (Ferman et al., 2005; Lucas et al., 2005a, 2005b, 2005c, 2005d; Rilling et al., 2005). Reviews of the advantages and disadvantages of establishing separate subcultural norms, along with a commentary addressing this topic with African Americans, have appeared, offering another approach that involves deconstruction of race and education in order to clarify the independent influences of race, culture, quality of education, and socioeconomic status on cognition and neuropsychological test performances. These are examples of the types of discussion and investigations needed with all types of subcultural, as well as cultural groups.

Cultural Concepts in Assessment

Often visuospatial, visuoperceptive, or visuoconstructive tests included in neuropsychological assessments are viewed as mostly "nonverbal," meaning less reliance on language. Such an assumption may be fallacious. Selection of a test instrument to minimize heavy reliance on language does not guarantee nonverbal response validity. For example, when an examination was conducted with Raven's Progressive Matrices in South Africa, and no correct responses were produced from the examinee, a postexamination interview provided the answer. When the examiner inquired about the bases for the examinee's responses, the reply was selections were made for the "pretty one," and not for logic required to complete a pattern (Nell, personal communication, June 24, 1999).

This example reemphasizes the obvious point that cultural values must be the same for both examiner and examinee in the assessment situation in order to obtain validity and reliability. For test instruments traveling freely from one culture to another, there must be universal agreement on value and merit of particular responses to particular questions and the same items must have the same meanings in different cultures (Greenfield, 1997). Cognitive abilities measures measured by neuropsychological tests represented culturally learned abilities. Different cultural contexts produce different patterns of abilities (Ardila, 1995). Furthermore, evidence is beginning to show culture-cognitive connections may become "hard wired." Different regions of brain activation as measured by fMRI were evident during Japanese and Caucasian observation of facial expressions of fear (Moriguchi et al., 2005).

An early cross-cultural study cited from Liberia illustrates the point. When 20 items were presented to Liberians to be evenly divided into four linguistic categories of foods, implements, food containers, and clothing, examiners were surprised by the appearance of functional pairings, which were not the expected taxonomic sorts. For example, an examinee placed a potato with a knife because "you take a knife and cut the potato." The pairings were justified by the Liberians as what a wise man would do, but were incongruent with the concepts of the examiners. When the examiners asked how would a foolish person sort the objects, they were amazed as examinees arranged items correctly in four western linguistic categories (Cole, Gay, Click, & Sharp, 1971). The Western and European expectations of the examiners were fulfilled, but not in the manner anticipated when underlying values and concepts were different between examiners and examinees during assessment. It would be easy for examiners from Western and European cultures to conclude that the Liberians had deficits in thought processes and were unable to sort similar objects in appropriate linguistic categories, had they not asked the examinees to perform the second task.

The example illustrates a number of problems in cross-cultural assessment. Test developers in creating cognitive and mental tests assume that the examiners and examinees are in agreement on a cultural level or social norm levels. Questions about the general consensus for intelligent responses raises profound questions in assuming cross-cultural validity of IQ tests. When a standardized interpretation means something different to examiners and examinees, then validity has been severely undermined for identifying cross-cultural similarities in neuropsychological abilities or for evaluating deficits in clinical assessment. Simply selecting items of similar content does not eliminate cultural biases because it does not necessarily address the kinds of cognitive processes valued in each culture. Following standardized administrative guidelines offers guidance during cross-cultural assessment if test instruments are standardized cross culturally. Herein lies the problem: Standardization across cultures is difficult. Our anthropology colleagues reportedly have not found a "culture-free" test, although a recent report states that Digit Symbol-Incidental Learning from the WAIS III may be a culture independent task useful for neuropsychological screening (Shuttleworth-Edwards, Donnelly, Reid, & Radloff, 2004).

Alternative possibilities include: selecting deviations from the standard method, such as the process approach; Luria's hypothesis testing with flexible methodology (Tupper, 1999), or creative assessment based on knowledge about cultural values being examined. These alternative techniques may be more useful during cross-cultural neuropsychological assessment. An interview following the examination is a must to inquire about the nature of responses when examiner and examinee have different cultural backgrounds. Otherwise, cross-cultural misunderstandings may go undetected during assessments. The greater the understanding of an examiner about why a response is made, the greater likelihood of true communication and the less likelihood of drawing erroneous conclusions.

Cross-Cultural Neurorehabilitation

Neuropsychologists who are aware of the influences of cultural factors tend to view their importance only in assessment, and not on neurorehabilitation. Cross-cultural neurorehabilitation is often overlooked. In fact,

1. GRASPING THE CROSS-CULTURAL REALITY

many neuropsychologists prefer to perform assessments only, leaving other nonneuropsychological professionals to address neurorehabilitation treatment needs. Yet, neuropsychologists with knowledge about brain–behavior relationships are best suited for neurorehabilitation. Those neuropsychologists engaging in neurorehabilitation need to understand and determine cross-cultural factors impinging on neurorehabilitation where the focus may be generally on a return of the brain-damaged individual to his or her culture within a family setting or full- or part-time work. Neuropsychologists in neurorehabilitation are professionally obligated to address and understand cultural and ethical factors in both assessment and neurorehabilitation situations.

Assessment for Neurorehabilitation

Assessment for neurorehabilitation includes attention to factors that are not necessarily included in assessments for strictly diagnostic or forensic purposes. The requirements during strictly diagnostic and forensic purposes are mainly to compare functional measurements with normative measures. Those performing assessment for neurorehabilitation are not only familiar with comparisons with normative measures of such functions as language, visuoperception, visuospatial integrity, executive skill, short-term memory, information processing speed, motor skills, but also qualitative data, obtained by observing behaviors of each patient during the assessment. For example, the methods each patient uses to cope with frustration, to perceive self or to develop problem-solving strategies. In other words, a task can be mastered or failed using various strategies, but the score or measurement may be the same. Examiners for rehabilitation patients collect data or measurements of strategies a patient utilizes in the assessment situation. For example, if a patient has difficulty with concepts of block rotations to achieve a desired red and white striped design during the Block Design task, how does he or she cope? Does the patient persist in trying to construct the design without rotation of each block or is there a systematic strategy followed to replicate a design pattern? How does the patient react to his or her performances on this and on other tasks? Is the patient unaware of his or her mistakes or successes? These and other qualitative data collected from observations by the examiner and others during assessment add another dimension critical for rehabilitation that is important for assessment with the intent to rehabilitate. It is important to be mindful that observed behaviors may be related to culture/ethnicity backgrounds.

Few studies have addressed cross-cultural factors during assessment for neurorehabilitation. However, one important concept for neurorehabilitation, self-awareness, has been examined cross culturally. Findings from examining traumatic brain-injured Maori in New Zealand or traumatic brain injured in Barcelona and Madrid, and Japanese with cerebral vascular accidents show that although cultural factors influence self-reports of competency, brain-damaged patients across cultures have reduced insight into their actual level of neuropsychological functioning (Prigatano et al., 1998; Prigatano & Leathem, 1993; Prigatano, Ogano & Amakusa, 1997). In other words, these studies show unawareness is present cross culturally following brain damage. The question is: are there similarities in how unawareness after brain damage is treated cross culturally?

In terms of language skills, aphasia is known to be present for languages after brain damage, but cross-cultural details of aphasia assessment are not always clear. For instance, are certain phonemes preserved in some languages, but not in others, because of the nature of the language? From the neurorehabilitation assessment point-of-view, what elements of language rehabilitation are specific to a given language by nature of its construction, and what elements are present cross culturally? Another dimension is more personal. What are the cultural similarities and differences in how individuals react to similar language losses cross culturally? Many studies are needed to examine factors from a cross-cultural neurorehabilitation perspective associated with other types of functional losses not only language, but visuospatial, attention/concentration, processing speed, memory, executive abilities, and constructional skills. Studies of these and other cognitive function are important for successful cross-cultural neurorehabilitation.

Cultural Concepts in Neurorehabilitation

Of importance when rehabilitating ethnic minority individuals is the degree to which they identify with the majority culture. Both assimilation and acculturation are important under these circumstances. Those less assimilated and acculturated are more likely attached to the cultural norms of their respective minority group and may find majority cultural interventions alien to their beliefs. Those more assimilated and acculturated may be more amenable to majority cultural intervention strategies (Parham & Helms, 1985). In a neurorehabilitation setting, the treating neuropsychologist must determine the degree of assimilation and acculturation before proceeding with appropriate treatment. The basis for these determinations may be made through education and through informal means consisting of observations of a patient and his or her interactions with the family on a rehabilitation unit and elsewhere, through reviews of hypothetical situations with the patient and the family, and through consultations with other professionals. The importance of neuropsychologists in initially recognizing the degree of assimilation and acculturation of a client or patient prior to treatment should be emphasized because it sets the tone for affective responses of all those involved, and ultimately the success of the rehabilitation program.

Neuropsychologists in a neurorehabilitation settings need to educate themselves so they develop an understanding about the cultural environments in which they offer neurotreatments. For example, about 61% of the total Hispanic population of the United States reportedly reside in Texas and California, perhaps due to the fact both states' southern borders are contiguous northern borders with Mexico and the prevalence of agriculture in Texas and California that requires seasonal farm workers. It is a must for neuropsychologists working in rehabilitation in those two states to become familiar with the customs and practices of their Hispanic population because this is a population they will likely treat. Due to limited availability of Mexican Spanish-speaking neuropsychologists in a rehabilitation setting, greater efforts must be made to recruit Hispanic neuropsychologists in rehabilitation facilities.

Family involvement is exceedingly important in a neurorehabilitation setting regardless of culture. Neuropsychologists in neurorehabilitation understand the importance of the family's involvement in the neurorehabilitation of a patient and include the family in formulating neurorehabilitation goals and practices during inpatient treatment and postdischarge plans. Continuing with the example of Mexican Americans, neuropsychologists in neurorehabilitation understand the extent of support and protection Mexican Americans provide to their family members who are ill. Because of these expectations, patients who have problematic, defiant, or resistive family members may be especially damaged by interpersonal experiences with those family members (Sharma & Kerl, 2001). More positively, personal experiences have shown Mexican American families visit the patient daily in a neurorehabilitation setting and remain present in a home setting of a brain-injured patient as long as necessary. Under those circumstances, it is critical to understand each family member's role, and to provide appropriate neurorehabilitation education for the family members. Evidence shows Hispanics do very well in a rehabilitation facility but have poor outcomes 1 year after discharge (Arango, 2006). Family involvement after 1 year may influence outcomes as well as other social factors.

Equally important for neurorehabilitation is the need for neuropsychologists to understand attitudes toward disabilities within the cultures they serve. Part of the attitudes toward individuals with disabilities depends on past experiences (Chan, Lee, Yuen, & Chan, 2002), physical and mental disabilities. As an example of how past experience influence a viewpoint is a report that Taiwanese college students have more past experience with physical disabilities than with mental ones (Wang, Thomas, Chan, & Cheing, 2003). Thus, Taiwanese college students may feel physical disabilities are more significant in everyday life than are mental disabilities. Another example of how culture influences the view of physical and mental abilities comes from a report that severe mental disabilities are a source of shame for parents within the Chinese culture, and thus, family members with mental disabilities are left in the home and not seen by others in the culture (Leung, 1990).

Models concerned with culture are beginning to appear for guiding neurorehabilitation interventions. One model has been designed to systematically integrate the literature on spinal cord injury with psychosocial adaptation among racial and ethnic groups (Henshenson, 1998). Another model, the Culturally Inclusive Ecological Model of Spinal Cord Adaptation has provided a framework for socioracial and ethnic factors potentially related to differential psychosocial outcomes (Neville, 2000). These models coming from trauma to the spinal cord, often including trauma to the brain as well, may be used as a springboard, so to speak, to develop a neurorehabilitation model that can be modified for a specific culture as required and applied. To develop a global model requires understanding of universals of brain functioning after insults, the motivations and feelings of the brain-injured person within the culture, cultural expectations and requirements of the patient as both an uninjured and injured person, and family members, particularly significant family members, feelings and expectations based on culture. The finally successful outcome of neurorehabilitation may be based on the culture in which the brain is damaged. Models developed by professional members of the culture can be useful, such as a Tribally Specific (Navajo) model for providing rehabilitation advanced by a psychologist of Navajo heritage (Lomay & Hinkebein, 2006).

Development of neurorehabilitation models is much needed in this area to provide guidance from a theoretical framework. Whereas the brain-damaged person, his or her neuropsychological assessment, and other factors, such as premorbid personality and medical history, education, gender and age are contained within the core of the neuropsychological rehabilitation model, culture is a predominant feature of the shell surrounding the brain-damaged core that influences the core. This shell contains many expressions of culture including, but not limited to family influences and beliefs, as well as presumptions about roles within the culture based on gender, age, education, work, or retirement. Of importance is how families and patients vary in holding steadfast to predominate cultural views in the culture in which they reside. Essential components of cross-cultural neuropsychology are shown in the Circle of Cross-Cultural Neuropsychology (See Fig. 1.1). The Circle begins with Ethnicity that is verbally expressed through Language, the next component. Leaving one's own ethnicity and joining a majority culture requires Acculturation and Assimilation. Services provided by neuropsychologists, namely, Neuroassessment and Neurorehabilitation, shown at the base of the Circle, are separated by Family Influences & Beliefs that exert a strong force on the process of cross-cultural neuropsychology. The Circle of Cross-Cultural Neuropsychology summarizes the major cross-cultural components.

CIRCLE OF CROSS-CULTURAL NEUROPSYCHOLOGY

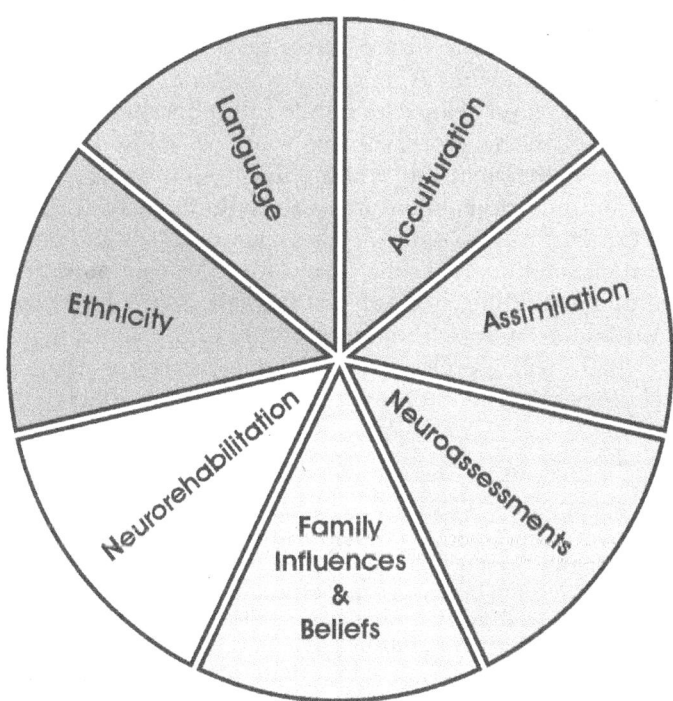

FIG. 1.1. Circle of Cross-Cultural Neuropsychology includes the major components of cross-cultural neuropsychology, starting with Ethnicity (reading clockwise), to Language, heavily intertwined with Ethnicity, onto Acculturation and Assimilation when moving from one culture to another. Neuroassessment and Neurorehabilitation, the chief functions of neuropsychology, are at the base of the Circle, separated by Family Influences & Beliefs because of the behaviors they shape in any given culture exert a strong force on the process of cross-cultural neuropsychology.

CONCLUSIONS

Although it has been stated many times in many cultures, death and taxes are an inevitable outcome in life, equally inevitable, but not always stated, so is culture. We are all shaped from birth to after death by the culture, or by the many cultures, in which we reside. We are shaped by cultures of neighboring cultures, or cultures geographically adjacent to our own. When we travel around the world we are often struck by aspects of culture that are similar and different to those of our own culture. As we become aware of the universals of human experiences and how some cultures manage these experiences better than others, we are also reminded of cultural differences. As we develop and gain understanding of cross-cultural neuropsychology, many questions are unanswered. Awareness of the cultural issues is now present more than it was a decade ago, but greater awareness is possible in the future. Because of the central role culture plays in the lives of individuals, many more decades may be required to reach the necessary level of knowledge and indispensable understanding. We have only begun the process. In no way does limited cross-cultural knowledge eliminate human and ethnic obligations of neuropsychologists as assessors and neurorehabilitators of those individuals with brain insults. Clearly, neuropsychologists around the world living in our present world of instant satellite, and other rapid forms of communications will gain more understanding, not only about their own culture, but about other cultures different from their own. Future predictions suggest a vast knowledge base will develop as the importance of cross-cultural neuropsychology to the field of neuropsychology is realized.

REFERENCES

Arango, J. C. (2006). *Cognitive rehabilitation and functional outcomes of Spanish-speaking TBI survivors.* Symposium presentation at the 34th International Neuropsychological Society, February 3, Boston, MA.

Ardila, A. (1995). Directions of research in cross-cultural neuropsychology. *Journal of Experimental and Clinical Neuropsychology, 17,* 143–150.

Berry, J. W., & Dasen, P. R. (1974). Introduction. In J. W. Berry & P. R. Dasen (Eds.), *Culture and cognition* (pp. 1–20). London: Methuen.

Berry, J. W., Poortinga, Y. H., Segall, M. H., & Dasen, P. R. (1992). *Cross-cultural psychology: Research and application.* New York: Cambridge University Press.

Chan, C. C. H., Lee, T. M. C., Yen, H.-Y., & Chan, F. (2002). Attitudes toward people with disabilities between Chinese rehabilitation and business students: An implication for practice. *Rehabilitation Psychology, 47,* 324–338.

Clark, C. M., DeCarli, C., Mungas, D., Chuo, H. I., Higdon, R., Nunez, J., et al. (2005). Earlier onset of Alzheimer's disease symptoms in Latino individuals is compared with Anglo individuals. *Archives of Neurology, 62,* 774–778.

Coffey, D. M., Marmol, L., Schock, L., & Adams, W. (2005). The influence of acculturation on the Wisconsin card sorting test by Mexican Americans. *Archives of Clinical Neuropsychology, 20,* 795–803.

1. GRASPING THE CROSS-CULTURAL REALITY

Cole, M., Gay, J., Glick, J., & Sharp, D. W. (1971). *The cultural context of learning and thinking.* New York: Basic Books.
Cuellar, I., Arnold, B., & Maldonado, R. (1995). Acculturation rating scale for Mexican Americans-II: A revision of the original ARSMA scale. *Hispanic Journal of Behavioral Science, 17,* 275–304.
Dashefsky, A., & Shapiro, H. (1976). Ethnicity and identity. In A. Dashefsky (Ed.), *Ethnic identity in society* (pp. 5–11). Chicago: Rand McNally.
Echemendia, R. J., & Harris, J. G. (2004). Neuropsychological test use with Hispanic/Latino populations in the U.S.: Part II of a national survey. *Applied Neuropsychology, 11,* 4–12.
Ferman, T. J., Lucas, J. A., Ivnik, R. J., Smith G. E., Willis, F. B., Petersen, R. C., et al. (2005). Mayo's older African American normative studies: Auditory verbal learning test norms for African American elders. *The Clinical Neuropsychologist, 19,* 214–227.
Ferraro, F. R., & McDonald, L. R. (2005). More culturally sensitive neuropsychological tests (and normative data) need. *Alzheimer's Disease and Associated Disorders, 19,* 53–54.
Fillenbaum, G. G., McCurry, S. M., Kuchibhatla, Masaki, K. H., Borenstein, A. R., Foley, D. J., et al. (2005). Performance on CERAD neuropsychology battery of two samples of Japanese-American elders: Norms for persons with and with dementia. *Journal of the International Neuropsychological Society, 11,* 192–201.
Fowers, B. J., & Richardson, F. C. (1996). Why is multiculturalism good? *American Psychologist, 51,* 609–621.
Gonzalez, H. M., Mungas, D., & Haan, M. N. (2005). A semantic verbal fluency test for English- and Spanish-speaking older Mexican Americans. *Archives of Clinical Neuropsychology, 20,* 199–228.
Greenfield, P. M. (1997). You can't take it with you: Why ability assessments don't cross cultures. *American Psychologist, 52,* 1115–1124.
Helms, J. E. (1994). Racial identity and career assessment. *Journal of Career Assessment, 2,* 199–209.
Henshenson, D. B. (1998). Systemic, ecological model for rehabilitation counseling. *Rehabilitation Counseling Bulletin, 42,* 40–50.
Hong, Y-Y., Morris, M. W., Chiu, C. Y., & Benet-Martinez, V. (2000). Multicultural minds: A dynamic constructivist approach to culture and cognition. *American Psychologist, 55,* 709–720.
Kennepohl, S., Shore, D, Nabors, N & Hanks, R. (2004). African American acculturation neuropsychological test performance following traumatic brain injury. *Journal of the International Neuropsychological Society, 10,* 566–577.
Leung, P. (1990). Asian Americans and psychology: Unresolved issues. *Journal of Training & Practice in Professional Psychology, 4,* 3–13.
Llorente, A. M., Taussig, I. M., Satz, P., & Perez, L. M. (2000). Trends in American immigration. In E. Fletcher-Janzen, T. L. Strickland, & C. R. Reynolds (Eds.), *Handbook of cross-cultural neuropsychology* (pp. 000–000). New York: Kluwer Academic/Plenum Publishers.
Lomay, V. T., & Hinkebein, J. H. (2006). Cultural considerations when providing rehabilitation services to American Indians. *Rehabilitation Psychology, 51,* 36–42.
Lucas, J. A., Ivnik, R. J., Smith, G. E., Glenn, E., Ferman, T. J., Willis, F. B., et al. (2005). A brief report on WAIS-R normative data collection in Mayo's older African American normative studies. *The Clinical Neuropsychologist, 19,* 184–188.
Lucas, J. A., Ivnik, R. J., Willis, F. B., Ferman, R. J., Smith, G. E., Parfitt, F. C., et al. (2005). Mayo's older African Americans normative studies: Normative data for commonly used clinical neuropsychological measure. *The Clinical Neuropsychologist, 19,* 162–183.

Lucas, J. A., Ivnik, R. J., Smith, G. E., Ferman, T. J., Willis, F. B., Petersen, R. C., et al. (2005). Mayo's older African Americans normative studies: WMS-R norms for African American elders. *The Clinical Neuropsychologist, 19,* 189–213.

Lucas, J. A., Ivnik, R. J., Smith G. E., Ferman, T. J., Willis, F. B., Petersen, R. C., et al. (2005). Mayo's older African American studies: Norms for Boston naming test, controlled oral word association, category, fluency, animal naming, token test, WRAT-3 reading, trail making test. Stroop test and judgment of line orientation. *The Clinical Neuropsychologist, 19,* 243–269.

Moriguchi, Y., Ohnishi, T., Kawachi, T., Hirakata, M., Yamada, M., Matsuda, H., et al. (2005). Specific brain activation in Japanese and Caucasian people to fearful faces. *Neuroreport: For Rapid Communication of Neuroscience Research, 16,* 133–136.

Neville, H. A. (2000). Psychological adaptation among racial and ethnic minority individuals following spinal cord injury: A proposed culturally inclusive ecological model. *Rehabilitation Psychology, 45,* 89–100.

Parham, T. A., & Helms, J. E. (1985). Attitudes of racial identity and self-esteem of black students: An exploratory investigation. *Journal of College Student Personnel, 26,* 143–147.

Pontón, M. O., & Ardila, A. (1999). The future of neuropsychology with Hispanic populations in the United States. *Archives of Clinical Neuropsychology, 14,* 565–580.

Pontón, M. O., Satz, P., Herrera, L., Ortiz, F., Urrutia, C. P., Young, R., et al. (1996). Normative data stratified by age and education for neuropsychological screening battery for Hispanics (NeSBHIS): Initial report. *Journal of the International Neurological Society, 2,* 96–104.

Prigatano, G. P., & Leathem J. M. (1993). Awareness of behavioral limitations after traumatic brain injury: A cross-cultural study of New Zealand Maoris and non-Maoris. *The Clinical Neuropsychologist, 7,* 123–135.

Prigatano, G.P., Ogano, M., & Anderson, B. (1997). The cross-cultural study of impaired self-awareness in Japanese patients with brain dysfunction. *Neuropsychiatry, Neuropsychology & Behavioral Neurology, 10,* 135–143.

Prigatano, G. P., Bruna, O., Mataro, M., Munoz, J. M., Fernandez, S., & Junque, C. (1998). Initial disturbances of consciousness and resultant impaired awareness in Spanish patients with traumatic brain injury. *Journal of Head Trauma Rehabilitation, 13,* 29–38.

Rilling, L. M., Lucas, J. A., Ivnik, R. J., Smith, G. E., Willis, F. B., Ferman, T. J., et al. (2005). Mayo's older African American studies: Norms for the Mattis dementia rating scale. *The Clinical Neuropsychologist, 19,* 229–242.

Rothbaum F., Weisz, J., Pott, M., Miyake, K., & Morelli, G. (2000). Attachment and culture: Security in the United States and Japan. *American Psychologist, 55,* 1093–1104.

Schurr, T. G. (2000). Mitochondrial DNA and the peopling of the new world. *American Scientist, 88,* 246–253.

Segall, M. H. (1979). *Cross-cultural psychology: Human behavior in global perspective.* Monterey, CA: Brooks/Cole.

Segall, M. H., Lonner, W. J., & Berry, J. W. (1998). Cross-cultural psychology as a scholarly discipline: On the flowering of culture in behavioral research. *American Psychologist, 53,* 1101–1110.

Sharma, P., & Kerl, S. B. (2001). Suggestions for psychologists working with Mexican American individuals and families in health care settings. *Rehabilitation Psychology, 46,* 230–239.

Shuttleworth-Edwards, A. B., Donnelly, M. J. R., Reid, I., & Radloff, S. E. (2004). A cross-cultural study with culture fair normative indications on WAIS-III digit symbol-incidental learning. *Journal of Clinical and Experimental Neuropsychology, 26,* 921–932.

Shuttleworth-Edwards, A. B., Kemp, R. D., Rust, A L., Muirhead, J. G. L., Hartman, N. P., & Radloff, S. F. (2004). Cross-cultural effects of IQ test performance: A review and preliminary indications on WAIS-III test performances. *Journal of Clinical and Experimental Neuropsychology, 26,* 903–920.

Tupper, D. E. (1999). Introduction: neuropsychological assessment après Luria. *Neuropsychology Review, 9,* 57–61.

Uswatte, G., & Elliott, T. R. (1997). Ethnic and minority issues in rehabilitation psychology. *Rehabilitation Psychology, 42,* 64–71.

Wang, M.-H., Thomas, K. R., Chan, F., & Cheing, G. (2003). A conjoint analysis of factors influencing American and Taiwanese college students' preferences for people with disabilities. *Rehabilitation Psychology, 48,* 195–201.

Wilde, M. C. (2005). Racial discrepancies on the repeatable battery for assessment of neuropsychological status in a mixed clinical sample. Poster presentation at the International Neuropsychological Society.

Wong, T. M. (2000). Neuropsychological assessment and intervention with Asian Americans. In E. Fletcher-Janzen, T. L. Strickland, & C. R. Reynolds (Eds.), *Handbook of cross-cultural neuropsychology* (pp. 43–53). New York: Kluwer Academic/Plenum Publishers.

Wong, T. M., Strickland, T. L., Fletcher-Janzen, E., Ardila, A., & Reynolds, C. R. (2000). Theoretical and practical issues in the neuropsychological assessment and treatment of culturally dissimilar patients. In E. Fletcher-Janzen, T. L. Strickland, & C. R. Reynolds (Eds.), *Handbook of cross-cultural neuropsychology* (pp. 3–18).

Chapter **2**

The Impact of Culture on Neuropsychological Test Performance

Alfredo Ardila
Florida International University

> ... a very limited kind of neuropsychology, appropriate to only a fraction of the world's population, is presented to the rest of the world as if there could be no other kind of neuropsychology, and as if the education and cultural assumptions on which ... neuropsychology is based were obviously universals that applied everywhere in the world.
>
> —*Matthews (1992, p. 421)*

In neuropsychology, cognitive disturbances associated with brain pathology of a limited subsample of the human species—contemporary Western, and most often, urban middle-class and literate brain-damaged individuals—have been relatively well analyzed. Our understanding about the brain's organization of cognitive abilities, and the disturbances in cases of brain pathology, is therefore not only partial but, undoubtedly, culturally biased (Ardila, 1995; Fletcher-Janzen, Strickland, & Reynolds, 2000). Cultural and linguistic diversity is an enormous, but frequently, overlooked moderating variable. Several thousands of different cultures have been described by anthropology (e.g., Bernatzik, 1957), and contemporary humans speak over 6,800 different languages (Grimes, 2000; *www.ethnologue.com*). Norms for performance in a sufficiently broad array of neuropsychological tests, and an extended analysis of cognitive disturbances in different cultural and ecological contexts are necessary for us to understand and serve the neuropsychological needs of our constituency. The need for the development of cross-cultural neuropsychology is evident.

A significant interest in understanding cultural variables in neuropsychology has been observed since the 1980s and particularly since the 1990s (e.g., Ardila, 1993, 1995; Ferraro, 2002; Fletcher-Janzen et al., 2000; Nell, 2000). Different questions have been approached including but not limited to: Bilingualism research; historical origins of cognition; studies on illiteracy; cross-linguistic analysis of aphasia, alexia, and agraphia; research about the influence of socioeducational factors in neuropsychological performance; norms in different national and cultural groups; studies on cultural variables on handedness; neuropsychological assessment and treatment in diverse human groups; analysis of neuropsychological test bias; cultural application of different neuropsychological test batteries; legal and forensic significance of cultural factors; and cognitive abilities in different cultural contexts.

In this chapter, I try to summarize the major cultural variables affecting neuropsychological test performance. I attempt to integrate some ideas previously presented in different publications. The reader can find previous versions of the sections included in this article in several journal articles and book chapters (Ardila, 1993, 1995, 1996, 1999, 2003; Ardila, Ostrosky-Solis, Rosselli, & Gomez, 2002a; Ardila, Ostrosky, & Mendoza, 2002b; Ardila, Rodriguez, & Rosselli, 2003; Harris, Echemendia, Ardila, & Rosselli, 2001; Ostrosky, Ardila, Rosselli, Lopez-Arango, & Uriel-Mendoza, 1998; Puente & Ardila, 2000).

WHAT IS CULTURE?

Culture refers to the set of learned traditions and living styles, shared by the members of a society. It includes the ways of thinking, feeling, and behaving (Harris, 1983). The minimal definition of culture could simply be, *culture is the specific way of living of a human group.*

Three different dimensions of culture can be distinguished: (1) The internal, subjective or psychological representation of culture, including thinking, feeling, knowledge, values, attitudes, and beliefs; (2) The behavioral dimension, including the ways to relate with others, ways of behaving in different contexts and circumstances, festivities and meeting, patterns of associations, and so forth; (3) Cultural elements or the physical elements characteristic of that human group such as symbolic elements, clothes, ornaments, houses, instruments, weapons, and so forth.

Culture represents a particular way to adapt to and survive in a specific context. Cultural differences are strongly related with environmental differences. Eskimo and Amazonian jungle cultural differences are to a significant extent due to the geographical and environmental differences between the Arctic region and the Amazonian jungle. Cultures, however, are usually in some contact and a significant cultural diffusion is generally observed. Cultural evolution and cultural changes are found throughout human history, depending on (a) new environmental conditions, (b) contact with other cultures, and (c) internal cultural evolution. For example, Gypsies in Russia and Gypsies in Spain have many cultural commonalties, but also many differences.

Cultures can be grouped into branches using different criteria, but are mainly grouped according to their origins (e.g., Latin cultures, Anglo-Saxon cultures, Islamic cultures, Amerindian cultures, etc.). When comparing two cultures, certain *relative distance* could be assumed. For instance, the cultural distance between Mediterranean cultures and Anglo-Saxon cultures is lower than the cultural distance between the Mediterranean cultures and the Amerindian cultures. This means that Mediterranean people have more attitudes, beliefs, behaviors, and physical elements in common with Anglo-Saxons than with Amerindians.

Certain cultural elements have been particularly successful and have tended to strongly diffuse across cultures. For instance, science and technology have been extremely successful in solving different human problems and have, in consequence, tended to spread throughout virtually all existing worldwide cultures. In this regard, contemporary man has tended to become more homogeneous and to share the culture of science and technology. To live in Peking and New York is not so different today as it was living in Tashkent and Rome several centuries ago. Furthermore, communication is faster today than it was any time in history and cultural diffusion has become particularly fast.

Formal education and school have played a crucial role in the diffusion of science and technology, and in the contemporary trend toward the relative cultural homogenization. In this regard, school can be considered as a subculture, the subculture of school (Ardila et al., 2000). School not only provides some common knowledge but also trains some abilities and develops certain attitudes. Cognitive testing is obviously based on those assumptions as well as on values of scientific and technologically oriented societies. Schooled children usually share more scientific and technologic values and attitudes than their lower educated parents, and schooled subjects significantly outperform illiterate individuals in cognitive testing (e.g., Ostrosky et al., 1998; Reis, Guerreiro, & Petersson, 2003; Rosselli, 1993).

Why Culture Affects Cognitive Test Performance

Cross-cultural cognitive testing has been a polemic matter, because cognitive assessment uses certain strategies and elements that are not necessarily shared by every culture (Laboratory of Comparative Human Cognition, 1983). Greenfield (1997) has pointed out that there are three different reasons to explain why cognitive ability assessments do not cross cultures: (1) values and meanings, (2) modes of knowing, (3) and conventions of communication.

Values and meanings means that there is not a general agreement on the value or merit of particular responses to particular questions. For example, some people may consider that in the Raven's Progressive Matrices test, it is a better response that one follow an aesthetic principle (i.e., the figure that looks better in that position) than a conceptual principle (i.e., the figure that continues the sequence). Furthermore, the same items do not necessarily have the same meaning in different cultures, regardless of how appropriate and accurate the translation is. An item referring to the protection of animals may have a rather different meaning in Europe than in a hunting society. "Why people should pay taxes?" may trigger quite different associations in a society where people consider that taxes are fairly expended, than in a society where people think that taxes are misused.

Knowing may be a collective endeavor, not an individual task. Many collective societies find it surprising that the testing situation requires individual's responses without the participation of the social group. If most activities are carried out in a collective way, why should answering a test be the exception? Many cultures, on the other hand, do not make a distinction between the process of knowing and the object of knowing. Therefore, questions such as "why do *you* think?" or "Why do *you* consider?" may be incomprehensible. The point is not what *I* think or *I* consider; the point is how *it is*.

Conventions of communication are highly culture dependent. The test questions assume that a questioner who already has a given piece of information can sensibly ask a listener for the same information. To ask or to answer questions can be highly variable among cultures. American children, for example, learn that they should not talk to strangers, but they also learn that they should answer questions from "the doctor," regardless if the doctor is a stranger. In many societies, adults rarely talk with children ("What could you talk with a child about?"), and it is not considered appropriate for children to participate in adults' conversations. Furthermore, relevant information is not always the same in every culture. Many types of questions can be difficult to understand. To copy nonsense figures (e.g., Rey-Osterrieth Complex Figure) can be suspicious for many people. It may be relevant item for an American school child, but absurd for somebody living in a nonpsychometrically oriented society. Certain question formats used in testing can be unfamiliar or less familiar in many cultures. For instance, a college Haitian student in the United States after his first multiple-choice test returned it to the instructor pointing out "I simply do not have the minimal idea of what I am supposed to do." Conversely, I have found that American university students score notoriously lower in open-question exams than in multiple-choice formats.

Effect of culture is not limited to verbal abilities, but is also clearly found in nonverbal abilities too (Rosselli & Ardila, 2003). When nonverbal test performance in different cultural groups is compared, significant differences are evident. Performance on nonverbal tests such as copying figures, drawing maps, or listening to tones can be significantly influenced by the individual's culture.

I emphasize five different cultural aspects potentially affecting neuropsychological test performance; (1) patterns of abilities, (2) cultural values, (3) familiarity, (4) language, and (5) education.

Patterns of Abilities. Whereas basic cognitive processes are universal, cultural differences in cognition reside more in the situations to which particular cognitive processes are applied than in the existence of the process in one cultural group and its absence in the other (Cole, 1975). Culture prescribes what should be learned, at what age, and by which gender. Consequently, different cultural environments lead to the development of different patterns of abilities. Cultural and ecological factors play a role in developing different cognitive styles (Berry, 1979).

Cognitive abilities usually measured in neuropsychological tests represent, at least in their contents, learned abilities whose scores correlate with the subject's learning opportunities and contextual experiences. Cultural variations are evident in test scores, as culture provides us with specific models for ways of thinking, acting, and feeling (Ardila, 1995; Berry, 1979). Some cultural differences in perception, spatial abilities and memory are reviewed in chapter 6 of this book.

Cultural Values. Culture dictates what is and what is not situationally relevant and significant. What is relevant, and worthy of learning or doing for an Eskimo does not necessarily coincide with what is relevant and worth learning or doing for an inhabitant of the Amazonian jungle. A culture provides specific models for ways of thinking, acting and feeling, and cultural variations in cognitive test scores are evident (Anastasi, 1988).

Current neuropsychological testing uses specific conditions and strategies that may not only be unfamiliar to many people, but may also violate some cultural norms. At least the following cultural values underlie psychometrically oriented cognitive testing (Ardila, 2005):

1. *One-to-one relationship.* There is a tester and there is a testee. Hence, it is a one-to-one relationship between two people that very likely never met before, are aliens, and will not meet again in the future.

2. *Background authority.* The testee will follow (obey) the instruction given by the tester, and hence, the tester has a background or situational authority. It is not so easy, however, to understand who and why this authority was conferred.

3. *Best performance.* The testee will perform at best. Performance "at best" is only done in those endeavors that are perceived and regarded as extremely important and significant. It is supposed in consequence that the testee has to perceive testing as a most important and significant endeavor. It may not be clear why it is so important and relevant to repeat a series of nonsense digits or to draw an absurd figure.

4. *Isolated environment.* Testing is done in an isolated room. Door is closed and even locked. Usually, nobody else is allowed to be present, and in this regard it is a private and intimate situation. Private appointments with aliens may be quite inappropriate in many cultures. The testee has to accept this type of unusual social relationship.

5. *Special type of communication.* Tester and testee do not maintain a normal conversation. Tester uses a stereotyped language, repeating over and over again the same phrases in a rather formal language. Testee is not allowed to talk about him or herself. Nothing points to a normal social relationship and usual conversation. This is a type of relationship that can be different from any type of relationship existing in the subject's past experience. For Hispanics, as an example, the personal relationship with the examiner may be more important than the test results (Geisinger, 1992). Dingfelder (2005) pointed out that "The detached professional relationship that many therapists cultivate with their clients may seem alien to those Latinos that adhere to the value of close interpersonal relationship. Therapist might consider sharing some minor details of their lives with these clients, to make the clients feel more comfortable and welcome." (p. 59)

6. *Speed.* In many tasks the tester warns that the testee must perform "as fast as possible" and even time is measured. In the middle of the task, however, the tester frequently interrupts saying, "stop!" For many cultural groups, speed tests are frankly inappropriate. Speed and quality are contradictory, and good products are the results of a slow and careful process. Speed, competitiveness, and high productivity are important cultural values in literate Anglo-American society, but that is not true in other cultural groups.

7. *Internal or subjective issues.* The tester may ask question that can be perceived as a violation of privacy. Questions about cognitive issues (e.g., "How is your memory?") are also questions about internal subjective representations, the most personal private sphere. Frequently, intellectual or cognitive testing may be perceived as aversive in some cultures. In Latin America, usually highly educated people dislike, and try to avoid

cognitive testing. Intellectual testing may even be perceived as a kind of humiliating situation and disrespectful of privacy.

8. *Use of specific testing elements and testing strategies.* The tester uses figures, blocks, pictures, and so forth, although the reason for presenting them may not be easy to understand. That is, the reason may be evident for the tester (e.g., to assess memory) but not for the testee. Sometimes the tester explains that it is like a game, but there is no evident reason to come to play with this alien tester. Sometimes the tester refers to "exercises," but exercises are by definition useless activities without any evident goal. "Exercises" are indeed "preparation for something." Preparation for what? Furthermore, if they are just "exercises," why to perform "at best"? In brief, it is not easy to understand (and to explain) the reason to memorize meaningless digits, or to say aloud "as many animal names as possible in one minute," and so forth.

In summary, the rationale and the procedures used in cognitive testing rely on a whole array of cultural values that in no way can be regarded as universal values. "When testers use tests developed in their own culture to test members of a different culture, testees often do not share the presumptions implicitly assumed by the test" (Greenfield, 1997, p. 1115). It is not surprising that the members of the culture where the test was developed usually obtain the highest scores.

Familiarity. Familiarity with the testing situation includes not only the elements used in testing (bikes, houses, figures, stories, etc.) but also the testing environment and the cultural relevance (meaningfulness) of the elements of the test (Ardila & Moreno, 2001). Familiarity also refers to the strategies needed to solve the task, and the attitudes required for success. Competitiveness, for example, in many societies is viewed with suspicion. Cooperation and social ability may be by far more important.

The Boston Naming Test (even the version adapted in Spain) includes naming a beaver and an acorn, an animal unfamiliar for people living in South America and a virtually unknown plant. North American people very likely would consider it unfair to be tested by naming South American animals and plants. The Boston Naming Test also includes a pretzel, a most typical American element but totally unknown in most countries. Obviously, it would also be frankly unfair to test naming ability in American subjects using tortillas or tacos as stimuli. Figures representing snow may be unfamiliar to people living in tropical and subtropical areas.

Cultural relevance (meaningfulness) may be another significant confounding factor in cross-cultural neuropsychological testing. Items developed in a particular cultural context do not have the same relevance when translated to another culture. Spelling out words (frequently included in the Mini-Mental State Exam) is not used in languages with phonological writing systems (such as Russian, Italian, or Spanish), and hence, it is perceived as an artificial task. In many world cities, people become oriented using cardinal points (North, South, West, and East) but this strategy is not found in every culture. I personally do not know where North, South, West, and East is in my Colombian hometown simply because I never used it. People in Barcelona (Spain) use spatial directions; "toward the sea" and "toward the mountain." People in Colombia frequently use "up" and "down," referring to the numbering system, but "up" and "down" in Guadalajara (México) mean "from downtown" and "toward downtown." The Picture Arrangement subtest from the Wechsler Intelligence Scale may have different levels of difficulty in different cultural contexts, depending on the familiarity with the story's elements. Something may be obvious in a culture, but unusual and weird in another.

Language. Language plays an instrumental role in cognition (Vygotsky, 1962, 1989). As a matter of fact, it represents the major cognitive instrument. Different languages differ in phonology, lexicon (semantic field of the words), grammar, pragmatic, and reading system. These differences may affect language test performance. These differences are analyzed in chapter 6 of this book. Different languages conceptualize the world in a different way (Whorf, 1956). For instance, the notion of time is quite different in Latin languages than in English. Latin languages have a significantly high number of tenses pointing to some temporal nuances. Slavic languages use perfective and nonperfective tenses in verbs. Space and casualty are also coded differently in different languages.

Language usage differs according to the cultural (and subcultural) background and strongly correlates with the subject's educational level. Sometimes, test instructions (and in general, the language used in testing) are given in a formal language, which may be very difficult to understand for individuals with limited education. Formal language represents a sort of academic language, most often found in a written form that many people neither use nor completely understand. A permanent effort is required to make test instructions and, in general, test language, understandable for less educated people and appropriate for different cultural and subcultural groups.

Education. Education plays a double role in test performance: School, on the one hand, provides some contents frequently included in cognitive tests; and on the other hand, trains some learning strategies and develops positive attitudes toward intellectual matters and intellectual testing. As a consequence, school could be considered as a subculture into itself. Greenfield (1997) has emphasized that "A major (probably the major) factor that makes a culture more or less different from the cultural conventions surrounding ability testing is the degree of formal education possessed by the participants" (p. 1119).

Learning to read reinforces certain fundamental abilities, such as verbal memory, phonological awareness, and visuospatial discrimination (Ardila, Ostrosky, & Mendoza, 2000b). It is not surprising that illiterate people underscore in cognitive tests tapping these abilities. Furthermore, attending school also reinforces certain attitudes and values that may speed the learning process, such as the attitude that memorizing information is important, knowledge is highly valuable, learning is a stepwise process moving from the simpler to the more complex, and so forth. It has been emphasized that schooling improves an individual's ability to explain the basis of performance on cognitive tasks (Laboratory of Comparative Human Cognition, 1983). The fundamental aims of schools are equivalent for all schools and school reinforces certain specific values regardless of where they are located. Hence, school could be seen as a culture unto itself, a transnational culture, the culture of school. School not only teaches, but also helps in developing certain strategies and attitudes that will be useful for future learnings. Ciborowski (1979) observed that schooled and nonschooled children can learn a new rule equally well, but once acquired, schooled children tend to apply it more frequently in subsequent similar cases.

Interestingly, education is not related with the ability to solve everyday problems. Cornelious and Caspi (1987) found that educational level has a substantial relationship with performance on verbal meaning tests but was not systematically related to everyday problem solving (i.e., functional criterion of intelligence). Craik, Byrd, and Swanson (1987) observed that differences in memory loss during aging are related to socioeconomic status. Ardila and Rosselli (1989) reported that during normal aging, the educational variable was even more influential on neuropsychological performance than the age variable. Albert and Heaton (1988) argued that, when education is controlled, there is no longer evidence of an age-related decline in verbal intelligence.

A significantly decreased neuropsychological test performance has been documented in illiterate individuals (Ardila, 2000; Ardila, Rosselli, & Rosas, 1989; Goldblum & Matute, 1986; Lecours et al. 1987a, 1987b, 1988; Manly et al., 1999; Matute et al., 2000; Ostrosky et al., 1998; Reis & Castro-Caldas, 1997; Reis et al., 2003). Rosselli, Ardila, & Rosas, 1990). Lower scores are observed in most cognitive domains, including naming, verbal fluency, verbal memory, visuoperceptual abilities, conceptual functions, and numerical abilities. Language repetition can be normal for meaningful words, but abnormal for pseudowords (Reis & Castro-Caldas, 1997; Rosselli et al., 1990). Similarly, copying meaningful figures can be easier than copying nonsense figures (Ostrosky et al., 1998). Furthermore, having illiterate people use concrete situations can be notoriously easier than using unreal and abstract elements. When the information is related to real life, it can be significantly easier to understand. Thus, for the illiterate person, it is easier to solve the arithmetical operation "If you go to the market and initially buy 12 tomatoes and place them in a bag and later on, you decide to buy 15 additional tomatoes, how many tomatoes will you have in your bag?" than the operation: "How much is 12 plus 15?" Semantic verbal fluency is easier than phonological verbal fluency (Reis & Castro-Caldas, 1997; Rosselli et al., 1990), seemingly because phonological abstraction is extremely difficult for the illiterate person. Semantic verbal fluency requires the use of concrete elements (animals, fruits) whereas phonological fluency is tapping a metalinguistic ability. The very low scores observed in neuropsychological tests in illiterates can be partially due to differences in learning opportunities of those abilities that the examiner considers most relevant, although they are not the really relevant abilities for illiterates' survival. They can also be due to the fact that illiterates are not used to being tested. Furthermore, testing itself represents a nonsense situation that illiterate people may find surprising and absurd. This lack of familiarity with the testing situation represents a confounding variable when testing individuals with limited education.

This educational effect has been supported by a diversity of studies since long time ago (e.g., Ardila, Rosselli & Ostrosky, 1992; Bornstein & Suga, 1988; Finlayson, Johnson, & Reitan, 1977; Heaton, Grant, & Mathews, 1986; Leckliter & Matarazzo, 1989; Ostrosky et al., 1985, 1986). However, some tests are notoriously more sensitive to educational variables (e.g., language understanding tests) than others (e.g., orientation tests).

This educational effect, nonetheless, is not a linear effect, but rather it is a negatively accelerated curve, ending in a plateau. Differences between zero and 3 years of education are highly significant; differences between 3 and 6 years of education are lower; between 6 and 9 are even lower; and so forth. And virtually no differences are expected to be found between, for example, 12 and 15 years of education. The reason is simple: The ceiling in neuropsychological tests is usually low (Ardila, 1998). Table 2.1 presents the differences in some cognitive tests between illiterates and subjects with 1–2 and 3–4 years of education.

Although it is well established that there is a significant correlation between cognitive test scores (e.g., IQ) and school attendance (e.g., Matarazzo, 1972), interpreting this correlation has been polemic (Brody, 1992; Neisser et al., 1996). The really crucial question is: Do cognitive (intelligence) tests indeed predict school performance? Or rather, does

TABLE 2.1
Effect of Education on Test Performance in the NEUROPSI
Neuropsychological Test Battery ($n = 807$)

	Years of education		
Test	0	1–2	3–4
Digits backwards	2.4	2.6	2.7
Verbal memory	4.2	4.2	4.3
Copy of a figure	7.5	8.8	9.4
Naming	7.3	7.3	7.5
Comprehension	3.7	4.4	4.6
Semantic fluency	13.5	14.6	15.4
Phonologic fluency	3.3	6.5	7.0

Note. Mean scores are presented. Adapted from "NEUROPSI: A Brief Neuropsychological Test Battery in Spanish," by F. Ostrosky, A. Ardila, and M. Rosselli, 1999, *Journal of the International Neuropsychological Society, 5,* p. 413–433.

school train those abilities appraised in intelligence tests? To answer these questions is not easy, even though frequently the interpretation has been that IQ predicts school performance (e.g., Hunter, 1986). Other researchers, however, consider that IQ scores are, to a significant extent, a measure of direct and indirect school learning (e.g., Ardila, 1999; Ceci, 1990, 1991).

Ceci and Williams (1997) presented an impressive and detailed review of the available data in this area. Seven types of historical evidence for the effect of schooling on IQ were examined: (1) The effect of intermittent school attendance. Several studies have provided a converging evidence that the longer youngsters stay out of school, the lower their IQs; (2) The effect of delayed school start-up: Different studies have demonstrated that children whose schooling was delayed experienced a decrement in several IQ points for every year that their schooling was delayed. (3) The effect of remaining in school longer: As a result of extra schooling (to avoid military service), men born on a particular date (July 9 instead of July 7) earned approximately a 7% rate of return on their extra years of schooling. The authors pointed out that this figure of 7% is very close to the estimate of the return on an extra year of schooling derived from studies of being born early or late in a given year. (4) The effect of discontinued schooling: There is a well-established detrimental effect of dropping out of school before graduating. For each year of high school not completed, a loss of 1.8 IQ points has been observed. (5) The summer school vacations: A systematic decline in IQ scores occurs during summer months. With each passing month away from school, children lose ground from their end-of-year scores on both intellectual and academic scores. (6) The effect of early-year birth dates: Given the age limits to enter school in the United States, within a given year, the number of years of schooling completed is the same for those born during the first 9 months of the year. But the amount of school attendance drops off for those born during the final 3 months of the year. After coming of age, some individuals leave school, and students with late-year births are more likely to stay in school 1 year less than students with early-year births. It has been observed that for each year of schooling that is completed, there is an IQ gain of approximately 3.5 points. (7) Cross-sequential trends: A correlation between the length of schooling completed and intellectual performance among same-age, same-SES children has been observed.

The general conclusion is that school attendance accounts not only for a substantial portion of variance in children's IQ but also apparently some, although not all, of the cognitive processes that underpin successful performance in IQ tests. The magnitude of this influence ranges between 0.25 to 6 IQ points per year of school (Ceci, 1991). Therefore, the association between IQ and education cannot be interpreted assuming that IQ predicts school success. Intelligence and schooling have complex bidirectional relationships, each one influencing variations in the other (Ceci & Williams, 1997).

According to our results (e.g., Ardila et al., 2000b), even though bidirectional relationships between intellectual test performance and schooling may exist, the real significant relationship is between schooling and cognitive test performance. That is, attending school significantly impacts cognitive test performance.

Minorities From Inside

Cognitive testing of so-called "minority groups" represents a special situation in neuropsychology assessment. Minority groups constitute a culture or subculture within a mainstream culture. Quite often, the tester belongs to the majority culture and may have a limited understanding of the minority culture or subculture. Testing is likely interpreted from the majority culture perspective. To be a member of a minority group, however, has significant implications that can affect the testing situation and the testing results.

There are over 120 million people living in a country different from that one where they were born. They are "minorities" in the new host country: Turks in Germany, Moroccans in Spain, Hindus in England, Colombians in

2. CULTURAL IMPACT ON TEST PERFORMANCE

Venezuela, Greeks in Switzerland, Rwandans in Zaire, Mexicans in United States, Greeks in France, and so forth. There are also some ethnic groups that are "minorities" in their own countries: African Americans in United States, Kurds in Turkey, Amerindians in Colombia (and virtually in every country), and so forth. Finally, there are some groups that are "minorities" everywhere because they do no have a country. Currently, Gypsies are the best example, but until recently, Jews were also a peoplehood without a country.

To be different from the mainstream people has a significant psychological impact. Patterns of behavior, beliefs, and attitudes may be different. Language can impair normal communication with the majority group. Even physical appearance and dressing can separate and distinguish the minority people. In the United States there are hundreds of groups that can be regarded as "minorities."

At least six different variables can potentially distinguish the minorities groups. They may also affect intellectual test performance and the "psychology of minority":

1. *Nationality*. Is that person regarded or not as an alien? Intermediate possibilities can exist. For instance, Hispanics in the United States have five different possibilities: U.S. born from the mainland or from Puerto Rico), acquired citizenship, legal immigrant, and illegal immigrant. It makes a significant difference if the country in which you are living is legally your country or whether you are a noninvited alien.

2. *Culture* (relative distance): Irish immigrants in United States have a closer culture to the mainstream American way of life than Ethiopians. The larger the cultural distance, the more separated you are to understand the new culture and appropriately behave in it.

3. *Language* (relative distance). Minorities may speak a different language, they may speak a dialect of the majority language, or they may simply speak the same language. The ability to communicate, and hence, participate (e.g., to have a job) in the host culture depends highly on the ability to speak. Language distance between English and German is lower than language distance between English and Spanish. Language distance between English and Chinese is huge. Age also plays a crucial role in the ability to learn the new language. Young Moroccan people in Spain can easily learn Spanish and improve in social status, whereas adults have to accept low qualified and low paying jobs.

4. *Normality* (how frequent—normal—is your group in your living environment). To be different depends on the community in which you live. Hispanics are the "normal people" in Miami, but very unusual people in Fargo. To be unusual may be associated with suspiciousness in the majority group and paranoia in the minority people.

5. *Reference group* (How many people are like you are). It depends on with which specific group one identifies. Hispanics, for instance, can consider that their reference group is Latin America or other U.S. Hispanics. In the fist case, the reference group is even larger than the majority U.S. group. In the second one, it is a notoriously smaller and weaker social reference group.

6. *Social image*. This refers to the positive or negative attitudes in the majority group toward the minority people. Even though minorities generally have a low social image (e.g., they are poor, with low education, inappropriate behaviors, etc.) sometimes positive attitudes are also associated with the minority group. For instance, in the United States, Oriental people are frequently regarded as "intelligent and hard-working people."

Being a member of a minority group obviously is associated with some psychological features. Furthermore, if you speak a different language, or you are an alien, or you have certain physical characteristics that make it easy to recognize you as a minority everywhere, certain psychological consequences can be anticipated. Some of these characteristics are:

1. *Paranoia*. You maybe feel you are different, and other people may identify you with the majority stereotype about your group. If you belong to a different culture, obviously you are not sure how to behave in many daily life situations. Any error can be particularly serious. Moreover, if you are an illegal immigrant, the slightest error can be fatal.

2. *Decreased self-esteem* may result and may be associated with the feeling that there is a barrier between you and the rest of the people. Your self-esteem will be permanently challenged if you are perceived as behaving (and/or speaking) in a foolish and childish way. Many minority people feel that they could do better if they were not minority people, but they are going to remain in a marginal social position.

3. *Isolation*. Quite often, belonging to a minority group is associated with a decreased social support (i.e., lack of family and friends). Often, the social support group is far away, maybe in another country.

4. *Cultural solitude*. To be different from the majority of people results in a feeling of "cultural solitude"—nobody can understand you because you are different. There is a permanent and unbreakable barrier between you and the rest of the people. For Hispanics in the United States, this cultural solitude is unlikely in Los Angeles, but quite likely in Seattle.

5. *Frustration* is mainly associated with two factors; the inability to appropriately deal with the environment, and the inability to do in the majority environment that which you could do if you were not a minority. Despite laws against discrimination, many (maybe, most) minority people feel they are discriminated against in one way or another.

6. *Anger* is the obvious result of frustration.

7. *Depression* as anger is associated with frustration but also with the feelings of isolation and cultural loneliness.

8. *Homesickness.* If you are living in a foreign country, a predictable "cycle of homesickness" can be anticipated. Homesickness is not significant at the beginning but becomes important about 2 or 3 years after you have moved to the new country. After this point, some adaptation to the new living conditions is usually observed, and new social links are established. Nonetheless, homesickness reappears about the age of retirement and frequently becomes so unbearable that the person has to return to his or her native place. That is the "return migration." But frequently, returning is not possible. Homesickness is also obviously associated with the age of migration. Sometimes (usually when migrating young but not too young) people feel that they belong nowhere because they are between two cultures and no one is really his or her own culture.

9. *Feelings of failure and/or success.* Frustration is frequent in minority people. Frustration, however, can coexist with the feeling of success. Minor successes can be perceived as very significant. These minor successes can be interpreted as "despite so many difficulties, I got it." Minor (and, unusually, major) successes are also highly reinforced and rewarded by the minority social reference group. Minority groups frequently display with pride the names of those people who have succeeded.

Neuropsychological testing of minority groups have progressively become a more and more important question in neuropsychology, particularly in some countries with a significant immigration flow (e.g., some European countries). It is not easy for a Spanish neuropsychologist to test a Moroccan patient, or for a Danish neuropsychologist to test a Somalian client. There are no obvious answers to questions such as how to carry the testing, what specific tests to use, and what conclusions can potentially be drawn from the testing results.

Norms in Different National and Cultural Groups

A tremendous effort has been devoted in neuropsychology to obtaining test performance norms (e.g., Ardila, Rosselli, & Puente, 1994; Lezak, 2004; Spreen & Straus, 1998). Currently, many neuropsychological tests possess relatively solid and reliable norms. Nonetheless, norms have been obtained in most cases in white English-speaking, middle-class subjects with a high school or college level of education.

In cognitive testing, it is usually assumed that norms are always required. Otherwise, no comparison is reliable. This idea, however, is more a desideratum than a reality. Furthermore, it does not seem to be a completely realistic idea. As a matter of fact, in the future, the search for norms may be coordinated with the search for understanding the sources of variation. Two evident problems with norms are readily observed:

1. Language. To obtain norms in English or Spanish (each one with about 400 million speakers) seems realistic. But English and Spanish are just two out of the three largest existing languages accounting together for no more than 15% of the world's population. Worldwide, there are about 6,800 different languages *(http://www.ethnologue.com/)*, most of them with a limited number of speakers. As an example, in Mexico, 288 Amerindian languages are currently spoken *(http://www.ethnologue.com/)*. In the United States, over 300 languages are found, when counting both Amerindian and immigrant languages *(http://www.ethnologue.com/)*. To obtain norms for all these 6,800 different languages is simply unrealistic. Furthermore, most of the world languages are small languages, and obtaining a reliable database would mean testing a high percentage of the speakers. If we assume that the average language has one million speakers (the real number is lower), and we wanted to normalize the neuropsychological instruments using just 200 stratified subjects in each language, it would mean that about one and half million participants would be required. This is a nonrealistic endeavor for contemporary neuropsychology. It seems more realistic to determine the linguistic factors potentially affecting cognitive test performance. A diversity of languages could be selected, comparison established, and significant variables distinguished. Language idiosyncrasies seem most important in understanding potential sources of variations. Obtaining norms is a realistic endeavor in English, Spanish, Quechua, or Bengali, but does not seem realistic for the 288 Amerindian languages spoken in Mexico.

2. Culture. There are solid bases to assume significant cultural variations in psychological and neuropsychological test performance (e.g., Ardila, 1995; Fletcher-Janzen et al., 2000; Nell, 2000). Thus, the question becomes, how many cultural groups should be separated? Although several thousand different cultures have been described by anthropology (e.g., Bernatzik, 1957), obviously there is not a definitive answer to this question. Cultures frequently represent a continuum and cultures are partially overlapped. For example, if asked whether separate norms should be used when testing Caucasians and Hispanics in the United States, most neuropsychologists might answer "yes." Nonetheless, a diversity of conditions may separate Caucasians and Hispanics; primary language (for many Hispanics, their primary language is English; most Hispanics are bilinguals, some are monolingual; the degree of mastery of Spanish and English is tremendously variable), "acculturation" (degree of assimilation of the modal American culture values is highly variable),

and so forth. So, there does not seem to be an obvious and direct answer. To be "Hispanic" or "Caucasian" is not a dichotomy. Another question: In the United States, can the norms obtained in San Francisco be used to test people in Boston, San Antonio, Honolulu, or Anchorage? San Francisco is a heterogeneous city and the question becomes what specific San Francisco norms are going to be used with what specific population in Boston, San Antonio, Honolulu, or Anchorage? The same type of question can be raised everywhere. For instance, can we use in Spain the norms obtained in Barcelona to test people in Canaria Islands, Santiago de Compostela, or Bilbao? The answer in all these cases may be, partially yes, partially no. This is indeed an endless question. If we move to the worldwide situation (with thousands of cultural variations!), we may conclude that this is also a nonrealistic endeavor for psychology and neuropsychology. I am proposing that this question has to be restated, and instead of looking for norms in every existing human group, we should try to understand why and how culture impacts cognitive testing, that is, what are the specific cultural variables that may affect the performance in a psychological or neuropsychological tests (Ardila, 2005). For this purpose, it seems more reasonable to select a series of rather different cultural groups, representing enough cultural dispersion, in an attempt to pinpoint those cultural variables potentially affecting cognitive test performance.

In brief, understanding the variables that can affect cognitive test performance seems to be as important as obtaining a large number of norms in different linguistic and cultural groups. (Ardila, Ostrosky, & Bernal, unpublished).

There does not seem, for example, any reason to find differences in verbal fluency in preschool and school-aged children when using an equivalent semantic category in Spanish and English. If the familiarity with the testing condition is equivalent (both are small children with little or no familiarity with testing), the level of education is the same (none or whatever), the age is the same, and the semantic category has the very same semantic field in both languages, no differences in performance are expected. Table 2.2 presents the norms obtained by Halperin, Healy, Zeitchik, Ludman, & Weinstein (1989) in the United States and Ardila and Rosselli (1994) in Colombia. Even though the age groups were divided differently (Halperin et al. used 1-year range; Ardila & Rosselli used 2-year range) it is evident that performance was virtually identical.

Table 2.3 compares performance on two verbal fluency tests (phonological and semantic verbal fluency) in Spanish and English monolingual speakers. As anticipated, performance is virtually identical if confounding variables are controlled. English speakers do a little better when using some

TABLE 2.2
Semantic Verbal Fluency (ANIMALS) in the United States and Colombia

Halperin et al., 1989 (USA)				Ardila and Rosselli, 1994 (Colombia)			
Age (years)	n	M	SD	Age (years)	n	M	SD
6	34	10.74	2.40	5–6	49	9.33	3.65
7	40	12.43	2.90				
8	32	12.31	2.70	7–8	63	11.49	2.87
9	38	13.76	3.70				
10	22	14.27	3.70	9–10	56	14.09	3.99
11	28	15.50	3.80				
12	10	18.90	6.20	11–12	65	16.75	4.64

TABLE 2.3
Semantic Verbal Fluency (ANIMALS) in Spanish and English Monolinguals
(60–65 years; 13–16 years of education)

	English	Spanish
F	12.9 (5.4)	11.7 (4.1)
A	10.7 (5.1)	11.8 (4.6)
S	13.8 (5.4)	11.4 (3.8)
Animals	16.8 (5.2)	16.7 (3.8)

Note. Mean scores and standard deviations are presented. Adapted from "Verbal Fluency and Repetition Skills in Healthy Older Spanish-English Bilinguals," by M. Rosselli et al., 2000, *Applied Neuropsychology, 7*, p. 17–24.

letters; Spanish speakers do a little better when using other letters, very likely depending on the frequency of words beginning with that particular letter in each language, the potential ambiguity existing between homophone letters, and some other uncontrolled confounding variables. Performance in semantic verbal fluency using the category ANIMALS was virtually identical.

Nonetheless, unexpected confounding variables can exist. Digit span looks like a relatively culture-fair test, and similar performance might be anticipated in people from different human groups. Nonetheless, that is not the case. A significant variability has been observed. Digit span varies from 5.4 (Poland) to 9.0 (China; Dehaena, 1997; Nell, 2000). The reason for this variability is not totally clear, but both linguistic and training factors seem to exist (Dehaene, 1997). The phonological length of digits (number of phonemes included in digit words) as well as previous exposure to similar tasks (e.g., to say phone numbers using digit-by-digit strategy) may play a significant role in digit span. In the Sikuani language spoken in the Amazon jungle, digits are *kae* (one), *aniha-behe* (two), *akueyabi* (three), *penayanatsi* (four), *kae-kabe* (five), *kae-kabe kae-kabesito-nua* (six), *kae-kabe aniha-kabesito-behe* (seven), *kae-kabe aniha-kabesito-akueyabi* (eight), *kae-kabe aniha-kabesito-penayatsi* (nine). With such long words, it can be conjectured that digit span will be very low.

What I am proposing is that understanding the variables potentially affecting (and confounding) test performance may be as important as obtaining norms for different human groups.

No doubt, cross-cultural neuropsychology represents a critical new direction of research, and will challenge neuropsychologists during the 21st century.

REFERENCES

Albert, M. S., & Heaton, R. (1988). Intelligence testing. In M. S. Albert & M. B. Moss (Eds.), *Geriatric neuropsychology* (pp. 10–32). New York: Guildford.
Anastasi, A. (1988). *Psychological testing*. New York: Macmillan.
Ardila, A. (Ed.). (1993). On the origins of cognitive activity [Special issue]. *Behavioural Neurology, 6*, 71–74.
Ardila, A. (1995). Directions of research in cross-cultural neuropsychology. *Journal of Clinical and Experimental Neuropsychology, 17*, 143–150.
Ardila, A. (1996). Towards a cross-cultural neuropsychology. *Journal of Social and Evolutionary Systems, 19*, 237–248.
Ardila, A. (1998). A note of caution: Normative neuropsychological test performance: Effects of age, education, gender and ethnicity: A comment on Saykin *et al.* (1995). *Applied Neuropsychology, 5*, 51–53.
Ardila, A. (1999). A neuropsychological approach to intelligence. *Neuropsychology Review, 3*, 117–136.
Ardila, A. (2000). Evaluación cognoscitiva en analfabetos [Neuropsychological assessment in illiterates]. *Revista de Neurologia, 30*, 465–468.
Ardila, A. (2003). Culture in our brains: Cross-cultural differences in the brain-behavior relationships. In A. Toomela (Ed.), *Cultural guidance in the development of the human mind* (pp. 63–86). Westport, CT: Ablex.
Ardila, A. T. (2005). Cultural values underlying cognitive test performance. *Neuropsychology Review, 15*, 185–195.
Ardila, A., & Moreno, S. (2001). Neuropsychological evaluation in Aruaco Indians: An exploratory study. *Journal of the International Neuropsychological Society, 7*, 510–515.
Ardila, A., Ostrosky, F., & Bernal, B. (2005). Cognitive testing toward the future: The example of semantic verbal fluency (ANIMALS). Unpublished manuscript.
Ardila, A., Ostrosky, F., & Mendoza, V. (2000b). Learning to read is much more than learning to read: A neuropsychologically based learning to read method. *Journal of the International Neuropsychological Society, 6*, 789–801.
Ardila, A., Ostrosky-Solis, F., Rosselli, M., & Gomez, C. (2000a). Age related cognitive decline during normal aging: The complex effect of education. *Archives of Clinical Neuropsychology, 15*, 495–514.
Ardila, A., Rodriguez, G., & Rosselli, M. (2003). Current issues in the neuropsychological assessment with Hispanics/Latinos. In: F. R. Ferraro (Ed.), *Minority and cross-cultural aspects of neuropsychological assessment* (pp. 151–179). Lisse, The Netherlands: Swets & Zeitlinger Publishers.

Ardila, A., & Rosselli, M. (1989). Neuropsychological characteristics of normal aging. *Developmental Neuropsychology, 5,* 307–320.
Ardila, A., & Rosselli, M.. (1994). Development of language, memory and visuospatial abilities in 5- to 12-year-old children using a neuropsychological battery. *Developmental Neuropsychology, 10,* 97–120.
Ardila, A., Rosselli, M., & Ostrosky, F. (1992). Sociocultural factors in neuropsychological assessment. In A R. Puente & R. J. McCaffrey (Eds.), *Handbook of neuropsychological assessment: A biopsychosocial perspective* (pp. 181–192). New York: Plenum Press.
Ardila, A., Rosselli, M., & Puente, A. (1994). *Neuropsychological assessment of Spanish-speakers.* New York: Plenum Press.
Ardila, A., Rosselli, M., & Rosas, P. (1989). Neuropsychological assessment in illiterates: Visuospatial and memory abilities. *Brain and Cognition, 11,* 147–166.
Bernatzik, H. A. (1957). *Razas y pueblos del mundo* [World races and people] (Vols. 1–3). Barcelona: Ediciones Ave.
Berry, J. W. (1979). Culture and cognition style. In A. Marsella, R. G. Tharp, & T. J. Ciborowski (Eds.), *Perspectives in cross-cultural psychology* (pp. 117–135). New York: Academic Press.
Bornstein, R. A., & Suga, L. J. (1988). Educational level and neuropsychological performance in healthy elderly subjects. *Developmental Neuropsychology, 4,* 17–22.
Brislin, R. W. (1983). Cross-cultural research in psychology. *Annual Review of Psychology, 34,* 363–400.
Brody, N. (1992). *Intelligence* (2nd ed.). New York: Academic Press.
Ceci, S. J. (1990). *On intelligence ... more or less: A bioecological treatise on intellectual development.* Englewood, NJ: Prentice-Hall.
Ceci, S. J. (1991). How much does schooling influence general intelligence and its cognitive components? A reassessment of evidence. *Developmental Psychology, 27,* 703–722.
Ceci, S. J., & Williams, W. M. (1997). Schooling, intelligence and income. *American Psychologist, 52,* 1051–1058.
Ciborowski, I. J. (1979). Cross-cultural aspects of cognitive functioning: Culture and knowledge. In A. J. Marsella, R. G. Tharp, & I. J. Ciborowski (Eds.), *Perspectives in cross-cultural psychology* (pp. 101–116). New York: Academic Press.
Cole, M. (1975). An ethnographic psychology of cognition. In R. Brislin, S. Bochner, & W. Lonner (Eds.), *Cross-cultural perspectives of learning* (pp. 157–175). Beverly Hills, CA: Sage.
Cornelious, S. W., & Caspi, A. (1987). Everyday problem solving in adulthood and old age. *Psychology of Aging, 2,* 144–153.
Craik, F. M., Byrd, M., & Swanson, J. M. (1987). Patterns of memory loss in three elderly samples. *Psychology and Aging, 2,* 79–86.
Dehaene, S. (1997). *The number sense. How the mind creates mathematics.* New York: Oxford University Press.
Dingfelder, S. (2005). Closing the gap for Latino patients. *Monitor, 36*(1), 58–61
Ferguson, G. (1956). On transfer and the abilities of man. *Canadian Journal of Psychology, 10,* 121–131.
Ferraro, F. R. (Ed.). (2002). *Minority and cross-cultural aspects of neuropsychological assessment.* Lisse, The Netherlands: Swets & Zeitlinger Publishers.
Finlayson, N. A., Johnson, K. A., & Reitan, R. M. (1977). Relation of level of education to neuropsychological measures in brain damaged and non-brain damaged adults. *Journal of Consulting and Clinical Psychology, 45,* 536–542.
Fletcher-Janzen, E., Strickland, T. L., & Reynolds, C. R. (Eds.). (2000). *Handbook of cross-cultural neuropsychology.* New York: Kluwer Academic/Plenum Publishers.

Geisinger, K. (Ed.). (1992). *Psychological testing of Hispanics.* Washington, DC: American Psychological Association.
Goldblum, M. C., & Matute, E. (1986). Are illiterate people deep dyslexics? *Journal of Neurolinguistics, 2,* 103–114.
Greenfield, P. M. (1997). You can't take it with you: Why ability assessments don't cross cultures. *American Psychologist, 52,* 1115–1124.
Grimes, B. F. (Ed.). (2000). *Ethnolongue: Languages of the world* (14th ed.). Dallas, TX: SIL International.
Halperin, J. M., Healy, J. M., Zeitchik, E., Ludman, W. L., & Weinstein, L. (1989). Developmental aspects of linguistic and mnesic abilities in normal children. *Journal of Clinical and Experimental Neuropsychology, 11,* 518–528.
Harris, M. (1983). *Culture, people, nature: An introduction to general anthropology* (3rd ed.). New York: Harper & Row.
Harris, J. G., Echemendia, R., Ardila, A., & Rosselli, M. (2001). Cross-cultural cognitive and neuropsychological assessment. In J. W. Jac, J. C. W. Andrews, D. H. Saklofske, & H. L. Janzen (Eds.), *Handbook of psychoeducational assessment* (pp. 512–535). San Diego, CA: Academic Press.
Heaton, R. K., Grant, I., & Mathews, C. (1986). Differences in neuropsychological test performance associated with age, education and sex. In I. Grant & K. M. Adams (Eds.), *Neuropsychological assessment in neuropsychiatric disorders* (pp. 108–120). New York: Oxford University Press.
Hunter, J. (1986). Cognitive ability, cognitive aptitudes, job knowledge, and job performance. *Journal of Vocational Behavior, 29,* 340–363.
Laboratory of Comparative Human Cognition. (1983). Culture and cognitive development. In P. Mussen (Ed.), *Handbook of child psychology: Vol 1. History, theories and methods* (pp. 342–397). New York: Wiley.
Leckliter, I. N., & Matarazzo, J. D. (1989). The influence of age, education, IQ, gender, and alcohol abuse on Halstead-Reitan Neuropsychological Test Battery performance. *Journal of Clinical Psychology, 45,* 484–511.
Lecours, R. L., Mehler, J., Parente, M. A., Caldeira, A., Cary, L., Castro, M. J., et al. (1987a). Illiteracy and brain damage I: Aphasia testing in culturally contrasted populations (control subjects). *Neuropsychologia, 25,* 231–245.
Lecours, R. L., Mehler, J., Parente, M. A., Caldeira, A., Cary, L., Castro, M. J., et al. (1987b). Illiteracy and brain damage 2: Manifestations of unilateral neglect in testing "auditory comprehension" with iconographic material. *Brain and Cognition, 6,* 243–265.
Lecours, A. R., Mehler, J., Parente, M. A., Beltrami, M. C., Canossa de Tolipan, L., Castro, M. J., et al. (1988). Illiteracy and brain damage 3: A contribution to the study of speech and language disorders in illiterates with unilateral brain damage (initial testing). *Neuropsychologia, 26,* 575–589.
Lezak, M. D. (2004). *Neuropsychological assessment* (4th ed.). New York: Oxford University Press.
Manly, J. J., Jacobs, D. M., Sano, M., Bell, K., Merchant, C. A., Small, S. A., & Stern, Y. (1999). Effect of literacy on neuropsychological test performance in non-demented, education-matched elders. *Journal of the International Neuropsychological Society, 5,* 191–202.
Matarazzo, J. D. (1972). *Wechsler's measurement and appraisal of adult intelligence* (5th ed.). New York: Oxford University Press.
Matthews, C. G. (1992). Truth in labeling: Are we really an international society? *Journal of Clinical and Experimental Neuropsychology, 14,* 418–426.

Matute, E., Leal, F., Zarabozo, D., Robles, A., & Cedillo, C. (2000). Does literacy have an effect on stick construction tasks? *Journal of the International Neuropsychological Society, 6,* 668–672.
Nell, V. (2000). *Cross-cultural neuropsychological assessment: Theory and practice.* Mahwah, NJ: Lawrence Erlbaum Associates.
Neisser, U., Boodoo, G., Bouchard, T .J., Boykin, A. W., Brody, N., Ceci, S.J., et al. (1996). Intelligence: Knowns and unknowns. *American Psychologist, 51,* 77–101.
Ostrosky, F., Ardila, A., Rosselli, M., Lopez-Arango, G., & Uriel-Mendoza, V. (1998). Neuropsychological test performance in illiterates. *Archives of Clinical Neuropsychology, 13,* 645– 660.
Ostrosky, F., Ardila, A., & Rosselli, M. (1999). NEUROPSI: A brief neuropsychological test battery in Spanish. *Journal of the International Neuropsychological Society, 5,* 413–433.
Ostrosky, F., Canseco, E., Quintanar, L., Navarro, E., & Ardila, A. (1985). Sociocultural effects in neuropsychological assessment. *International Journal of Neuroscience, 27,* 53–66.
Ostrosky, F., Quintanar, L., Canseco, E., Meneses, S., Navarro, E., & Ardila, A. (1986). Habilidades cognoscitivas y nivel sociocultural [Cognitive abilities and sociocultural level]. *Revista de Investigación Clínica, 38,* 37–42.
Puente, A., & Ardila, A. (2000). Neuropsychological assessment of Hispanics. In E. Fletcher-Janzen, T. L. Strickland, & C. R. Reynolds (Eds.), *The handbook of cross-cultural neuropsychology* (pp. 87–104). New York: Plenum Press.
Reis, A., & Castro-Caldas, A. (1997). Illiteracy: A cause for biased cognitive development. *Journal of the International Neuropsychological Society, 5,* 444–450.
Reis, A., Guerreiro, M., & Petersson, K. M. (2003). A sociodemographic and neuropsychological characterization of an illiterate population. *Applied Neuropsychology, 10,* 191–204.
Rosselli, M. (1993). Neuropsychology of illiteracy. *Behavioral Neurology, 6,* 107–112.
Rosselli, M., & Ardila, A. (2003). The impact of culture and education on nonverbal neuropsychological measurements: A critical review. *Brain and Cognition, 52,* 226–233.
Rosselli, M., Ardila, A., Araujo, K., Weekes, V. A., Caracciolo, V., Pradilla, M., & Ostrosky, F. (2000). Verbal fluency and repetition skills in healthy older Spanish-English bilinguals. *Applied Neuropsychology, 7,* 17–24.
Rosselli, M., Ardila, A., & Rosas, P. (1990). Neuropsychological assessment in illiterates II: Language and praxic abilities. *Brain and Cognition, 12,* 281–296.
Spreen, O., & Strauss, E. (1991). *A compendium of neuropsychological tests* (2nd ed.). New York: Oxford University Press.
Vygotsky, L. S. (1962). *Thought and language.* Cambridge, MA: MIT Press.
Vygotsky, L. S. (1989). Historia del desarrollo de las funciones psíquicas superiores [History of the development of higher psychological processes]. In A. L. Vygotsky, A. Leontiev, & A. R. Luria (Eds.), *El proceso de formación de la psicología marxista* (pp. 156–163). Moscow: Progress.
Whorf, B. L. (1956). *Language, thought and reality.* Cambridge, MA: MIT Press.
www.ethnologue.com
Yamadori, A. (1975). Ideogram reading in alexia. *Brain, 98,* 231–238.

Chapter **3**

The Art of Clinical Neuropsychology

Nathaniel William Nelson
University of Minnesota

Marcel O. Pontón
Harbor-UCLA Medical Center

Good science is good art. It is elegant, simple, replicable, and sustained for the sake of culture. Good science challenges the observer to view the world in new and transformative ways and serves in turn to enrich society. Karl Popper (1982) suggested that "science may be described as the art of systematic over-simplification—the art of discerning what we may with advantage omit" (p. 44). When science successfully describes the universe in a parsimonious yet cogent manner, it becomes an artful endeavor.

Clinical neuropsychology is grounded in a unique form of "systematic oversimplification"; with reliable and valid measures, it describes individual human behavior and compares it to culturally relevant normative groups. Describing the complexities of human behavior in a concise fashion is itself a daunting task; all the more so in our ever-increasingly diverse society. To the extent that neuropsychologists succeed in describing brain–behavior relationships amidst the world's present cultural diversity, they will succeed as both scientists and as artists.

The present chapter discusses a number of topics pertinent to the practice of clinical neuropsychology in diverse cultural settings. First, a brief discussion of the epistemological assumptions that underlie the practice of clinical neuropsychology is made, with special attention given to two epistemological approaches (idiographic and nomothetic) that have prevailed over the last century. Second, we suggest that clinicians should have an awareness of the general issues that relate to test performances in all cultures. Third, we discuss the limitations of traditional measures in culturally diverse settings. Finally, through a brief review of the recent cross-cultural literature, we suggest that neuropsychologists' cultural sensitivity will be maintained only when measures and norms are made appropriate to the individual patient's cultural background. We conclude by suggesting that the progress of neuropsychology in the years to come will be highly dependent on supervisory relationships, and the need to expose clinicians-in-training to a variety of assessment techniques that are not limited to a single approach to the neuropsychological evaluation.

NEUROPSYCHOLOGY AS AN EPISTEMIC TASK

Neuropsychology, as practiced today, represents an epistemic task. Neuropsychologists seek to know and understand basic "truths" about cognitive functioning in individuals, and the conclusions we reach from our assessments provide the basis for diagnostic and treatment recommendations. Because we come to "know" the nature of a patient's condition as a function of obtained test results, neuropsychology may be regarded as an epistemic discipline.

Neuropsychology is also an epistemic discipline because it creates and warrants knowledge through research. It is a field requiring expertise and specialization. In the words of Lezak (1995), "Clinical Neuropsychology is an applied science concerned with the behavioral expression of brain dysfunction" (p. 7). There are specific principles that inform and guide the field's knowledge system and procedures. It is entrenched in knowledge institutions for its validation as a science, and it has a sanctioned machinery of knowledge (e.g., use of technology and tools, dissemination channels, alliance with capital sources, codes of practice) that furthers its epistemic base (Cetina, 1999). The dynamic relationship between the different branches of neuroscience and neuropsychology purport to contribute to society through the integration of knowledge into better diagnostic and treatment benefits to patients.

However, this knowledge is predicated on a number of assumptions and methodologies (chief among which is the use of norm-referenced tests) that may differ in relevance across cultures. The question then becomes: What is true about cognition across cultures? Seasoned clinicians will readily admit that they are limited by their training, their methodology, their school of thought (i.e., philosophical biases), and by the economics of service delivery in coming to conclusions that reflect what they know about patients. Patients, on the other hand, pose a variety of limitations to our task. Well-documented variables such as age and education affect test performance, but so do less understood variables such as cultural background, bilingualism, language mastery, acquiescence, motivation, and behavioral scripts for ethnic relations (Ponton & Ardila, 1999). The current *sitz em lieben*, which involves large migration patterns from East to West and South to North, makes the possibility of our clinical interaction with culturally different patients highly likely and at times equivocal. We don't need to travel far away to encounter clinical situations with groups from different ethnic and language backgrounds than the majority cultures of where we live. The world is next door.

To interact clinically across cultures with patients whose backgrounds may be dissimilar from the groups on which many tests are normed, poses an epistemological challenge to our task: What is the quality of the "knowledge" I have derived through these tests? Such challenge places a direct burden on our ethical mandates to do well for our clients and faces us with the imperative of obtaining more appropriate (ecologically valid, culturally relevant, functionally based) data. The "how" of this approach, however, may be farther away from the marketing urge permeating our profession in the United States. That is to say, we may not be able to package it, but we need to buy the notion (by virtue of its intellectual integrity) that modified, more culturally appropriate approaches are necessary for neuropsychology to remain relevant in a cross-cultural world where North American tests and norms may not apply. The prospect of such a transition is not a new one, and as is reviewed later in this chapter, recent studies have attempted to observe patients' performances through use of modified measures and norms. We encourage clinicians to recognize that our test results invariably dictate how we "know" our patients, and to appreciate that this represents only one way of understanding how our patients think, feel, and behave.

Throughout the history of psychology, a tension has existed between two epistemological sources: the nomothetic (law-based) and the idiographic (individual-based; Franck, 1982). As regards the nomothetic approach, psychology has emphasized the importance of what is shown to be "lawful" through theoretical predictions and their respective confirmatory observations, with replicability being the main objective (Gorsuch, 2002). Those theories that demonstrate especially consistent findings over time and testing become cornerstones on which future exploratory studies may build. Levav, Mirsky, French, and Bartko (1998) noted that "the quest for universal similarities of behavioral manifestations or performance continues to be a major theme in cross-cultural psychology" (p. 658). Clearly, this appeal to "universal similarities" is a notion representative of a nomothetic approach, and the theory behind this approach is that the construct of interest can be measured in a replicable and universal way. In neuropsychology, predominant emphasis on the quantitative method is a *sine qua non*, and it allows neuropsychologists to retain "objective" approaches to understanding human behavior. As Ivnik et al. (2001) stated, "Neuropsychological assessments are, by their nature quantitative. They move beyond potentially idiosyncratic judgments of patient features (symptoms) or crude estimates of important abilities, such as non-standardized clinical rating schemes" (p. 123).

Differently, idiographic emphases may include a description of the patient through behavioral observations or how the patient experienced the neuropsychological evaluation (e.g., was it tiring? what tests did the patient find especially difficult or easy?). Clinicians whose specialization in neuropsychology comes as a part of a more general training in clinical psychology develop psychotherapeutic skills that prove to be essential when interviewing a patient for the first time. Through self-directed questions (e.g., "what impression did the patient make on me") during the clinical interview, many clinicians rely heavily on the impressions they receive even before testing begins. The clinician may become aware that a patient "feels" a bit "frontal." As another example, the patient's description of his or her social history may cause the examiner to wonder to what extent the patient's Axis II characteristics might be the result of an underlying cognitive compromise. The patient's history and observed behaviors are as pertinent as formal test scores. This is because the latter, quantitative descriptor, while a necessary and valuable way of understanding the patient, can never definitively account for the patient's functioning or describe how the patient's culture interacts with the patient's presentation. Data derived from a quantitative approach and data taken on an idiographic, case-sensitive basis are essential if we are to understand the patient's functioning both in terms of the individual culture, and how he or she compares to others with similar conditions of similar cultural backgrounds. To the extent that either of these approaches is minimized, an accurate and culture-sensitive assessment of the individual patient is compromised.

Historically, some have expressed concern that the field of psychology has emphasized the nomothetic approach to patients over and against the idiographic. Gordon Allport, for example, understood more than most the limitations of the nomothetic method. As Franck (1982, p. 1) said, "It was Allport's oft-repeated complaint that psychology has given its attention only to universals, has neglected to study the individual, and has therefore been guilty of a serious failure in the fulfillment of its scientific task." Furthermore, Allport (1961) recognized that every individual life is in some ways like every other life, is in some ways like some other lives, and is in some ways like no other life. A staunchly nomothetic approach to an understanding of human behavior will not account for those times when the individual patient is in some ways like no one else. In other words, the nomothetic approach may or may not be congruent with the individual patient's unique experiences (Haynes, Kaholokula, & Nelson, 1999).

Some neuropsychologists have also expressed their concern that the field may have a limited ability to recognize individual differences in cognition. Ardila (1995, p. 143), for instance, stated that "we barely have dealt with individual differences in neuropsychological performance; and our understanding of cultural differences is, to be optimistic, very insufficient." Although Ardila does not deny the notion of certain universals in basic human cognition, he argued that "... different cultural environments lead to the development of different patterns of abilities" (p. 145). Thus, individuals whose cultures vary to a great extent from traditional normative samples will not necessarily demonstrate the same sorts of behaviors on present standardized tests. What is needed is an "anthropological neuropsychology" that attempts to improve on our knowledge of culture in the assessment setting, especially as it relates to the individual patient.

An artful, culturally sensitive approach to clinical neuropsychology entails striking a balance between the nomothetic and idiographic perspectives, a notion that Franck (1982, p. 3) has previously described as an "idiographic-nomothetic symbiosis." Or, as Allport (1960, p. 147) aptly stated: "Unless ... idiographic (particular) knowledge is fused with nomothetic (universal) knowledge, we shall not achieve the aims of science...." We suggest that a fusion between the particular and the universal characteristics of human behavior represents *the* task with which neuropsychology as a culturally sensitive science should be concerned. Arriving at this fusion, at a minimum, will include: (1) an awareness of the general issues that relate to test performances across all cultures; (2) a recognition of how culture may influence cognition and related test performances; and (3) the appropriate modification of neuropsychological measures or norms when they do not adequately represent the cultural background(s) of the individual patient.

Use of Neuropsychological Measures: General Considerations

There are a number of issues that invariably influence the clinician's interpretation of a patient's test performance, regardless of his or her cultural background. These include, but are not limited to, construct validity, one's conception of "normal" test performance, and basic underlying demographic variables.

Tests with questionable construct validity cannot be expected to be valid in diverse settings. Dodrill (1997, 1999) suggested that it is a "myth" that neuropsychologists "have a good knowledge of the constructs that our tests measure" (1997, p. 3). He found that neuropsychological measures drawn from within the same cognitive domains demonstrated only slightly greater correlational magnitudes than measures observed between differing cognitive domains, with similar findings observed in both control participants and clinical patients. These findings challenge the assumption that current neuropsychological measures adequately represent the constructs they purport to measure..

We are not suggesting that Dodrill's (1997) findings are necessarily representative of how well current neuropsychological measures embody intended constructs. Indeed, Bell and Roper (1998) presented literature to suggest otherwise. We only wish to emphasize that an awareness of measures' construct validity will lead to the improvement of test quality, and the minimization of harm to patients of all cultural backgrounds. As an example of how construct validity may relate to minimizing harm, consider the findings of Dulay et al. (2002). They examined the Family Pictures subtest of the Wechsler Memory Scale-III (WMS-III; Wechsler, 1997) in a sample of patients evaluated for epilepsy surgery. Although this subtest was originally designed as a contributor to the visual memory indices, the authors found the test to correlate highly with another measure that is typically understood to be verbal in nature (Logical Memory). In response to their findings, the authors concluded that Family Pictures may not be an appropriate predictor of visual memory ability. Neuropsychological measures such as these often play an important role in determining treatment of neurological conditions (e.g., epilepsy), and treatment of such conditions may involve very invasive procedures (e.g., temporal lobectomy). As such, the importance of construct validity becomes all the more essential to proper treatment of the individual patient, regardless of his or her cultural background.

Another general consideration relates to the clinician's understanding of "normal" versus "abnormal" test performances. Neuropsychologists are sometimes confronted with the challenging task of deciding whether "impaired" scores represent the individual patient's typical ability, or whether "normal" scores may represent relative impairments for the patient. Additionally, test performances that are not uniformly extreme (i.e., all within the "normal" or "severely impaired" ranges) may be especially difficult to interpret. Recognition of how healthy individuals commonly perform on neuropsychological measures will aid the clinician's ability to interpret individual test performances.

For instance, Palmer, Boone, Lesser, and Wohl (1998) observed frequencies of "impaired" performances in 132 healthy older adults who did not exhibit evidence of neurological disorder. Through administration of a number of commonly used neuropsychological measures, they found that nearly three-quarters (73%) of the sample showed at least one score that was within the borderline range (< 1.3 SD), and more than one third (37%) of the sample showed at least one score in the impaired range (< 2.0 SD). More recently, Schretlen, Munro, Anthony, and Pearlson (2003) observed the extent of "intraindividual" variability that healthy adults exhibited across a number of neuropsychological measures. They observed differences between each participant's highest and lowest scores to calculate a "maximum discrepancy" in each individual's performance. They found that the majority (66%) of their 197 healthy adults showed discrepancies of three or more standard deviations between their highest and lowest scores. Studies such as these highlight the importance of recognizing that even healthy or "normal" individuals can exhibit substandard performances and great variability on neuropsychological measures. Foreknowledge of "normal" test performances in mainstream samples will aid the clinician's ability to interpret individual patients' performances within diverse settings.

Demographic variables (e.g., age, education, gender) are often related to individual test performances, and numerous studies have previously described the nature of these relationships (e.g., Ardila & Rosselli, 1989; Gontkovsky, Mold, & Beatty, 2002; Heaton, Grant, & Matthews, 1986; Reitan & Wolfson, 1995). Although it is necessary for clinicians to continue examining these commonly studied variables, consideration of other, less commonly reported variables that can influence test performances should also be examined. O'Bryant, O'Jile, and McCaffrey (2004) reviewed literature from five of the most frequently read neuropsychology journals from the years 1995 to 2000. They found that whereas age, education, and gender are often included in studies, demographics such as race, ethnicity, level of acculturation, and primary language are reported infrequently, if at all. The authors argued that failing to report these demographics limits neuropsychologists' ability to apply research to their everyday practices; "... how can one know if the findings of a study are applicable to his/her practice if they do not know if the sample utilized in the study resembled what they see everyday in practice?" (p. 231). In short, although the field of neuropsychology has documented the relationships between demographics and neuropsychological tests, research that considers other culturally specific demographics (e.g., ethnicity) remains to be conducted with satisfactory frequency.

Generally, the current literature attests to the merit of neuropsychological tests and their role in describing cognition, and test limitations may sometimes be independent of culture. Consideration of these limitations, as well as of how culture may influence cognition, is especially important when neuropsychological measures are used with culturally diverse patients. In addition to obtaining an awareness of the general issues that relate to test performance across cultures, clinicians should be aware of how the patient's individual cultural background may influence cognition and related test performances.

Cognition and Culture

Numerous recent studies have explored the influence that culture may have over cognition (e.g., Benet-Martinez, Leu, Lee, & Morris, 2002; Norenzayan,

Smith, Kim, & Nisbett, 2002; Tavassoli, 2002). Benet-Martinez et al. (2002), for instance, found that attributional styles varied at different levels of perceived "bicultural identity integration" (BII). Chinese Americans with high levels of BII made more external attributions when presented with Chinese cultural primes (e.g., The Great Wall of China), and more internal attributions when exposed to American cultural primes (e.g., The White House). The reverse process was observed in Chinese American participants with low perceived BII, suggesting that one's perception of individual identity may be related to how he or she interprets the environment. Norenzayan et al. (2002) found that European Americans tend to prefer formal or "rule-based" styles of cognitive reasoning, whereas Chinese and Korean participants tend to prefer intuitive or experience-based styles of reasoning.

Other recent studies have suggested that environmental factors such as reading acquisition, language characteristics, and literacy may play a role in cognition (e.g., Conant et al., 2003; Folia & Kosmidis, 2003; Gonzalez da Silva, Petersson, Faisca, Ingvar, & Reis, 2004; Hedden et al., 2002; Levinson, Kita, Haun, & Rasch, 2002; McBride-Chang & Kail, 2002). Regarding reading acquisition, McBride-Chang and Kail (2002) found that while reading development itself was similar in participants from Hong Kong and the United States, the strongest predictor of reading acquisition was "phonological awareness" (in contrast to other constructs such as visual processing) in both cultures. Hedden et al. (2002) addressed how language differences may relate to differences in working memory (visual and verbal) and processing speed (visual and verbal). They found relatively similar visual working memory and processing speed performances in Chinese and American participants, regardless of their ages. However, younger Chinese participants outperformed the American participants on a verbal working memory test. The authors suggested that this finding may have been related to "linguistic differences," such as differences in the number of syllables used to represent digits, between the Chinese languages and English.

Regarding literacy and cognition, Gonzalez da Silva et al. (2004) found that although literate and illiterate groups performed comparably on a verbal fluency task involving naming of supermarket items, the illiterate group performed significantly worse on an animal naming task. Folia and Kosmidis (2003) observed verbal and visual list learning performances in a group of literate, semiliterate, and illiterate Greek women. The illiterate group performed significantly worse than the other two groups on most verbal learning indices, and showed worse performances in delayed visual free and cued recall. The authors suggested that the observed differences in the illiterate group may have been related to relatively less developed encoding abilities compared to the other two groups. However, differences between groups might also be related to the nature of the tasks themselves, and the authors emphasized the importance of developing ecologically valid measures when assessing illiterate individuals.

The results of the latter two studies speak to the importance of ecological validity in neuropsychological assessment, and it can be assumed that variations in test performances may be associated with variation in cultural relevance of tests. In other words, individuals from various cultures may experience the testing relationship in dissimilar ways, and not all who take these tests necessarily agree on the tests' relevance to their lives. Shepherd and Leathem (1999) observed the Maori population of New Zealand (which represents 12% of the total population in that region), a group who has previously shown especial difficulty in academic success. This cohort speaks English, and attends the same educational facilities as New Zealanders of European descent. However, the group's children consistently performed more poorly on standard measures of cognition. In order to explore possible reasons why the group showed declined scores relative to the majority culture, the authors were interested in Maori patients who suffered traumatic brain injuries and their personal experiences during their assessments. The authors administered questionnaires that solicited information regarding patients' experiences of the neuropsychological examination itself. Results showed that the "Maori were less satisfied ... with the service than the non-Maori respondents, especially in the areas concerning current Maori cultural practices, physical surroundings, type of service, and quality of service" (Shepherd & Leathem, 1999, p. 84). Others "found the clinic difficult to travel to as well as uncomfortable and intimidating" (p. 84). The authors concluded that cultural expectation differences between ethnic minorities and majority group examiners can adversely affect the patients' perceptions of the testing and their performance on tests. The authors recommended more effort be made to accommodate test-takers from minority groups by paying attention to "situational, procedural, and interpersonal variables," and these efforts might yield more valid results.

As an example of a group for whom Western measures may be particularly inappropriate or irrelevant, consider the findings of Ardila and Moreno (2001) who observed neuropsychological performances in an indigenous South American tribe, the Aruaco Indian culture in Colombia. The authors found Western tests to have limited usefulness within the cohort. Three of the participants were unable to draw simple or complex designs, and these participants "had never used a pencil before, nor had they engaged in drawing or copying anything before" (p. 513). Furthermore, although the authors anticipated that nonverbal measures would be more appropriate relative to verbal measures, results suggested this was not the case; in fact, they noted, "nonverbal tests are not necessarily more appropriate for cross-cultural testing than verbal tests." The authors conclude that "tests tapping abilities related to the everyday life (meaningful functional movements used in the everyday life, naming of animals, etc.) seem to be valid for every human group" (p. 514).

How others, such as family members, perceive a patient's cognitive impairment in daily living may also vary from culture to culture. For instance, in diagnosing dementia, Teng (2002) suggested that factors of language, education, ecological relevance of test items, and cultural attitudes be taken into account if neuropsychologists are to arrive at accurate descriptions of how impairments may relate to everyday living. The author noted that peoples from various ethnic or cultural groups may have different understandings of how cognition affects tasks related to everyday living. For instance, "for an older white couple who live by themselves in a modern city, many complex skills are needed in their daily life, such as cooking, driving or using public transportation, banking, shopping, using the telephone, and operating a variety of appliances. Impairment in any of these skills will draw attention and cause concern" (p. S78). In contrast, for an older couple living with extended family, perhaps others manage many of the chores. In this case, "mild or even moderate deteriorations in cognitive abilities or social behavior are either unnoticed, or simply accepted as signs of normal aging" (p. S78). Thus, an individual patient's symptom-related behaviors can only be regarded in light of cultural perceptions of the same.

The studies reviewed here are only a small representation of the literature that has recently addressed relationships between culture and cognition. We refer the reader to the APA Web site (www.apa.org/science/testclearinghs.html) for a more comprehensive review. A common theme of the present cross-cultural literature is that the growth of neuropsychology is dependent on its ability to make psychometric alterations that adequately correspond to the ever-changing international community. As van de Vijver (2002) noted, "Western societies continue to be multicultural and the issue of valid assessment in culturally heterogeneous groups will only become more prominent" (p. 559). Numerous efforts are being made in this regard currently, with some studies yielding more success than others. In response to these changes, modifications to traditional measures and norms will need to be made, and qualitative measures will need to be administered when the former endeavor does not live up to expectations.

Modifying Current Neuropsychological Measures and Norms for Cross-Cultural Use

The fusion between individual and universal understandings of human behavior involves modifying traditional measures or developing new measures to match the cultural backgrounds of individual patients. As Lezak (2002, p. 343) stated, "It should now be common knowledge among psychologists that some test norms developed for the dominant culture so skew their application to persons from other cultures that we cannot use them to evaluate ability levels in intact participants ..." To modify measures and norms, or to develop new ways of describing cognition, is both a scientific and an ethical responsibility. The APA Ethics Code (2002) Standard 9.06 (Interpreting Assessment Results) states that when psychologists make test interpretations, they should "take into account the purpose of the assessment as well as the various test factors, test-taking abilities, and other characteristics of the person being assessed, such as situational, personal, linguistic, and *cultural differences* [emphasis added], that might affect psychologists' judgments or reduce the accuracy of their interpretations." A respect for cultural differences in interpreting test results is a necessary step in avoiding harm and respecting the patient's autonomy (Harris, 2002). Clearly, then, use of traditional norms that do not adequately match the cultural background(s) of an individual patient would represent an ethical violation, as cognitive function may be described as "normal" or "impaired" when indeed this may not be the case. Thus, if neuropsychologists are to retain a respectful, scientific approach to describing individual behavior in cross-cultural settings, measures and norms will need to be modified appropriately, or qualitative approaches should be employed when the former methods do not suffice.

In light of the changing nature of Western cultures, appropriate modifications to measures and norms to meet these changes in the dominant culture are necessary. Among the most laudable examples of research that has appropriately modified norms to meet fluctuations in aging are the Mayo Older Americans Normative Studies (MOANS; Harris, Ivnik, & Smith, 2002; Ivnik et al., 1992a, b, c, d; Ivnik, 1996; Ivnik et al., 1997; Lucas et al., 1998; Malec et al., 1992; Schretlen & Ivnik, 1996; Smith et al., 1992). It is hoped that this line of research will continue in the future, with added modifications to normative data inclusive of the most recent revisions of standardized measures (e.g., WMS-III, 1997).

Further, the changing nature of Western culture's ethnic base makes development of ethnically appropriate norms a necessity, even for those who practice solely within the United States (e.g., Friedman, M. A., Schinka, J. A., Mortimer, J. A., & Graves, A. B., 2002; Moering, Schinka, Mortimer, & Graves, 2004; Patton et al., 2003). For instance, Patton et al. (2003) found group differences between African American and Caucasian participants on 10 of the 12 subtests of the Repeatable Battery for the Assessment of Neuropsychological Status (RBANS; Randolph, 1998). The authors provided normative data for the African American participants for each subtest of this measure. Moering et al. (2004) recently provided normative data for elderly African Americans on the Stroop Color and Word Test (Golden, 1978), a step that had not previously been taken.

Outside of Western culture, a plethora of studies have recently provided support for the use of modified versions of Western neuropsychological measures and norms in other cultural settings (e.g., Chan, Choi, Chiu, & Lam, 2003; Chan & Manly, 2002; Holding et al., 2004; Kojima et al., 2002; Kosmidis, Vlahou, Panagiotaki, & Kiosseoglou, 2004; Lee et al., 2002, 2004; Lee, Yuen, & Chan, 2002). Lee et al. (2002) translated the original Consortium to Establish a Registry for Alzheimer's Disease (CERAD) battery from English to Korean (CERAD-K), and Lee et al. (2004) provided norms for the CERAD-K. Chan, Lee, Fong, Lee, and Wong (2002) demonstrated the cross-cultural validity of a Chinese version of the Cognistat (Chan et al., 1999) in a sample of Chinese patients with stroke. Chan and Manly (2002) demonstrated the usefulness of Cantonese versions of the Dysexecutive Questionnaire (DEX; Wilson, Alderman, Burgess, Emsley, & Evans, 1996), the Cognitive Failures Questionnaire (CFQ; Broadbent, Cooper, FitzGerald, & Parkes, 1982), The Modified Six Elements Test (Wilson et al., 1996), and The Tower of Hanoi (Humes, Welsh, Retzlaff, & Cookson, 1997) in a group of TBI patients from Hong Kong. Results from this study suggested that executive symptoms in the Chinese sample did not differ markedly from those that had been obtained from a like sample in the United Kingdom. Kojima et al. (2002) found a Japanese version of the Beck Depression Inventory-II (BDI-II; Beck, Steer, & Brown, 1996) to be sensitive to symptoms of depression in a large Japanese sample. Chan et al. (2003) found a Chinese version of the Mattis Dementia Rating Scale (DRS; Mattis, 1988) to effectively discriminate Chinese elderly patients with Alzheimer's disease from normal controls. Lee et al. (2002) provided normative data across a number of commonly used neuropsychological measures in a Hong Kong Chinese sample. These studies provide only a sample of the many new cross-cultural studies that are coming to the fore, and judging from the results of most of these studies, it appears that use of traditional measures cross culturally is oftentimes warranted.

Despite recent progress, Western measures are sometimes limited for use in non-Western cultures (e.g., Almagor & Koren, 2001; Azocar, Arean, Miranda, & Munoz, 2001; Dugbartey, Townes, & Mahurin, 2000). Dugbartey et al. (2000) were interested in observing the Color Trails Test (D'Elia, Satz, Uchiyama, & White, 1996) and Trail Making Test in a sample of 64 bilingual Turkish university students. The authors were interested in identifying the extent to which the Color Trails is "culture-fair," a claim that has previously been suggested. The authors found that participants' performances on Color Trails 1 and Trails A were virtually the same, indicating that these measures represent functionally equivalent tasks. In contrast, Color Trails 2 and Trails B (and their interference indices) showed significant differences. The authors concluded that the Color Trails 2 task, "may not necessarily be the 'culture reduced' equivalent" of Trails B (as suggested by D'Elia et al., 1996), "but that they measure different underlying cognitive skills" (Dugbartey et al., p. 428). The authors further suggested that "simply substituting the obviously verbally mediated alphabetical elements with colors may not necessarily be sufficient to ensure the universality of a test" (p. 429).

In times when normative data are either unavailable or inappropriate for particular cultural groups, neuropsychologists may need to identify other qualitative methods of describing individual behavior. As one example, Christensen's (1975) Luria Neuropsychological Investigation (LNI) has shown diagnostic merit in the past, and may be a viable option when quantitative measures are unavailable. Christensen and Caetano (1999) provided a number of case studies that elucidate the method's effectiveness with individual patients. They suggested that the method is particularly useful in rehabilitation settings. In response to the criticism that the LNI lack normative data, the authors argued that its qualitative approach is the method's strength. Further, the qualitative method is "no less scientific than the prevalent psychometric tradition; it just follows traditions evolved in neurology and medicine more closely than traditions evolved in experimental psychology" (Christensen & Caetano, 1999, p. 76). Lurian methods still afford a place in describing brain–behavior relationships when quantitative approaches are not readily available. Luria continues to be "honored as a founder of neuropsychology" (Cole, 2002, p. 7), and a revival of qualitative methods (Lurian or otherwise) seems in order amidst the current cultural landscape.

IN CLOSING

We argue that the task of cultural neuropsychology involves striking a balance between individual and universal understandings of human cognition and behavior. This fusion will be attained most efficiently when neuropsychologists educate themselves on the limitations of current measures and norms, and remain flexible in describing cognition through the use of alternative measures and norms when necessary. A scientific, artful approach to patients' behavior should contextualize the behavior in light of his or her culture. Alasdair MacIntyre stated that, "It is only when theories are located in history, when we view the demands for justification in highly particular contexts of a historical kind, that we are freed from either dogmatism or capitulation to skepticism" (MacIntyre, 1989, p. 157). Neuropsychologists can avoid "dogmatism" by remaining open to new approaches to the patient's immediate cultural context. We can avoid "capitulation" by acknowledging the remarkable contributions our tradition has yielded and continue to access those practices that have proved to be useful in the past. Achieving this freedom involves the successful integration of traditional approaches with newly developing, culturally relevant approaches to neuropsychological assessment.

The future of clinical neuropsychology depends significantly on collaborative relationships. Among the "myths" proposed by Dodrill (1997) was the assumption that "relationships among our neuropsychological colleagues are not sufficiently important that they require our attention" (p. 15). In contrast to this myth, he stated that relationships between professionals "are of the greatest importance, and I urge us all to spend the effort that is needed to advance our profession ..." (p. 16). His advice cannot be ignored. None are as critical as training relationships. Behind every great neuropsychologist there has been an equally important supervisor. Indeed, how would anyone become a successful clinician without the guidance of an experienced mentor?

In his essay, *The Essential Tension,* Thomas Kuhn (1977) described the importance of both convergent and divergent thinking within a scientific field. The tendency for educators in the sciences is to emphasize what is convergent, often at the expense of those divergent thinkers who might be inclined to discover new and revolutionary ideas and practices within their respective fields. Students, in Kuhn's words, need to be provided with "an arsenal of techniques for approaching these future problems; and they must learn to judge the relevance of these techniques and to evaluate the possibly partial solutions which they can provide" (p. 229). Culturally diverse students and young faculty will grapple with a vastly different world from that of their predecessors. This new world requires relevant answers to the age-old question of how brain–behavior relationships are accurately assessed.

As neuropsychologists, it is our responsibility to give meaning to Luria's desire for a "psychology that [is] relevant, that would give some substance to our discussions about building a new life" for the patient (Luria, 1979, p. 29). To do so will require an eclectic approach that is good science as much as it is good art.

REFERENCES

Almagor, M., & Koren, D. (2001). The adequacy of the MMPI-2 Harris-Lingoes subscales: A cross-cultural factor analytic study of scales D, Hy, Pd, Pa, Sc, and Ma. *Psychological Assessment, 13,* 199–215.

Allport, G. W. (1961). *Pattern and growth in personality.* New York: Holt, Rinhart & Winston.

Allport, G. W. (1960). *Personality and social encounter.* Boston: Beacon Press.

American Psychological Association. (2002). Ethical principles of psychologists and code of conduct. *American Psychologist, 57*(12), 1060–1073.

Ardila, A. (1995). Directions of research in cross-cultural neuropsychology. *Journal of Clinical and Experimental Neuropsychology, 17,* 143–150.

Ardila, A., & Moreno, S. (2001). Neuropsychological test performance on Aruaco Indians: An exploratory study. *Journal of the International Neuropsychological Society, 7,* 510–515.

Ardila, A., & Rosselli, M. (1989). Neuropsychological characteristics of normal aging. *Developmental Neuropsychology, 5,* 307–320.

Azocar, F., Arean, P., Miranda, J., & Munoz, R. F. (2001). Differential item functioning in a Spanish translation of the Beck Depression Inventory. *Journal of Clinical Psychology, 57,* 355–365.
Beck, A. T., Steer, R. A., & Brown, G. K. (1996). *Manual for the Beck Depression Inventory—2.* San Antonio, TX: Psychological Corporation.
Bell, B. D., & Roper, B. L. (1998). Myths of neuropsychology: Another view. *The Clinical Neuropsychologist, 12,* 237–244.
Benet-Martinez, V., Leu, J., Lee, F., & Morris, M. W. (2002). Negotiating biculturalism: Cultural frame switching in biculturals with oppositional versus compatible cultural identities. *Journal of Cross-Cultural Psychology, 33,* 492–516.
Broadbent, D. B., Cooper, P. F., FitzGerald, P., & Parkes, K. R. (1982). The Cognitive Failures Questionnaire (CFQ) and its correlates. *British Journal of Clinical Psychology, 21,* 1–16.
Cetina, K. K. (1999). *Epistemic cultures.* Cambridge, MA: Harvard University Press.
Chan, A. S., Choi, A., Chiu, H., & Lam, L. (2003). Clinical validity of the Chinese version of Mattis Dementia Rating Scale in differentiating dementia of Alzheimer's type in Hong Kong. *Journal of the International Neuropsychological Society, 9,* 45–55.
Chan, R. C. K., & Manly, T. (2002). The application of 'dysexecutive syndrome' measures across cultures: Performance and checklist assessment in neurologically healthy and traumatically brain-injured Hong Kong Chinese volunteers. *Journal of the International Neuropsychological Society, 8,* 771–780.
Chan, C. C. H., Lee, T. M. C. Lee, Fong, K. N. K., Lee, C. & Wong, V. (2002). Cognitive profile for Chinese patients with stroke. *Brain Injury, 16,* 873–884.
Chan, C. C. H., Lee, T. M. C., Wong, V., Fong, K., & Lee, C. (1999). Validation of Chinese version Neurobehavioral Cognitive Status Examination (NCSE). *Archives of Clinical Neuropsychology, 14,* 71.
Christensen, A. L. (1975). *Luria's Neuropsychological Investigation.* New York: Spectrum.
Christensen, A. L., & Caetano, C. (1999). Luria's neuropsychological evaluation in the Nordic countries. *Neuropsychology Review, 9,* 71–78.
Cole, M. (2002). Alexander Luria, cultural psychology, and the resolution of the crisis in psychology. *Journal of Russian and East European Psychology, 40,* 4–16.
Conant, L. L., Fastenau, P. S., Giordani, B., Boivin, M. J., Chounramany, C., Xaisida, S., Choulamountry, L., & Phlsena, P. (2003). Environmental influences on primary memory development: A cross-cultural study of memory span in Lao and American children. *Journal of Clinical and Experimental Neuropsychology, 25,* 1102–1116.
D'Elia, L. F., Satz, P., Uchiyama, C. L., & White, T. (1996). *Color Trails Test. Professional manual.* Odessa, FL: Psychological Assessment Resources.
Dodrill, C. B. (1997). Myths of neuropsychology. *The Clinical Neuropsychologist, 11,* 1–17.
Dodrill, C. B. (1999). Myths of neuropsychology: Further considerations. *The Clinical Neuropsychologist, 13,* 562–572.
Dugbartey, A. T., Townes, B. D., & Mahurin, R. K. (2000). Equivalence of the Color Trails Test and Trail Making Test in nonnative English-speakers. *Archives of Clinical Neuropsychology, 15,* 425–431.
Dulay, M. F., Schefft, B. K., Testa, S. M., Fargo, J. D., Privitera, M., & Yeh, H.-S. (2002). What does the family pictures subtest of the Wechsler Memory Scale-III Measure? Insight gained from patients evaluated for epilepsy surgery. *The Clinical Neuropsychologist, 16,* 452–462.
Folia, V., & Kosmidis, M. H. (2003). Assessment of memory skills in illiterates: Strategy differences or test artifact? *The Clinical Neuropsychologist, 17,* 143–152.

Franck, I. (1982). Psychology as a science: Resolving the idiographic-nomothetic controversy. *Journal for the Theory of Social Behavior, 12,* 1–20.
Friedman, M. A., Schinka, J. A., Mortimer, J. A., & Graves, A. B. (2002). Hopkins Verbal Learning Test—Revised: Norms for elderly African Americans. *The Clinical Neuropsychologist, 16,* 356–372.
Golden, C. J. (1978). *Stroop Color and Word Test.* Chicago: Stoelting.
Gontkovsky, S. T., Mold, J. W., & Beatty, W. W. (2002). Age and educational influences on RBANS index scores in a nondemented geriatric sample. *The Clinical Neuropsychologist, 16,* 258–263.
Gonzalez da Silva, C., Petersson, K. M., Faisca, L., Ingvar, M., & Reis, A. (2004). The effects of literacy and education on the quantitative and qualitative aspects of semantic verbal fluency. *Journal of Clinical and Experimental Neuropsychology, 26,* 266–277.
Gorsuch, R. L. (2002). The pyramids of sciences and of humanities. *American Behavioral Scientist, 45,* 1822–1838.
Harris, J. G. (2002). Ethical decision making in individuals of diverse ethnic, cultural, and linguistic backgrounds. In S. Bush (Ed.), *Studies on neuropsychology, development, and cognition: Vol 4. Ethical issues in clinical neuropsychology* (pp. 103–133). Lisse, Netherlands: Swets & Zeitlinger.
Harris, M. E., Ivnik, R. J., & Smith, G. E. (2002). Mayo's Older American Normative Studies: Expanded AVLT recognition trial norms for ages 57 to 98. *Journal of Clinical and Experimental Neuropsychology, 24,* 214–220.
Haynes, S. N., Kaholokula, J. K., & Nelson, K. (1999). The idiographic application of nomothetic, empirically based treatments. *Clinical Psychology: Science & Practice, 6,* 456–461.
Heaton, R. K., Grant, I., & Matthews, C. G. (1986). Differences in neuropsychological test performance associated with age, education, and sex. In I. Grant & K. Adams (Eds), *Neuropsychological assessment of neuropsychiatric disorders* (pp. 100–120). New York: Oxford University Press.
Hedden, T., Park, D. C., Nisbett, R., Ji, L-J, Jing, Q., & Jiao, S. (2002). Cultural variation in verbal versus spatial neuropsychological function across the life span. *Neuropsychology, 16,* 65–73.
Holding, P. A., Taylor, H. G., Kazungu, S. D., Mkala, T., Gona, J., Mwamuye, B., Mbonani, L., & Stevenson, J. (2004). Assessing cognitive outcomes in a rural African population: Development of a neuropsychological battery in Kilifi District, Kenya. *Journal of the Neuropsychological Society, 2,* 246–260.
Humes, G. E., Welsh, M. C., Retzlaff, P., & Cookson, N. (1997). Towers of Hanoi and London: Reliability and validity of two executive function tasks. *Assessment, 4,* 249–257.
Ivnik, R. J., Malec, J. F., Smith, G. E., Tangalos, E. G., & Petersen, R. C. (1996). Neuropsychological tests' norms above age 55: COWAT, BNT, MAE Token, WRAT-R Reading, AMNART, Stroop, TMT, and JLO (1996). *The Clinical Neuropsychologist, 10,* 262–278.
Ivnik, R. J., Malec, J. F., Smith, G. E., Tangalos, E. G., Petersen, R. C, Kokmen, E., & Kurland, L. T. (1992a). Mayo's Older Americans Normative Studies: WAIS-R Norms for ages 56 to 94. *The Clinical Neuropsychologist, 6,* 1–30.
Ivnik, R. J., Malec, J. F., Smith, G. E., Tangalos, E. G., Petersen, R. C, Kokmen, E., & Kurland, L. T. (1992b). Mayo's Older Americans Normative Studies: Utility of corrections for age and education for the WAIS-R. *The Clinical Neuropsychologist, 6,* 31–47.
Ivnik, R. J., Malec, J. F., Smith, G. E., Tangalos, E. G., Petersen, R. C, Kokmen, E., & Kurland, L. T. (1992c). Mayo's Older Americans Normative Studies: WMS-R Norms for ages 56 to 94. *The Clinical Neuropsychologist, 6,* 49–82.

Ivnik, R. J., Malec, J. F., Smith, G. E., Tangalos, E. G., Petersen, R. C, Kokmen, E., & Kurland, L. T. (1992d). Mayo's Older Americans Normative Studies: Updated AVLT Norms for ages 56 to 97. *The Clinical Neuropsychologist, 6,* 83–104.

Ivnik, R. J., Smith, G. E., Cerhan, J. H., Boeve, B. F., Tangalos, E. G., & Petersen, R. C. (2001). Understanding the diagnostic capabilities of cognitive tests. *The Clinical Neuropsychologist 15,* 114–124.

Ivnik, R. J., Smith, G. E., Lucas, J. A., Tangalos, E. G., Kokmen, E., & Petersen, R. C. (1997). Free and cued selective reminding test: MOANS norms. *Journal of Clinical and Experimental Neuropsychology, 19,* 676–691.

Kojima, M., Furukawa, T. A., Takahashi, H., Kawai, M., Nagaya, T., & Tokudome, S. (2002). Cross-cultural validation of the Beck Depression Inventory-II in Japan. *Psychiatry Research, 110,* 291–299.

Kosmidis, M. H., Vlahou, C. H., Panagiotaki, P., & Kosseoglou, G. (2004). The verbal fluency task in the Greek population: Normative data, and clustering and switching strategies. *Journal of the International Neuropsychological Society, 10,* 164–172.

Kuhn, T. S. (1977). *The essential tension.* Chicago: University of Chicago Press.

Lee, J. H., Lee, K. U., Lee. D. Y., Kim, K. W., Jhoo, J. H., Kim, J. H., Lee, K. H., Kim, S. Y., Han, S. H., & Woo, J. I. (2002). Development of the Korean version of the Consortium to Establish a Registry for Alzheimer's Disease Assessment Packet (CERAD-K): Clinical and Neuropsychological Assessment Batteries. *Journal of Gerontology Series B: Psychological Sciences and Social Sciences, 57,* 47–53.

Lee, D. Y., Lee, K. U., Lee. J. H., Kim, K. W., Jhoo, J. H., Kim, S. Y., Yoon, J. C., Woo, S. I., Ha, J., & Woo, J. I. (2004). A normative study of the CERAD neuropsychological assessment battery in the Korean elderly. *Journal of the International Neuropsychological Society, 10,* 72–81.

Lee, T. M. C., Yuen, K. S. L., & Chan, C. C. H. (2002). Normative data for neuropsychological measures of fluency, attention, and memory measures for Hong Kong Chinese. *Journal of Clinical and Experimental Neuropsychology, 24,* 615–632.

Levav, M., Mirsky, A. F., French, L. M., & Bartko, J. J. (1998). Multinational neuropsychological testing: Performance of children and adults. *Journal of Clinical & Experimental Neuropsychology, 20,* 658–672.

Levinson, S. C., Kita, S., Haun, D. B. M., & Rasch, B. H. (2002). Returning the tables: Language affects spatial reasoning. *Cognition, 84,* 155–188.

Lezak, M. D. (1995). *Neuropsychological assessment* (3rd ed.). New York: Oxford University Press.

Lezak, M. D. (2002). Responsive assessment and the freedom to think for ourselves. *Rehabilitation Psychology, 47,* 339–353.

Lucas, J. A., Ivnik, R. J., Smith, G. E., Bohac, D. L., Tangalos, E. G., Graff-Radford, N. R., & Petersen, R. C. (1998). Mayo's Older Americans Normative Studies: Category fluency norms. *Journal of Clinical and Experimental Neuropsychology, 20,* 194–200.

Luria, A. R. (1979). *The making of mind: A personal account of Soviet psychology.* Cambridge, MA: Harvard University Press.

MacIntyre, A. (1989). Epistemological crises, dramatic narrative, and the philosophy of science. In S. Hauerwas & L. Jones (Eds.), *Why Narrative?* (pp. 138–157). Grand Rapids, MI: Eerdmans.

Malec, J. F., Ivnik, R. J., Smith, G. E., Tangalos, E. G., Petersen, R. C., Kokmen, E., & Kurland, L. T. (1992). Mayo's Older Americans Normative Studies: Utility of corrections for age and education for the WAIS-R. *The Clinical Neuropsychologist, 6,* 31–47.

Mattis, S. (1988). *Dementia Rating Scale professional manual.* Odessa, FL: Psychological Assessment Resources, Inc.

McBride-Chang, C., & Kail, R. V. (2002). Cross-cultural similarities in the predictors of reading acquisition. *Child Development, 73*, 1392–1407.

Moering, R. G., Schinka, J. A., Mortimer, J. A., & Graves, A. B. (2004). Normative data for elderly African Americans for the Stroop Color and Word Test. *Archives of Clinical Neuropsychology, 19*, 61–71.

Norenzayan, A., Smith, E. E., Kim, B. J., & Nisbett, R. E. (2002). Cultural preferences for formal versus intuitive reasoning. *Cognitive Science, 26*, 653–684.

O'Bryant, S. E., O'Jile, J. R., & McCaffrey, R. J. (2004). Reporting of demographic variables in neuropsychological research: Trends in the current literature. *The Clinical Neuropsychologist, 18*, 229–233.

Palmer, B. W., Boone, K. B., Lesser, I. M., & Wohl, M. A. (1998). Base rates of 'impaired' neuropsychological test performance among healthy older adults. *Archives of Clinical Neuropsychology, 13*, 503–511.

Patton, D. E., Duff, K., Schoenberg, M. R., Mold, J., Scott, J. G., & Adams, R. L. (2003). Performance of cognitively normal African Americans on the RBANS in community dwelling older adults. *The Clinical Neuropsychologist, 17*, 515–530.

Ponton, M. O., & Ardila, A. (1999). The future of neuropsychology with Hispanic populations. *Archives of Clinical Neuropsychology, 14*, 565–580.

Popper, K. R. (1982). *The open universe*. Totowa, NJ: Rowman & Littlefield.

Randolph, C. (1998). *Repeatable battery for the assessment of neuropsychological status manual*. San Antonio, TX: The Psychological Corporation.

Reitan, R. M., & Wolfson, D. (1995). Influence of age and education on neuropsychological test results. *The Clinical Neuropsychologist, 9*, 151–158.

Schretlen, D., & Ivnik, R. J. (1996). Prorating IQ scores for older adults: Validation of a seven-subtest WAIS-R with the Mayo Older Americans Normative Sample. *Assessment, 3*, 411–416.

Schretlen, D. J., Munro, C. A., Anthony, J. C., & Pearlson, G. D. (2003). Examining the range of normal intraindividual variability in neuropsychological test performance. *Journal of the International Neuropsychological Society, 6*, 864–870.

Shepherd, I., & Leathem, J. (1999). Factors affecting performance in cross-cultural neuropsychology: From a New Zealand bicultural perspective. *Journal of the International Neuropsychological Society, 5*, 83–84.

Smith, G. E., Ivnik, R. J., Malec, J. F., Kokmen, E., Tangalos, E. G., & Kurland, L. T. (1992). Mayo's Older Americans Normative Studies (MOANS): Factor structure of a core battery. *Psychological Assessment, 4*, 382–390.

Tavassoli, N. T. (2002). Spatial memory for Chinese and English. *Journal of Cross-Cultural Psychology, 33*, 415–431.

Teng, E. L. (2002). Cultural and educational factors in the diagnosis of dementia. *Alzheimer Disease & Associated Disorders, 16*, S77–S79.

van de Vijver, F. J. R. (2002). Cross-cultural assessment: Value for money? *Applied Psychology: An International Review, 51*, 545–566.

Wechsler, D. (1997). *Wechsler Memory Scale* (3rd ed.). San Antonio, TX: The Psychological Corporation.

Wilson, B. A., Alderman, N., Burgess, P. W., Emsley, H., & Evans, J. (1996). *Behavioural assessment of the dysexecutive syndrome*. Bury St. Edmonds, England: Thames Valley Test Company.

Chapter 4

Environmentalists and Nativists: The IQ Controversy in Cross-Cultural Perspective[1]

Victor Nell
University of South Africa

This chapter sets out to answer two deceptively simple questions: Why do intelligence test scores vary from one culture to another? And are these variations the result of real differences in intelligence, or are they caused by the tests that are used to measure intelligence?

Let's begin by asking, Why did publication of *The Bell Curve* (Herrnstein & Murray, 1994) provoke the most bitter controversy in recent psychology? The simple answer is that the book pitted *environmentalists* against *nativists*, and came out in favor of the nativist view. The result was the most controversial book of the decade, with literally hundreds of articles in the popular and scientific press attacking the nativist position.[2]

---

[1]This chapter was first published in a different form in my book, *Cross-Cultural Neuropsychological Assessment: Theory and Practice*, 2000, Mahwah, NJ: Lawrence Erlbaum Associates, and appears here by permission of the publisher. It draws mainly on chap. 4 of the book, "The Nature of Intelligence: The IQ Controversy in Cross-Cultural Perspective," with additional material from chap. 1, "Westernization and the Politics of Culture," and chap. 9, "Buds, Flowers, Fruits: Potential, Performance, and Test Administration."

[2]A curious aspect of this polemic is that it has been focused on ethnic differences in cognitive ability. But the book's central thesis is that American society is today stratified not by social class, but by intelligence—a development that has significant policy implications, but has been largely ignored in the brouhaha about the politically much more sensitive issue of race and IQ.

Both environmentalism and nativism have a long history in psychology. The environmentalists have three fundamental beliefs: The first is universalism, which holds that mind, like brain, is one, and therefore unitary in all humans. The second is that culture makes mind,[3] and that differences between individuals and across cultures arise from cultural and not genetic differences. The third is that IQ is not immutable, but will respond—perhaps dramatically—to environmental enrichment and improved learning opportunities.

The principle argument against environmentalist optimism is the nativist view, which holds that only some 40% (perhaps as little as 20%) of each individual's intelligence is shaped by the environment; the remaining 60-80% is genetically determined, and therefore immutable. Let us now consider the historical development of these positions in more detail.

ENVIRONMENTALISM TRIUMPHANT, NATIVISM RESURGENT

IQ measurement had its beginnings in an era that willingly accepted many racist beliefs that found their most virulent expression in Nazi doctrines directed at extermination of "inferior" races—Jews, gypsies, and Negroes. By 1945, as the concentration camps were liberated and the horror of the Nazi genocide dawned on the outside world, the tide turned, and customary racism, at least in scientific circles, was treated with the obloquy it deserved. Moreover, anything that smacked of genetic determinism was perceived as an odious throwback to racism. For decades, the environmentalist view has therefore held sway, and mainstream psychology has paid only sporadic attention to the nativists.

In this new intellectual climate, shaped by memories of Nazi racism, by the triumphs of the Civil Rights movement in the United States, and by the growing success of the colonial struggle for liberation in Africa and Asia, a 1969 paper by Arthur Jensen, "How much can we boost IQ and scholastic achievement?", burst like a bombshell. In the opening sentence, Jensen gave his view of the effectiveness of the compensatory education programmes mandated by the U.S. government's Head Start Project: "Compensatory education has been tried and it apparently has failed." The reason for the failure, he argued, is that genetic factors are more important than the environment in determining intelligence: Environment accounts for about 20% of the mean IQ scores of a population, and heredity for the other 80%. The weightiest evidence for this 1969

---

[3]For an account of this position in its historical context, see chap. 3, "Radical Environmentalism: Vygotsky, Luria, and the Historical Determination of Consciousness," in Nell, 2000.

conclusion are the studies of identical twins reared apart[4]—because, as Jensen put it, "if their environments are uncorrelated, all they have in common are their genes" (p. 51). Cyril Burt, discredited after his death by allegations of forgery, found the IQ correlation between 53 such pairs of twins to be .77.[5] Heredity also determines race, continued Jensen—and then comes the hard part: "On the average, Negroes test about 1 standard deviation (15 IQ points) below the average of the white population in IQ, and this finding is fairly uniform across ... 81 tests of intellectual ability" (1969, p. 81). In a major 1980 book, *Bias in Mental Testing,* Jensen argued his position on both these themes in greater detail—that intelligence is largely heritable, and that standardized psychometric tests were free of bias against minority groups in the United States.

So it is not surprising that a book supporting the nativist position was the target of bitter attacks. But before dismissing *The Bell Curve,* we first need to understand it. Herrnstein and Murray (1994) wrote that by the 1980s, the state of received wisdom about IQ testing was that

> intelligence is a bankrupt concept. Whatever it might mean—and nobody really knows even how to define it—intelligence is so ephemeral that no-one can measure it accurately. IQ tests are of course culturally biased, and so are all other "aptitude" tests, such as the SAT [Scholastic Aptitude Test].... The tests are nearly useless as tools ... [and] do not predict anything except success in school.... All that tests really accomplish is to label youngsters ... creating a self-fulfilling prophecy that injures the socioeconomically disadvantaged in general and blacks in particular. (pp. 12–13).

The Bell Curve argued on the contrary that IQ and what it measures are real. The authors cited data showing that IQ scores vary substantially across ethnic and cultural groups: Chinese living in Hong Kong have a mean IQ of about 110, Jews living in the United States have a mean of between 108 and 115, and for Latinos living in the United States, the mean is about 85. For African Americans, they report that even when rigorous selection criteria are applied to eliminate methodologically suspect studies, the Black–White difference of just over 1 standard deviation holds up; the National Longitudinal Study of Youth (NLSY), which administered an apparently bias-free

---

[4]The methodological problem with these studies, as Taylor (1980) and others have pointed out, is that when twins are separated (following the death of both parents, for example), they almost always remain within the same family so that the environmental differences are not very large. If the environments differed dramatically, with one twin going to the home of Harvard professors and the other to an inner city single mother on welfare (or to subsistence farmers in a developing country), the 80/20 heredity/environment loading the identical-twins-reared-apart studies have found might be very different.

[5]Herrnstein and Murray (1994) cited the Minnesota twin study (Bouchard, Lykken, McGue, Segal, & Tellegen, 1990) as yielding a correlation of .78, almost identical to Burt's disputed finding.

IQ test, the Armed Forces Qualification Test, to 6,502 whites and 3,022 blacks, found a Black–White difference of 1.21 standard deviations.

HEREDITY AND THE SOCIAL CONSTRUCTION OF HOPE

These data have profound human welfare implications. I can only begin to imagine the hurt and bewilderment I would have experienced had I been born a Latino or African American, and as a child I had been placed in the D-stream in my school regardless of my test scores (a practice called "racial tracking"), had been assigned to bored teachers who expected me to be dumb and treated me accordingly, and then, as I matured, having to carry this burden of customary expectations that made it near impossible for me to get into a good college.

The debate becomes even more heated because the claim that IQ is immutable strikes at a profoundly held western belief—the notion of human progress and perfectibility. The Protestant Ethic and the triumph of free market capitalism rest on the conviction that each individual has limitless potential: Bellhops become hotel magnates, and a man born in a log cabin becomes President of the United States. The reach of this limitlessness is set by effort, not by inheritance.[6] If on the other hand intelligence is fixed by race and by birth, fundamental social beliefs are strained. Predestination rules, and the liberal-democratic dream lies in tatters. Worse, an immutable barrier to the individual's progress threatens social stability by threatening the social construction of hope.

THE PROBLEM OF BIAS

The environmentalist rejoinder to these conclusions is that IQ tests are biased against African Americans and Hispanics. One of many U.S. studies pointing to this conclusion is by Jane Mercer (1984), comparing the WISC-R performances of 627 Black, 617 Hispanic, and 669 White students, all native-born and all at California public schools. Her conclusion was "that the WISC-R discriminates systematically in favor of white students at the item level, the subtest level, and the scale level.... Inferences based on those test scores are racially and culturally discriminatory."

Herrnstein and Murray, on the contrary, concluded that "no one has found statistically reliable evidence of predictive bias against blacks" (pp.

---

[6]Among the hallmarks of western culture are the ascendancy of individualism over collectivism (Triandis, 1995), and the centrality of the achievement motive (McClelland, 1961) in western culture. Westerners have a driven, competitive attitude not only to psychological tests, but also to all other opportunities for the demonstration of individual excellence. The origin of many of these values is the Protestant Ethic (Albee, 1977; Weber, 1904/1965), a secular religion that brings salvation in the next world and high status in this through hard work and unremitting effort.

281, 627). Moreover, "the cultural content of test items is not the cause of group differences in scores" (p. 282). These sweeping statements sit strangely with a paragraph from the last chapter of *The Bell Curve:*

The gaping cultural gap between the habits of the underclass and the habits of the rest of society, far more impassable than a simple economic gap between poor and not poor, or the racial gap of black and white, will make it increasingly difficult for children who have grown up in the inner city to function in the larger society even when they want to. (Herrnstein & Murray, 1994, p. 524)

In a strictly technical sense, this acknowledgment of cultural difference can be reconciled with the denial of bias. This is because IQ tests predict the school and university achievements of Black Americans no less accurately than those of Whites: In other words, when *The Bell Curve* says that IQ tests are unbiased, it is not bias *in the tests* it is talking about, but *external bias*, measured against the criteria of school and college success.

Of course, the criterion might be as biased as the test[7]. After all, the educational system and the test system are devised and implemented by a single intellectual elite that shares a wide range of work-related and cultural values, and the two systems are two sides of the same coin: Just as one can predict academic success by IQ test results, so should one be able to predict IQ by extrapolating from academic success. It is therefore tautologous to say that tests are unbiased when measured against a very similar kind of yardstick.

The Pernicious Consequences of *Inflating* IQ Scores

The damage done to individuals whose IQ scores are artificially lowered by test bias is clear. But giving some people artificially higher scores also has a pernicious effect. Commenting on the Spanish version of the WAIS published in 1968 and still in use in the United States for the assessment of Spanish-speaking adults, Melendez (1994) noted that it inflates full-scale IQ scores by about 20 points in comparison with the American versions of this test. This has the effect of labeling impaired individuals as normal and thus depriving them of social benefits and services to which they would be entitled if their IQs were correctly computed. Melendez goes on to note that at the time this version was standardized,

> the concept that a large segment of the Puerto Rican population had significantly lower IQs than the comparative sample of the WAIS must have been both scientifically and politically unsettling.... However, it is both demeaning and patronizing toward Hispanics to use a test ... which artificially boosts the IQ results.... The transformations caused by the [Spanish version of the

---

[7]Herrnstein and Murray acknowledge this possibility (pp. 285–286), but go on to dismiss it as a possible source of test bias.

WAIS] may be an egalitarian's dream, but they can also be a clinician's nightmare. (p. 392)

Similar difficulties have been noted (Nell, 1994) for the South African version of the Wechsler Adult Intelligence Scale (which is not in fact the WAIS but the Wechsler-Bellevue, an earlier and cruder version that predates the WAIS by 16 years, and the WAIS-R by nearly half a century): the South African test inflates full-scale IQ by close to a standard deviation, and also has the effect of depriving people with significant brain injuries of the compensation to which they are entitled.

The Hispanic WAIS and the South African Wechsler-Bellevue inflate IQ scores unintentionally. But setting norms at a spuriously low level can take on a sinister aspect, for example, if an insurance carrier promotes unduly flattering norms in order to "prove" that individuals who have been significantly compromised by head injury are still normal!

Broadening the Canvas

For neuropsychologists working in South America, Africa, and Asia, the most curious aspect of *The Bell Curve* debate is its insularity. It is conducted as if the United States of America were the whole world.[8] What might happen to the IQ controversy if the canvas were broadened to take account of a nearly a century of cross-cultural psychological assessment? The following sections of this chapter—organized around the psychometric and information processing paradigms of psychological assessment—provide additional perspectives on culture and intelligence. Don't be put off by the detailed material on test performances in culturally different settings that follows—read it as an extended commentary on the IQ controversy, and as leading toward a thoughtful balance between the environmentalist and nativist positions.

THE PSYCHOMETRIC AND INFORMATION-PROCESSING PARADIGMS

A useful way of distinguishing between psychometrics and information processing is to see the psychometrists as classicists and the information-processing school as revisionists (Herrnstein & Murray, 1994). The *classicists* see intelligence as structure: They work within the tradition of Spearman, whose 1904 paper identified a general intelligence factor, g, that stands at the center of this structure. "Despite numerous theoretical attacks on

---

[8]America is in any case a poor laboratory for the study of the effects of culture on intelligence. Looking at the available evidence, Hunt (1995) observed that there is "surprisingly little evidence for influences of cultural experiences on intelligence" (p. 365)—very likely because such evidence has not been seriously sought in a society that prides itself on universal adherence to core cultural values.

4. ENVIRONMENTALISTS AND NATIVISTS

Spearman's basic notion of a general factor, g has stood like a rock of Gibralter in psychometrics, defying any attempt to construct a test of complex problem solving which excludes it," wrote Jensen (1969, p. 9), who is the foremost of modern classicists.

The *revisionists*, on the other hand, emphasize process rather than structure. Their focus is on information processing, on what people do when acting intelligently. Jean Piaget was the first of the revisionists, and Robert Sternberg is the leading contemporary worker within this paradigm.

However, like all dichotomies, the distinction between the psychometric and the information-processing paradigms is initially helpful, but becomes forced and artificial if pushed too far. Ultimately, there is no dividing line. The literal meaning of psychometrics is the measurement of intellectual processes, and this by definition includes all forms of mental measurement. There is in fact an inexorable movement from psychometrics to information processing: Psychometric structuralists become information-processing revisionists as they seek explanations for their findings.

This interparadigmatic movement is well illustrated by Jensen himself. In the concluding section of his conventionally structuralist 1969 paper, he accounted for test performance anomalies by proposing a two-level structure of intellect. *Associative ability* (Level 1) is tapped by tests such as digit span, serial order learning, the learning of paired associates, or free list recall. Lower class children—white, Black, or Hispanic—perform as well on these tests as middle-class children. However, *conceptual ability* (Level 2) requires self-initiated transformation of the input before the response is made. Raven's Progressive Matrices, with its high loading on g, is a good example.

Jensen goes on to note that a slight variation in the test procedure can change a free recall task from Level 1 to Level 2. For example, if a 20-word list made up of five items from each of four categories—animals, furniture, clothing, and foods—was used, the lower class children did no better than they did on the uncategorized lists, whereas the middle-class children did much better—their mean scores were about a standard deviation above those of the lower class group, with far more clustering by category (Jensen, 1969, p. 113): In other words, the middle-class children are able to apply a conceptual transformation to the input material. This is of course no longer structuralism, but squarely within the information processing paradigm.

I. The Psychometric Paradigm

In a 1935 address to the American Association for the Advancement of Science, Florence Goodenough remarked that intelligence tests are not measuring devices, but sampling devices: Everyday life is multifactorial, and so are psychometric tests, which sample broad swatches of behavior, such as engaging in a drawing-room conversation (the Information Subtest in the Wechsler), or explaining why a particular course of action should be taken (Comprehension), assembling a jigsaw puzzle (Object Assembly), or working out in one's head if a shopkeeper's bargain is such a bargain after all (Arithmetic). These behavioral *samples* have turned out to be most closely related to school situations, and for this reason they have very high predictive validity for success in the educational system.

But precisely because these tests are broad spectrum, they tell us very little about the component process out of which each of these samples of behavior is constructed. For example, in order to do well at Object Assembly, one needs to have visuomotor coordination and manual dexterity, to construct a mental model of what one is about to build, and to categorize it by giving it a name ("a child," "a camel"), to develop an edge alignment or internal detail strategy (Kaplan, 1988), to make effective use of error feedback in order to scrap false starts and begin again, and to show the ongoing drive and future orientation needed to persevere.

The score alone tells one nothing about each of these separate components. Neuropsychology's response has been twofold—to retain psychometric tests because of their proven diagnostic utility, but to resort increasingly to qualitative test interpretation; and to supplement psychometric tests by information processing probes.

Two aspects of the psychometric paradigm are of special importance in the testing of culturally different subjects—*education* and *practice*.

Education and Urbanization. Formal schooling plays a major part in all test performance, and overwhelmingly so in psychometric tests. Kendall, Verster, and Von Mollendorf (1988) specify the elements of classroom skill that contribute to test performance; practice in using a pencil, familiarity with the use of booklets, facility with letters, numbers, and other symbols, an appreciation of the importance of paying attention, obeying instructions, and sitting still as contributors to speed and accuracy of work, and, in general, an appropriate orientation to the examination situation:

> No other cultural learning experience is as concentrated and as fundamental than that which is provided, systematically, through the formal education system. (p. 310)

Powerful education effects recur with unfailing regularity in the testing of nontest-wise subjects, demonstrated for example by Crawford-Nutt's (1977 a, b, c) work on the Symmetry Completion Test, administered to 1,151 Black subjects whose educational level ranged from virtually none (mean 1.6 years, SD 2.2) to university students with a mean of 14 years of education (SD 0.7). Their scores varied in almost linear fashion with education. Similarly, among South African paint factory workers (Nell, Myers,

Colvin, & Rees, 1993) and farm laborers (Nell, Kruger, Taylor, Myers, & London, 1995), years of education was the single largest moderator of test performance.

An interesting sidelight on education effects is that in the youngest age groups, where no education effects exist, scores in different cultures converge more than at a later age. Verster and Prinsloo (1988) reported no differences between English and Afrikaans speakers aged 3 to 5 years on the Junior South African Intelligence Scale; but from age 6, differences began emerging, suggesting that before the commencement of formal schooling, differences are smaller. Similarly, Richter and Griesel (1988) compared 722 Black South African children aged between 2 months and 30 months with the 1969 American reference group on the Bayley Scales of Mental and Motor Development. The South African children significantly outperformed the Americans at the ages of 4, 5, 6, 8, 10, 12, and 15 months on the mental scale scores, and at 2, 3, 4, 5, 6, 8, and 10 months on the motor scale scores ($p < .01$ on all groups except 10 months, $p < .05$). In view of the long-standing claim that African infants are precocious in relation to western children, it is worth noting that when the South African and American samples were simultaneously compared with British and Baganda infants tested on the same tests, there were no significant differences between the four groups (Richter-Strydom & Griesel, 1984).

Formal education effects greatly overshadow the consequences of urbanization when both are controlled, although there is nonetheless an acculturation construct that traces a hierarchy from rural illiterate to urban illiterate to rural literate to urban literate (Kendall et al., 1988, p. 312)—much as Gilbert (1986), Berry (1988) and other rural researchers have demonstrated.

Between them, these factors of formal education and urbanization override ethnicity as a contributor to test performance variance in culturally different settings, and are also more important than the traditional sources of variance found in age, sex, and socioeconomic status: The "cultural variable," in which education and urbanization are subsumed, therefore, makes far and away the largest contribution to performance variance on psychometric tests. Until shown otherwise, one must assume that these large cultural differences also occur between different groups in western societies.

Practice Effects

In 1976, M. A. Verster described how the test performances of a group of 1,200 Black miners were affected by exposure to the technologically sophisticated mine environment on the one hand, and repeated testing on the other. The test instrument was the Classification Test Battery developed by the National Institute for Personnel Research of the South African Council for Scientific and Industrial Research. One group of subjects was retested four times at 3-month intervals to maximize test practice; another was retested only once, 12 months after the initial test administration, in order to maximize the effects of exposure to the highly westernized mine environment; intermediate groups were retested two and three times, respectively.

Exposure to the mine environment did not make a significant contribution to test performance, but repeated test exposure did. The greatest mean increase, of the order of one half of a standard deviation,[9] occurred between the first and second testing, with diminishing increments thereafter, of the order of a quarter to a fifth of a standard deviation on the third and fourth retesting. Score increments thus describe a classic learning acquisition curve (Verster, 1976, Fig. 3), with rapid initial learning that approaches asymptote after the fourth retest (Kendall et al., 1988, p. 307). Test score improvements did not vary significantly with initial test performance, indicating that in this largely illiterate group, the brighter subjects benefited as much from repeated test exposure as the duller.

In a reexamination of these data to examine the sources contributing to this strong learning curve, J. M. Verster and Muller (1985) considered five possible contributors. They found that test items, test format, and mental operations involved in the underlying construct all contributed significantly to improvements, but not test procedure and environmental stimulation. Another finding of note was that the educational level of subjects also influenced the amount they gained from retest exposure, with the least educated and most educated groups showing the highest gains.

For neuropsychologists working with subjects who have had very little previous test exposure, the question that arises is whether "in any one test exposure, one is measuring [a fully developed ability, or] at a point on the acquisition curve for the ability being measured?" (Kendall et al.,1988, p. 308). This question was addressed in an important study by Desmond Crawford-Nutt (1976), who showed that modifying the instructional phase in the presentation of Raven's Progressive Matrices eliminated the often-reported "inferiority" of Black subjects on this test.

"Retarded" Westerners

But the conclusion to be drawn from the psychometric test enterprise with the Black people of southern Africa that spans 80 years, from 1915 to the present, is wider: "We are still far from a scientifically defensible understanding of the manner in which people from different cultures process the same information" (Kendall et al., 1988, p. 328). Psychometric tests in Africa and in other developing countries have focused on industrial selection.

---

[9]Equivalent to 7 or 8 scale points on an IQ test, for example scoring 96 at the first testing and 104 at the second.

Indeed, a perennial frustration of knowledgeable cross-cultural psychologists has been that procedures based entirely on well-known local activities and skills would have had no predictive value for industrial applications. There has thus seemed to be no need to determine indigenous concepts of "smartness": Sarcastically, Kendall et al. (1988) asked how well Westerners would do at discerning rhythms and counterrhythms in African music, constructing arguments that cannot be logically refuted, or deriving secondary meaning from various forms of visual symbolism:

> Psychologists would do well to consider just how "simple" and "retarded" Westerners would appear to black people conducting imaginary investigations of "intelligence" using African-designed techniques of evaluation.... The surest solution to the "problem" would be to accelerate the process of Africanization of Westerners over successive generations of contact with an African culture. (p. 328)

II. The Information Processing Paradigm

The strength of the information-processing paradigm is in the decomposition of complex behaviors into their constituent parts, and the separate investigation of each of these constituents. For such investigations, the computer is both a processing model, and also a device that allows for response quantification along otherwise inaccessible dimensions, such as reaction time, movement time, or variations in response latency. Because laboratory tasks can be simplified to a point where all intact individuals can do all the items (see "Speed and Power"), it is these dimensions, rather than success or failure, that are the dependent variable. Such single factor, low-ceiling laboratory tasks are needed in order to tease out the different variance components that enter into a score to determine its level.

Of the multitude of currently available information processing models of complex problem-solving behavior, one above all has exceptional power in elucidating the precise nature of the differences between test-wise and naive subjects, and in accounting for the large differences in test scores between countries and cultures: This is Robert Sternberg's triarchic theory of intelligence (1984, 1986). The triarchic theory is analyzed in considerable detail later because of the lucidity and theoretical elegance it brings to the understanding of test score variations across cultures.

Linking Psychometrics and Information Processing: Sternberg's Triarchic Theory of Intelligence

An appealing feature of the triarchic theory is that it takes into account both universal features of human intelligence, identical from one culture to another, and also fundamental variations in the nature of intelligence and the ways in which it is appropriate to measure it from one culture to another (Sternberg, 1988). Also, the theory avoids trivializing "intelligence" out of existence as a human adaptive capacity, as it is both in a pure information processing approach, and by those theories that equate it with cortical speed (see the comments by Eysenck and by Jensen in the issue of *Behavioral & Brain Sciences* in which Sternberg's 1984 paper appears).

The three components of the triarchic theory allow the construction of a cognitive science framework within which neuropsychological tests can be deconstructed and interpreted. They are a *contextual subtheory* that relates intelligence to adaptive mental activity in the person's real-world environment; an *experiential subtheory* that is two faceted, relating novelty and automatization to task performance; and a *componential subtheory* that specifies the mental mechanisms or component processes through which intelligent behavior is effected.

1. The Contextual Subtheory. This subtheory "addresses the question of which behaviors are intelligent for whom, and where these behaviors are intelligent" (Sternberg, 1984, p. 269). As Irvine has pointed out in another context, counting to the base of 12 and 20 was an essential skill in England when its currency was pounds, shillings (20 to the pound), and pence (12 to the shilling); today, after decimalization, the capacity to count to such bases remains as a cognitive competence, but cannot be defined as intelligent, nor included in tests that measure contextual intelligence. Defining contextual intelligence against an external standard—"purposive adaptation to, shaping of, and selection of real-world environments relevant to one's life" (1984, p. 271)—not only accommodates the Marxist view that mind is shaped by environment, but achieves a larger purpose: It gives formal recognition to cultural relativism, making it possible, without theoretical strain, to predict for example that performance on a supposedly universal measure of ability to educe rules, such as the Halstead Category Test, is anything but universal. In cultures in which these eductive skills are used to adapt, shape and select environments, one can assume that people have cognitive competence in eduction, and that this competence is there to be measured; in cultures to which these criteria do not apply, low scores on the Category Test will have a quite different meaning, or no meaning at all.

2. The Experiential Subtheory. This two-faceted subtheory is concerned with skills at the interface between individuals and tasks: The ability to deal with novel kinds of task and novel situational demands on the one hand, and the ability to automatize information processing on the other. Automatization is a central concept in cognitive psychology. It means the ability to perform a complex task without thinking about it. Experienced surgeons can graft a vein while telling jokes to one another, and experienced drivers can dictate a business letter or listen with full comprehension to the morning news while at the same time (if the driver in question is one of the diehard purists who prefer a manual shift) executing the intricate serial actions of release accelerator/depress clutch/change gear/clutch out/decelerate for curve and so on. Full conscious attention (what Sternberg called "the global processor") is given to the former task, and none to the automatized driving task. Novice drivers, on the contrary, must dedicate the global processor to driving, and have no attentional capacity left for anything else.

Of the three subtheories, the experiential is the most important for psychologists working with subjects who are not test-wise. Readers of the material that follows will recognize in it a reformulation, in more rigorous terms, of the question raised by Kendall and his coauthors (1988) in the context of practice effects: Whether the test score of a subject from a different culture reflects a fully developed ability, or "a point on the acquisition curve for the ability being measured" (Kendall et al., 1988, p. 308).

2.1. *Novelty.* Novel tasks are not automatized; to use Sternberg's evocative term, they are "non-entrenched." In this sense, Part A of the Trail Making Test, which requires a subject to connect circles numbered 1, 2, 3, and so forth, calls on entrenched knowledge, whereas Trail B, which requires the subject to connect 1 to A, A to 2, 2 to B, B to 3, and so forth, deliberately sets up a conflict between two highly entrenched kinds of information, the number series, and the alphabet. Similarly, to reflect further on the neuropsychological armamentarium, the first two parts of the Stroop Colour-Word Interference Test call on entrenched knowledge, that is the reading of single-syllable words and the naming of colors; Part 3, the interference task, requires the subject to say aloud the color of the ink in which a word is printed rather than the word itself: If the word RED is printed in green ink, the subject must say "green," again setting up a deliberate conflict between an entrenched process (reading the word you see printed on the page) with a nonentrenched task (naming an ink color and not the word printed in that color).

The two-facet subtheory thus measures intelligence "precisely at those points where the relation between the individual and the task or situation is most rapidly changing" (1984, p. 276). The change arises because the individual automatizes every novel task as rapidly as possible, so that one is measuring learning on a steep acquisition curve. This curve will reach asymptote at different points for more and for less intelligent individuals so that the difference in information-processing speed early and later in the task, after asymptote has been approached or attained, will in fact be a measure of the time the individual needs to convert novelty to automatization. This in turn suggests that the measure of interest on a novel task, whether this is Part 3 of the Stroop, Trails B or learning to change gears, will be the extent to which response latency decreases as a function of the number of items completed, or the number of gear changes practiced. Neuropsychologists, on the contrary, have hitherto concerned themselves only with elapsed time to task completion, or the number of responses in a stipulated time. Sternberg's theory suggests that a more interesting measure on Trails B would be to average response time from 1 to A, A to 2, 2 to B, and so forth, in the first time epoch (this might be 10 or 15 sec), and compare it with average response time per item in the second epoch, third epoch, and so forth. Time decreases from epoch to epoch would provide a numerical index of automatization, indicating how much automatization was taking place and its rate of increase or decrease.

Both tasks and situations can be novel. Novel or nonentrenched *tasks* require information processing outside of people's ordinary experience (thus, on a novelty–familiarity dimension, the Wechsler Verbal Scale consists of familiar classroom-type tests, whereas the Performance Scale items are novel, some more than others; thus, Block Design is almost completely novel, whereas Object Assembly calls on jigsaw puzzle skills familiar to western subjects). Sternberg noted that if a task is so novel that it is totally outside the individual's past experience (such as a syllogism for a Uzbeki peasant or calculus for a 5-year-old) it has no assessment value.

Situations can also be novel or familiar, as with an examination taken in one's own classroom or in the hall of another school under a strange invigilator. It will be recalled that the psychological test-taking situation calls on a range of skills familiar from the classroom situation, such as sitting still, paying attention, and using booklets (Kendall et al., 1988), which are unfamiliar to unschooled adults, thus adding a dimension of situational novelty to the high degree of task novelty.

A further distinction can now be made within the area of task novelty, and that is between the skills necessary to understand the task (task comprehension) and those needed to execute it (task solution). To measure *task comprehension*, Sternberg presented subjects with a "concept projection" task: An object could be presented either as a blue dot or a green dot, or described as one of four colors, *green, blue, grue, or bleen*. In the year 2000, the color might change, so that an object that is green now might appear blue in the year 2000: The name of its color in that year would be "grue"; similarly, what is blue now and green then would be called "bleen." The novelty demand of this task is to understand what is wanted (task comprehension) rather than to produce the novel words (task solution): Having just read this section of Sternberg's paper several times in order to present the previous brief description of the task, I can attest to the fact that the task comprehension demand is indeed stringent!

Task solution is assessed, for example, by a time-rate problem: If there are 3 windmills that each fill one tank in 2 days, how long will 12 windmills take to fill 3 tanks? Here, in contrast to the bleen–grue problem, task compre-

4. ENVIRONMENTALISTS AND NATIVISTS

hension is easy for well-schooled subjects, but task solution is difficult because of the novel execution demands set by the problem. Sternberg calls these insight problems, and by manipulating problem content, he and his colleagues were able to isolate three different kinds of insight subjects used to generate solutions: Selective encoding, selective combination, and selective comparison.

2.2. Automatization. As noted earlier, familiar complex tasks such as reading or driving are completely automatized. However, novel tasks require fully conscious control by the global processor or central executive. This cognitive manager plans, monitors, and revises information processing, gets direct feedback from automatized nonexecutive processes, and makes available to them the individual's total knowledge base stored in long-term memory (1984, pp. 277–278).

But the global processor is not needed for entrenched tasks, such as speaking one's own language or doing the jobs a busy executive carries out every day. For example, a sales executive dials a customer's number and greets the switchboard operator while at the same time filling out a factory work order on a familiar form. Here, the central executive calls two local production systems into operation, one for making the telephone call and the other for filling in an order form, both drawing on their own stores of locally applicable knowledge, while a third local system, talking, proceeds in parallel with both other sets of activities. Such automated processing is of virtually unlimited capacity and does not require focused attention. But introducing a single element into this scenario that calls for the use of full conscious attention—for example, the company buyer comes on the line to discuss the details of a new order—brings the other local processes to a complete halt: The notorious bottleneck in processing capacity caused by the use of full conscious attention (Kahneman, 1973) has come into play.

Why the Wechsler Intelligence Scales Cannot Rule Out Brain Damage.

Sternberg's analysis gives a novel answer to a troublesome problem in neuropsychological assessment, which is why the Wechsler tests cannot rule out brain damage. This is because the Wechsler verbal scale stands on the automatization side of the interface between novelty and automatization. As a result, there can be startling contrasts between apparently preserved global intelligence on the verbal scale on the one hand, and grossly compromised life skills on the other.

A troublesome shortcoming of Wechsler-type tests is that because they do not distinguish between entrenched and nonentrenched skills, they are blind to the adaptive syndrome produced by frontal injuries. Five of the six subtests on the Wechsler verbal scale (Information, Comprehension, Arithmetic, Similarities, and Vocabulary) draw heavily on old learning and classroom-type skills that are well entrenched and relatively more resistant to central nervous system insult than the novel and relatively unfamiliar skills required by the five subtests of the performance scale.

The Australian neuropsychologist Kevin Walsh tells an anecdote to illustrate the consequences of prefrontal injuries for adaptive behavior. The story concerns a judge of the Australian High Court, to whom the excellent Wechsler-type IQ scores of a grossly hypofrontal traumatic brain injury survivor had been presented. The psychologist for the plaintiff then explained the nature of the man's adaptive deficit, to which the judge responded: "I see. You mean he has the intelligence, but he can't use it."

2.3. *Expertise.* The disadvantage of the local production system is that it has available only a limited knowledge base that previous experience has packed into it. This limited knowledge base can be enormously expanded by experts in their field of expertise.[10] For example, a chess grandmaster has packed a huge amount of information into a local system and can use it in an automatized mode to handle 20 simultaneous chess games, and win them all. Part of the efficiency of such local systems derives from their nonhierarchical nature, integrating executive and process functions into a single system; if the local system is inadequate for a given condition, control is passed back to the attention-demanding global processor, which decides how to handle the task. The benefit is that the new learning acquired during this exit to centrally controlled global processing is packed back into the local system (1984, p. 278) so that there is no need to exit the local system next time around.

A useful model for the acquisition of expertise is thus created: It is "the successively greater assumption of information processing by local resources" (Sternberg, 1984, p. 278). Accordingly, novices are overwhelmed by new information when they enter an expert area, such as an upmarket hi-fi shop (or a neuropsychological case conference), and lose most of the new information as it is presented. Experts in the area have already stored a great deal of information in local systems, and have more global resources free—including selective attention—in order to effortlessly learn the context-bound new information, such as the wattage of the amplifier, the impedance of the speakers, and the oversampling ratio of the CD player; the novice, on the other hand, would still be puzzling out which of the black boxes is the amplifier and which the CD player, and taking in no information about wattage or impedance.

2.4. *Automatization and test wiseness.* The more efficient the individual is in dealing with novelty, the more resources are available for automatized per-

---

[10] In arguing for the utility of mental speed as a principal contributor to intelligence, Jensen (1984) made a similar point: Because of the limited capacity of conscious attention, speed allows more operations per unit time to be executed without overloading the system, and before rapid decay has destroyed incoming traces. Thus, the most discriminating test items would be those that "threaten the information-processing system at the threshold of breakdown" (p. 295), which in turn could be predicted for more complex tasks by reaction time measures.

4. ENVIRONMENTALISTS AND NATIVISTS

formance, notes Sternberg. The trade-off between global and local processing takes place along an experiential continuum, and this has an important implication for the measurement of intelligence. For this purpose, two points of most interest on this continuum are the time when the task is first encountered, and the time on the experience acquisition curve when novelty wears off and automatization begins. For some subjects on some tasks, for example for test-wise students taking a multiple-choice synonyms test, task comprehension is automatized. For others, task execution is automatized, as in a letter recognition or letter matching task. For both kinds of task, some automatization on the other, nonautomatized aspect will be acquired while performing the task.

For ability measurement, Sternberg advocated selecting tasks that involve a blend of automatized and novel behaviors by presenting a task that is novel, but giving enough practice for performance to become "differentially automatised across subjects over the length of the practice period: Such a task will thereby measure both response to novelty and a degree of automatization, although at different times during the course of the testing" (Sternberg, 1984, p. 280). This formulation allows test performance to be related to cultural variables:

> Individuals who have been brought up in a test-taking culture are likely to have had much more experience with [both verbal tests and test of non-verbal reasoning] than individuals not brought up in such a culture.... Even if the processes of solution are the same, the degrees of novelty and automatization will be different, and hence the tests will not be measuring the same skills across populations.... Between-group comparisons may [thus] be defective and unfair. A fair comparison between groups would require comparable degrees of novelty and automatization in test items as well as comparable processes and strategies." (1984, p. 280).

For the neuropsychologist, the implications of this statement are dazzling. Even on apparently culture-fair tasks such as Object Assembly or the WISC-R Mazes or the Austin Maze (Walsh, 1985, p. 236) western subjects can use automatized task comprehension. Not so for subjects from other cultures. On the Austin Maze, for example, the arrays of switches and signal lights are familiar to western subjects because they have analogues in such common objects as a puzzle toy or an instrument display panel. Automatized task comprehension will also be applied to the instructions for the test (in essence, "find a pathway through the array"), which is analogous to tracing through a maze, trouble-shooting in an electrical system, and the like. This leaves global resources free for automatization of the initial phases of task execution, so that on each repetition of the maze, a larger number of correct moves has been moved into local memory.

The unsophisticated subject, on the other hand, can bring no automatic task comprehension to bear. The switch array on the board may be the first they have encountered. The instructions about finding a safe pathway across the buttons are obscure, even in amplified form, so that task comprehension requires full global processing capacity, leaving none to spare for automatization of task solution. For this hypothetical subject, then, in the first several trials, one is measuring not a visuomotor analogue of a supraspan learning task, but apparatus familiarization and instruction acquisition tasks. An unknown number of initial trials is thus used on tasks other than learning the pathway.

The experiential subtheory therefore specifies what a task or a situation must measure in order to assess intelligence: Tasks follow from the subtheory rather than the theory attempting a post hoc explanation of task demands. This in turn links intelligence to the real world rather than to tasks. Behavior is intelligent when it involves either adaptation to novelty, or automatization of performance, or both.

The issue of practice and test-wiseness that has been a perennial puzzle to ability assessment in the developing countries is also elegantly resolved. Practice facilitates both task comprehension and task solution, and is therefore an integral part of the task itself. All subjects must be given enough practice to allow for differential automatization of performance across subjects over time, so that the task will measure both response to novelty and degree of automatization at different times during the course of testing (1984, p. 280; there are echoes in this formulation of Vygostskian notion of the zone of proximal development).

3. The Componential Subtheory. The basic unit of analysis in Sternberg's theory of intelligence is the information-processing component, namely "an elementary information process that operates on internal representations of objects or symbols" (1984, p. 281); this process replaces the unit of analysis in earlier theories, such as the "factor" or the "stimulus-response bond." An information-processing component may translate a sensory input into a conceptual representation, may transform such representations, or may translate them into motor outputs. The three properties associated with components are *duration* (time to execution), *difficulty* (probability of being executed erroneously), and *probability of execution* (the likelihood that an individual will arrive at an answer, whether or not it is correct).

Components perform three kinds of function: *Metacomponents* plan, monitor, and make decisions; *performance components* are processes used in task execution; and *knowledge-acquisition components* are used to learn new things.

3.1. *Metacomponents* are of special interest to neuropsychologists because of their explanatory power in getting into neuropsychology's "black box," referred to in previous typologies as the brain's third functional unit (Luria,

4. ENVIRONMENTALISTS AND NATIVISTS 81

1973), the executive processes (Lezak, 1995), or the three components of adaptive behavior (Walsh, 1985). Sternberg defined metacomponents as "specific realizations of control processes that are sometimes collectively (and loosely) referred to as the 'executive' or the 'homunculus'" (Sternberg, 1984, p. 282): This is an endearing image, suggesting a tiny human being sitting in a cabin somewhere in the brain, steering the cerebral motor car along familiar or strange roads, accelerating down the straight and braking at the caution signs.

During automatized processing, metacomponents operate at the same level as process components and lose their executive character (this distinction at once draws attention to a puzzling phenomenon in high-functioning individuals who sustain a frontal injury, namely their complaint that "everything takes twice as long." This is because previously automatized process components now require the full attention of the global processor, thus ruling out the possibility of time-saving parallel functioning of a number of local processors simultaneously). Sternberg identified seven metacomponents (Sternberg, 1984, p. 282), not as an exhaustive catalogue but as exemplars of those most often encountered in intellectual functioning. Five of these are now reviewed.

3.1.1. *What is the problem.* The task here is to decide what the problem is that needs to be solved. For example, a group of intern clinical neuropsychologists at the doctoral level consistently "rigidifies" brain-injured clients against therapeutic interventions. Does this rigidification arise from incorrect joining with the client system or because of overly decisive information giving or did the intake selection process pick a bunch of poor trainees?

3.1.2. *Selection of lower-order components.* For example, some syllogistic tasks are best solved by using spatial representation, and others by linguistic encoding; some tasks require that more time be allocated to encoding and less to stimulus combination and response. Selecting an inappropriate set of components will give rise to errors or inefficient performance. For example, an appropriate set of strategies on the Wisconsin Card Sorting Test is flexible error utilization to move away from one sorting principle to another. Some clients, however, give all their energy to the eduction of a single bizarre and over-complex sorting principle such as, "If there are two on top and one below, the next match must be with one below and two on top, then the next one must be four on top and none below ..."; in fact, no cards exist that can match this fanciful question being asked; following Mundy-Castle's (1983) distinction between social and technological intelligence, the Baoul also attached importance to skills of observation, attention, fast learning, and memory skills. But when the children who had performed the Piagetian tasks were ranked by adults on these indigenous conceptions of intelligence, most correlations were negative, leading Dasen

(1984) to conclude "that the Baoul concept of intelligence is basically different from concrete operational reasoning [and] that spatial skills are not valued in this culture" (pp. 428–429).

In essence, these studies confirm Irvine's view that intelligent acts are of a conforming kind. However, with increasing westernization, there is a marked shift away from slowness and carefulness as the criteria of intelligent behavior toward the desirability of quickness. Mundy-Castle (1983) captured this movement in the distinction he drew between "social intelligence" and "technical intelligence." Berry (1988) reported further studies of lay concepts of intelligence in Guatemala, Malaya, China, Taiwan, Australia, and the United States.

Can this large body of knowledge about intelligent acts in different societies be converted to an integrated universal theory of intelligence? Such frameworks have been proposed (Berry, 1984, Fig. 2) but the goal is unlikely to be realized: one would have to demonstrate the ecological validity and equivalence of a huge set of derived etics[11] across the full range of human cultures. "In practice, this implies a research programme of unrealizable scope" (Verster, 1986, p. 28).

A significant additional difficulty with the notion of *cognitive* competence is that it devalues the range of emotionally based adaptive behavior—tact, considerateness, conversational pragmatics, and intact affectivity (Damassio, 1994; Prigatano, 1991). Neuropsychologists in particular require a wider definition of competence that includes all of adaptive behavior, and not only its intellectual aspects. It is interesting in this context that Sternberg, Conway, Ketron, and Bernstein (1981) found that a "social competence" factor emerged when lay people rated intelligent behavior.

Can competence testing live up to the hopes it aroused in the 1970s? Barrett and Depinet (1991) concluded that it has not been more successful than traditional intelligence and aptitude testing in predicting job success or in avoiding prejudice to minorities; there is little evidence that "competency testing has the potential to make a unique contribution to the field of testing" (p. 1021).

However, in culturally different settings, the need for alternative approaches to the quantification of ability remains urgent. *Competence* as a construct is heir to the conceptual ills of intelligence. One of the reasons for this failure is that the cognitive content given to theories of competence has focused exclusively on the culture-laden executive processes, which are only one component of intelligent behavior. On the other hand, the measurement of *cognitive potential* may offer a viable alternative method of ability assessment.

---

[11]Cross-cultural psychologists make a useful distinction between the etic (or universal) and the emic (or particular). These terms derive from the words phonETICS, which is the study of the general and universal aspects of sound in language, and phonEMICS, the science of sounds which are meaningful and employed within a single linguistic system.

One of the most intriguing challenges in modern psychometrics is to develop a measure of cognitive or learning potential that has good predictive validity. But since the 1950s, this has remained tantalizingly out of reach. For example, Dague (1972) cited the work of Ombredane and his colleagues in the 1950s in which the gains on repeated test administration were taken to measure learning potential among young Congolese in the 10–14 age group. But far from predicting educability, correlations of educational success with difference scores were poor. Schochet (1986, cited in Boeyens, 1989) adapted Feuerstein's learning potential method (Feuerstein, 1979, 1980; Feuerstein, Rand, Hoffman, & Miller, 1979) to investigate this potential among disadvantaged first year bachelor of arts students at the University of the Witwatersrand in Johannesburg, South Africa. Test gains from pretest through to a posttest following intensive coaching failed to correlate with any measures of academic performance. Boeyens (1989) noted that this and many other studies of learning potential "evidence a complete disregard for the problems of reliability" (p. 40); for Schochet's study the mean difference score was so low as to be uninterpretable. Taylor (1994) distinguished between Type 1 potential, achieved through the teaching of thinking skills, and Type 2 potential, measured by tests of learning, and speculated that Type 1 potential, measured as test–retest gains on novel tasks, may eliminate differences that arise from test-wiseness and culture.

A Case Study as a Footnote: English–Afrikaans IQ Differences

As a final step in broadening the canvas, it is useful to consider the marked intelligence score differences between White English and Afrikaans speaking South Africans. There are no race differences between these groups; they share a cultural heritage, are brought up within a unitary state, and are compelled to acquire a working knowledge of one another's language; their socioeconomic status is equivalent, and so is their education. The force of the following material is thus to show that even very subtle cultural differences that in this case relate only to social values and norms can have a substantial effect on IQ scores, and that such scores cannot therefore reliably reflect an innate, universal "intelligence." Let us see what might be learned from this state of affairs that is helpful in understanding IQ differences between White and Black Americans, and other intergroup disparities.

An introductory word about South Africa's two White tribes will be helpful. Afrikaners are descendants of the Dutch, who settled the Cape from 1652. English settlement began with the first British occupation of the Cape in 1806, and expanded greatly with the arrival of a large British settler group in 1820 in the wake of the Napoleonic wars. To escape British rule, groups of Afrikaners moved north and east into South Africa's interior, fighting a series of bloody skirmishes with African tribes: This Great Trek has been mythologized (Hofmeyr, 1991) as the birth of the Afrikaner nation, simultaneously facing a White enemy, the British, and African. After the discovery of diamonds and gold in the late 19th century, the Afrikaners fought and lost a bitter war of independence against the British in 1899–1902.

Afrikaner ascendancy in South African politics began with the election victory of the Nationalist Party—the architect of apartheid—in 1948, and was symbolically consolidated by South Africa's withdrawal from the British Commonwealth in 1956. The late 1950s were thus marked by the consolidation of Afrikaner political power, the extension of this power into heavy industry, growing government control of universities and other state funded research institutions, and a repressive political climate.

Against this background, a more emotional and politically sensitive issue than a report in 1959 that Afrikaners were of lower intelligence than English speakers could hardly be imagined.

A Difference of Six Scale Points. Standardization of the Wechsler-Bellevue Intelligence Scale for White South Africans began in the 1940s, and used a sample of 1,500 English-speaking and 1,500 Afrikaans-speaking South Africans ranging in age from 18 to 59. In 1959, Biesheuvel and Liddicoat reported that a reanalysis of data from a sample of 305 English speaking and 299 Afrikaans speaking subjects from this norm group showed that English speakers scored on average 6 scale points higher than Afrikaans speakers (nearly half a standard deviation, significant at the .01% level). When the sample was stratified by socioeconomic standard (SES), no significant difference was found at the lowest SES category, which, argued the authors, showed "lack of responsiveness due to low intelligence and an environment catering for little more than the necessities of life [which] would leave little scope for differential cultural development" (p. 5). At the highest SES level, the difference, although still significant, was lower than in the intermediate SES range, implying that developmental conditions might converge for both language groups at the highest and lowest income levels.

Stratifying the sample by both socioeconomic standard and subtest performance showed that English and Afrikaans speakers had virtually equal scores on the Arithmetic subtest, because, argued the authors, "arithmetic is a subject in which all scholars are drilled alike, and in which a specific cultural effect is therefore least likely to occur" (p. 8). Block Design and Digit Symbol Substitution, although supposed to be free of cultural bias, also yielded a significant English-speaking advantage in the highest and intermediate SES categories, suggesting a difference in fluid intelligence levels.

4. ENVIRONMENTALISTS AND NATIVISTS

Biesheuvel and Liddicoat (1959) concluded that these persistent differences in favor of English speakers pointed to "a more general and fundamental influence, operative in all the tests, and most probably affecting the level of g" (p. 11). Given the political climate in South Africa in the 1950s, their conclusions are remarkably hard-hitting:

> The possibility must at least be considered that the lower stimulus value of the Afrikaans-speaking environment (in terms of parental education and interests, diversity of aspirations, material culture in the home, frequency and intensity of contacts with people, ideas, and intellectually challenging situations) has drawn out the intellectual potentialities of its members to a lesser extent than the English-speaking environment. (p. 12).

Partly as a result of this publication, Biesheuvel's position as director of the South African National Institute of Personnel Research came under siege, and in 1962 he resigned his post. Biesheuvel died in 1991 at the age of 83, and his son-in-law, John Verster, writes in his obituary notice that the Afrikaner establishment had in the 1950s read into Biesheuvel's work "an attempt to denigrate Afrikaans South Africans as intellectually inferior" (Verster, 1991, p. 269), and responded defensively. In 1960, for example, H. P. Langenhoven argued that the conclusions drawn about the comparative "intellectual potentialities" of different cultural groups were premature (Langenhoven, 1960, p. 152), and suggested that the difference in test performance could be ascribed to a lack of test sophistication rather than to performance differences in real life situations.

The Continued But Diminishing Gap. Reanalysis of the South African Wechsler-Bellevue data by Verster and Prinsloo (1988) showed a steady increase in the magnitude of the difference in favor of English speakers from the age of 45 onward. This is not because of differential aging effects on intelligence, but rather the result of differential cohort experiences: "The cultural distance between the two populations is likely to be greater in the older cohorts [born in the decade of the 1890s] than in the younger" (p. 541).

Another large investigation of English-Afrikaner test score differences was a Human Sciences Research Council survey that compared 21,000 English-speaking with 41,000 Afrikaans-speaking children who were in Std 6 (the 8th year of formal schooling) in 1965, and retested these cohorts in 1967 and 1969. In all comparisons, English speakers outperformed Afrikaans speakers, and more markedly so on the fluid intelligence nonverbal scale of the New South African Group Test. Among Std 6 pupils, English speakers fared significantly better than Afrikaans speakers on tests of paragraph memory, memory for words and symbols, number ability, and reasoning.

This gross difference masks a far more interesting process, namely that in comparison with the Biesheuvel and Liddicoat data, there has been "a progressive decrease in ability score discrepancies with increasing cultural convergence over successive generations[12] of white South Africans" (p. 544).

In an extension of this series of studies, Verster (1974) found significant differences between English- and-Afrikaans speaking graduate research scientists at the Council for Scientific and Industrial Research, again in favor of English speakers. Factor analysis of the six tests he used showed that five loaded on what he called a common reasoning factor, akin to g_f, in which inductive and deductive variance merged, whereas the sixth loaded on spatial reasoning for English speakers, but on both space and reasoning for Afrikaans speakers (p. 546). To what can these continued differences in the 1970s be attributed? Verster suggested that they are due "to stylistic differences in approach to intellectual tasks [and differences] on personality dimensions such as over-regimentation and conservatism, authoritarianism, and ethnocentrism" (pp. 546–547). In a subsidiary analysis of the same data, Sussenguth found that a battery of self-report items showed higher scores for the Afrikaans speakers on such dimensions as "rigidity versus versatility in thinking, ideational conformity versus ideational independence, and low performance potential versus high performance potential" (p. 546), thus confirming that there are indeed underlying stylistic differences in approaches to problem-solving tasks:

> These findings suggest the need for extreme caution when wishing to infer equivalence of psychological meaning in tests [even] when psychometric criteria for equivalence have been met. Mean population differences on ability tests are at least as likely to reflect the stylistic or other differences in approach to the tests as differences on the presumed underlying "ability." (Verster & Prinsloo, 1988, p. 554)

The Bell Curve in Cross-Cultural Perspective

It is untrue to say that the explanation for these differences is either genetic or cultural. Ordinary people don't have to go to college to know that bright parents usually have bright kids, and that siblings have similar intellectual endowments; there is a proverb in English and many other languages, "The

---

[12] A similar process has been at work in the United States. Data from the National Assessment of Educational Progress (NAEP) show that over a 20-year period, there has been an overall narrowing of the Black–White IQ gap equal to .28 of a standard deviation, or about 5 IQ points. Some age-specific subject gains are much higher—for example, for 17-year-olds, reading scores improved by .44 of a standard deviation over this period. Speculating on the reasons, Herrnstein and Murray (1994) noted that the quality of Black schooling has improved, nutrition and health care have improved, travel opportunities have increased, and media exposure has reduced the impact of environmental differences.

apple never falls far from the tree." There is an overwhelming commonsense and scientific case for a large genetic contribution to intelligence, just as genetics contributes to every other characteristic that marks individuals as members of the species, as the children of their parents, and as individually unique.[13]

There is also an overwhelming case for the cultural molding of intelligence. Herrnstein and Murray, the archnativists, acknowledged as we have just seen the effects of school quality, nutrition, health care, travel opportunities, and media exposure on IQ; their comment on "the gaping cultural gap" between rich and poor was cited earlier. Jensen wrote that if the first IQ tests had been devised in a hunting culture, "'general intelligence' might well have turned out to involve visual acuity and running speed, rather than vocabulary and symbol manipulation" (1969, p. 14). But even more telling, because it comes from a different place and time, is the attribution Biesheuvel and Liddicoat made nearly 40 years ago—that Afrikaners score lower on IQ tests as a result of "parental education and interests, diversity of aspirations, material culture in the home, frequency and intensity of contacts with people, ideas, and intellectually challenging situations" (1959, p. 12).

These data show that there is a general tendency for developing country populations to score lower on psychological tests than western subjects; some enclave cultures embedded within larger populations—African Americans, Hispanics, Jews, English-speaking South Africans—also score lower or higher than the population mean. The lesson to be learned from close on a century of cross-cultural psychological assessment is that until language proficiency, educational quality, test-wiseness, cognitive style, and socially mediated definitions of what it means to be smart have been shown beyond any reasonable doubt to be equivalent for the groups whose scores are being compared, score differences cannot be attributed to genetic differences. Sandra Scarr cited evidence "that black children are being reared in circumstances that give them only marginal acquaintance with the skills and knowledge being sampled by the tests" (1978, p. 335; see also Mercer, 1984). For these and other lower scoring groups, the test as given may not be the test as received, invalidating score comparisons.

Similar reasoning applies to groups that do better than the population average: Genetic attributions for the higher scores of Jews and Asians are suspect until due weight has been given to the foundational assumptions of the culture that determine achievement motivation, among these the value placed on speed and classroom learning. So, even after careful validation

---

[13]It is "ridiculous to suppose that abolishing intellectual measurement will revolutionize anyone's life chances," or that "biological diversity must be denied to defend universal civil liberties" (Scarr, 1978, p. 327).

and norming, psychological tests are a chancy way of getting through to the underlying construct of adaptive capacity in subjects from other cultures.

But for the time being, they are the *only* way. The good news is that in the hands of cross-culturally sophisticated neuropsychologists, many psychological tests created within the matrix of western values can be sensitively and usefully applied to the bearers of other cultures.

REFERENCES

Albee, G. W. (1977). The Protestant Ethic, sex and psychotherapy. *American Psychologist, 32*, 150–161.

Anastasi, A. (1988). *Psychological testing* (6th ed.). New York: Macmillan.

Barrett, G. V., & Depinet, R. L. (1991). A reconsideration of testing for competence rather than for intelligence. *American Psychologist, 46*, 1012–1024.

Berry, J. W. (1976). *Human ecology and cognitive style*. New York: Wiley.

Berry, J. W. (1984). Towards a universal psychology of cognitive competence. *International Journal of Psychology, 19*, 335–361.

Berry, J. W. (1988). Cognitive and social factors in psychological adaptation to acculturation among the James Bay Cree. In G. K. Verma & C. Bagley (Eds.), *Cross cultural studies of personality and cognition* (pp. 111–142). London: Macmillan Press.

Biesheuvel, S., & Liddicoat, R. (1959). The effects of cultural factors on intelligence-test performance. *Journal of the National Institute for Personnel Research, 8*, 3–14.

Boas, F. (1911). *Handbook of American Indian languages*. Washington, DC: Government Printing Office.

Boeyens, J. (1989). *Learning potential: A theoretical perspective*. (Report Pers-432). Pretoria, South Africa: Human Sciences Research Council.

Bouchard, T. J., Lykken, D. T., McGue, M., Segal, N. L., & Tellegen, A. (1990). Sources of human psychological differences: The Minnesota study of twins reared apart. *Science, 250*, 223–228.

Carroll, J. B. (1993). *Human cognitive abilities: A survey of factor analytical studies*. New York: Cambridge University Press.

Crawford-Nutt, D. H. (1976). Black scores on Raven's Standard Progressive Matrices: An artefact of method of test presentation. *Psychologia Africana, 16*, 201–206.

Crawford-Nutt, D. H. (1977a). Assessing the intellectual capacity of subjects in cultural transition. In J. H. Poortinga (Ed.), *Basic problems in cross-cultural psychology* (pp. 49–59). Amsterdam & Lisse: Swets & Zeitinger.

Crawford-Nutt, D. H. (1977b). The effect of educational level on the test scores of people in South Africa. *Psychologia Africana, 17*, 49–59.

Crawford-Nutt, D. H. (1977c). *The Symco Test: Research report and guide to its administration and scoring*. (Pers-165). Johannesburg: National Institute for Personnel Research Council for Scientific and Industrial Research.

Dague, P. (1972). Development, application and interpretation of tests for use in French-speaking black Africa and Madagascar. In L. J. Cronbach & P. J. D. Drenth (Eds.), *Mental tests and cultural adaptation* (pp. 63–74). The Hague: Mouton.

Damassio, A. R. (1994). *Descartes' error: Emotion, reason, and the human brain*. New York: Avon.

Dasen, P. R. (1984). The cross-cultural study of intelligence: Piaget and The Baoulé. *International Journal of Psychology, 19*, 407–434.

Feuerstein, R. (1979). *The dynamic assessment of retarded performers.* Baltimore, MD: University Park Press.

Feuerstein, R. (1980). *Instrumental enrichment: An intervention programme for cognitive modifiability.* Baltimore, MD: University Park Press.

Feuerstein, R., Rand, Y., Hoffman, M., & Miller, R. (1979). Cognitive modifiability in retarded adolescents: Effects of instrumental enrichment. *American Journal of Mental Deficiency, 83,* 539–550.

Gilbert, A. J. (1986). *Psychology & social change in the third world: A cognitive perspective.* Unpublished doctoral dissertation, University of South Africa, Pretoria.

Grant, G. V. (1970). Spatial thinking: A dimension in African intellect. *Psychologia Africana 13,* 222–239.

Grant, G. V. (1972). Conceptual reasoning: Another dimension of African intellect. *Psychologia Africana, 14,* 170–185.

Herrnstein, R. J., & Murray, C. (1994). *The bell curve: Intelligence and class structure in American life.* New York: Free Press.

Hofmeyer, I. (1991). Popularising history: The case of Gustav Preller. In R. Hill, M. Miller, & M. Trump (Eds.), *African studies forum.* Pretoria, South Africa: Human Sciences Research Council.

Hudson, W. (1960). Pictorial depth perception in sub-cultural groups in Africa. *Journal of Social Psychology, 52,* 183–208.

Hunt, E. (1995). The role of intelligence in modern society. *American Scientist, 83,* 356–368.

Irvine, S. H. (1969). Figural tests of reasoning in Africa: Studies in the use of the Raven's Progressive Matrices across cultures. *International Journal of Psychology, 4,* 217–228.

Irvine, S. H., & Berry, J. W. (1988). The abilities of mankind: A revaluation. In S. H. Irvine & J. W. Berry (Eds.), *Human abilities in cultural context* (pp. 3–59). Cambridge, England: Cambridge University Press.

Jahoda, G. (1981). Pictorial perception and the problem of universals. In B. Lloyd, & J. Gay (Eds.), *Universals of human thought* (pp. 25–45). Cambridge, England: Cambridge University Press.

Jensen, A. R. (1969). How much can we boost IQ and scholastic achievement? *Harvard Educational Review, 39,* 1–123.

Jensen, A. R. (1980). *Bias in mental testing.* London: Methuen.

Jensen, A. R. (1984). Mental speed and levels of analysis. *The Behavioural and Brain Sciences, 7,* 295–296.

Kahneman, D. (1973). *Attention and effort.* Englewood Cliffs, NJ: Prentice-Hall

Kaplan, E. (1988). A process approach to neuropsychological assessment. In T. Boll & B. K. Bryant (Eds.), *Clinical neuropsychology and brain function: Research, measurement, and practice.* Washington, DC: American Psychological Association.

Kendall, I. M., Verster, M. A., & von Mollendorf, J. W. (1988). Test performance of Black in Southern Africa. In S. H. Irvine, & J. W. Berry (Eds.), *Human abilities in cultural context* (pp. 239–299). Cambridge, England: Cambridge University Press.

Laboratory of Comparative Human Cognition. (1982). Culture and intelligence. In R. J. Sternberg (Ed.), *Handbook of human intelligence* (pp. 642–719). Cambridge, England: Cambridge University Press.

Langenhoven, H. P. (1960). Comments on "The effects of cultural performance on intelligence test performance." *Journal of the National Institute for Personnel Research, 8,* 150–152.

Lezak, M.D. (1995). *Neuropsychological assessment* (3rd ed.). New York: Oxford University Press.

Luria, A. R. (1980). *Higher cortical functions in man*. New York: Basic Books Inc. (Original work published 1962)
Luria, A. R. (1973). *The working brain: An introduction to neuropsychology*. London: Penguin.
McClelland, D. C. (1961). *The achieving society*. New York: Free Press.
Melendez, F. (1994). The Spanish version of the WAIS: Some ethical considerations. *The Clinical Neuropsychologist, 8,* 388–393.
Mercer, J. R. (1984). What is a racially and culturally nondiscriminatory test? A sociological and pluralistic perspective. In C. R. Reynolds & R. T. Brown (Eds.), *Perspectives on "Bias in Mental Testing."* New York: Plenum.
Mundy-Castle, A. (1983). Are Western psychology concepts valid in Africa? A Nigerian review. In S. H. Irvine & J. W. Berry (Eds.), *Human assessment of cultural factors*. New York: Plenum.
Nell, V. (1988). *Lost in a book: The psychology of reading for pleasure*. New Haven, CT: Yale University Press.
Nell, V. (1994). Interpretation and misinterpretation of the South African Wechsler-Bellevue Adult Intelligence Scale: A history and a prospectus. *South African Journal of Psychology, 24,* 100–109.
Nell, V. (1999). Luria in Uzbekistan: The Vicissitudes of cross-cultural neuropsychology [Special Luria issue]. *Neuropsychology Review, 9,* 45–52.
Nell, V. (2000). *Cross-cultural neuropsychological assessment: Theory and practice*. Mahwah, NJ: Lawrence Erlbaum Associates.
Nell, V., Kruger, D. J, Taylor, T. R., Myers, J. E., & London, L. (1995). *Bypassing culture: A performance process approach to the neuropsychological assessment of nonwestern subjects*. Unpublished manuscript, University of South Africa Health Psychology Unit.
Nell, V., Myers, J., Colvin, M., & Rees, D. (1993). Neuropsychological assessment of organic solvent effects in South Africa: Test selection, adaptation, scoring and validation issues. *Environmental Research, 63,* 301–318.
Prigatano G. (1991). *Awareness of deficit after brain injury: Clinical and theoretical issues*. New York: Oxford University Press.
Reitan, R. M. (1972). Verbal problem-solving as related to cerebral damage. *Perceptual and Motor skills, 34,* 515–524.
Richter, L. M., & Griesel, R. D. (1988). *Bayley Scales for infant development*. Pretoria, South Africa: University of South Africa.
Richter-Strydom, L. M., & Griesel, R. D. (1984). *African infant precocity: A study of a group of South Africa infants from two to fifteen months of age*. Pretoria, South Africa: University of South Africa.
Rogan, J. M., & MacDonald, A. M. (1983). The effect of schooling on conversation skills. *Journal of Cross-cultural Psychology,14,* 309–322.
Sacks, O. (1989). *Seeing voices*. Berkeley: University of California Press.
Scarr, S. (1978). From evolution to Larry P., or what shall we do about IQ tests? *Intelligence, 2,* 325–342.
Sternberg, R. J. (1984). Toward a triarchic theory of human intelligence. *The Behavioural and Brain Sciences, 7,* 269–315.
Sternberg, R. J. (1986). *The triarchic mind*. New York: Viking.
Sternberg, R. J. (1988). A triarchic view of intelligence in cross-cultural perspective. In S. H. Irvine & J. W. Berry (Eds.), *Human abilities in cultural context* (pp. 60–85). Cambridge, England: Cambridge University Press.
Sternberg, R. J., Conway, B. E., Ketron, J. L., & Bernstein, M. (1981). People's conceptions of intelligence. *Journal of Personality and Social Psychology, 41,* 37–55.

Taylor, H. F. (1980). *The IQ game: A methodical inquiry into the heredity–environment controversy*. New Brunswick, NJ: Rutgers University Press.
Taylor, T. R. (1994). A review of three approaches to cognitive assessment and a proposed integrated approach based on a unifying theoretical framework. *South African Journal of Psychology, 24,* 184–193.
Triandis, H. C. (1995). *Individualism & collectivism*. Boulder, CO: Westview Press.
Verster, J. M. (1974). A study of intellectual structure in two groups of South African scientists. *Psychologia Africana, 15,* 169–190.
Verster, J. M. (1986). *Cognitive competence in Africa and models of information processing: A research prospectus* (pers-411). Pretoria, South Africa: Human Sciences Research Council.
Verster, J. M. (1991). Simon Biesheuvel. *South African Journal of Psychology, 21,* 267–270.
Verster, J. M., & Muller, M. W. (1985). *Further investigation of the effects of multiple exposure to the classification test battery: Hypotheses and proposed research design* (Confidential report c/pers 231). Johannesburg: National Institute for Personnel Research.
Verster, J. M., & Prinsloo, R. J. (1988). The diminishing test performance gap between English speakers and Afrikaans speakers in South Africa. In S. H. Irvine, & J. W. Berry (Eds.), *Human abilities in cultural context* (pp. 534–559). Cambridge, England: Cambridge University Press.
Verster, M. A. (1976). *The effect of mining experience and multiple test exposure on test performance of Black mine workers*. Pretoria, South Africa: University of South Africa.
Walsh, K. W. (1985). *Understanding Brain Damage: A primer of neuropsychological evaluation*. Edinburgh, Scotland: Churchill Livingstone.
Walsh, K. W. (1987). *Neuropsychology: A clinical approach*. Edinburgh: Churchill Livingstone.
Weber, M. (1965). *The Protestant Ethic and the spirit of capitalism*. London: Unwin. (Original work published 1901)

Chapter 5

Qualitative Assessment Within and Across Cultures

Carla Caetano
*Center for Rehabilitation of Brain Injury
University of Copenhagen, Denmark*

Neuropsychological assessment has traditionally focused on measures of cognition. Although cognition and culture are closely connected, implications of the relationship between the two have often been neglected. The assessment of cognition originally referred primarily to the concept of intelligence, with an emphasis on a traditional, western, quantitative approach, requiring literacy and skills in test taking, (e.g., using writing materials, symbols; being attentive, following instructions, working with speed and accuracy, etc) typically achieved through a formal educational system. Nell (2000) notes that both formal education and urbanization contribute more to test performance variance, than does ethnicity or the traditional variables of age, sex, and socioeconomic status.

Neuropsychological assessments have, however, also come to measure cognitive processes in a more specific manner such as in the information processing approach. In addition to their use in diagnosis, neuropsychological assessments have also come to be used in rehabilitation planning. With the advent of holistic neuropsychological rehabilitation programs (e.g., Ben-Yishay & Larkin, 1989; Christensen & Caetano, 1999; Christensen & Danielsen, 1987; Prigatano et al., 1986), a more holistic view of the individual has been incorporated into neuropsychological assessments. As such, neuropsychological assessments are meant to evaluate the individual more comprehensively, that is, to include a broader range of psychological variables such as emotional responses, coping strategies, and so forth. Cross-cultural studies have shown, however, that as with cognitive processes, emotion, and experience of self are not necessarily universal concepts. See, for example, Schweder and Bourne (1984) and Cole (1996).

A cross-cultural application of neuropsychological assessments requires an approach to functioning that addresses the interaction of that which is unique and variable with that which is universal (i.e., irrespective of individuality and culture). Although two primary approaches exist for interpretation of data (i.e., quantitative and qualitative), this chapter describes the value of qualitative assessment by postulating that this form of assessment is rooted in an epistemological framework (i.e., phenomenology and systems theory) that differs fundamentally from quantitative assessment. The proposed framework allows for interpretation of data that emphasizes both culturally variable and individually unique aspects of functioning. Prior to discussing the characteristics of qualitative and quantitative methods, the relationship between culture and cognition is discussed briefly.

CULTURE AND COGNITION

As one of the many definitions of culture, LeVine (1984), states "culture represents a consensus on a wide variety of meanings among members of an interacting community approximating that of the consensus on language among members of a speech-community" (pp. 68), whereas cognition may be viewed as the organization of cognitive skills and abilities, namely, perception, language, actions, memory, and thought (McCarthy & Warrington, 1990). Whereas cross-cultural psychologists make a distinction between the etic (or universal) and the emic (or particular), certain perspectives in neuroscience have made the assumption that commonalities shared by all humans (such as genetic endowment) override environmental and cultural factors, whereas others have argued for the predominance of cultural influence over neurocognitive universals. This debate reflects earlier discussions of rationality contra relativism in exploring the foundations of neuropsychological functioning.

A close relationship exists between culture and cognition. Gardner (1984, 1993) postulates that cultural acquisition occurs by culture exiting as a historical and geographical unity thereby providing valued forms of knowledge through physical, social, and human made objects, which necessitate individuals acquiring this knowledge. Bruner, Olver and Greenfield (1966) viewed three elements as fundamental to cognitive growth and development, namely representation, adaptation, and evolution.

The first element relates to how individuals represent their experience of the world, that is, knowledge based on a constructed model of reality constrained by the human neuromuscular system where representations of the world develop from being enactive (habitual actions), to ikonic (imagery free of action), and finally symbolic (translating action and image into language). Gardner (1984, 1993), similarly refers to the individual's genetic inheritance and neurological and psychological proclivities toward learning as sources for competency in various domains. The second element related to cognitive growth pertains to the impact of culture. Models of representation are first adopted from the culture and then adapted to individual use. This process is dependent on the modes of transmission in a culture, the lifestyle of the individual, and the extent to which the individual is encouraged to explore concordance/discordance among the three modes of knowing, (i.e., action, image, and symbol). Gardner (1984, 1993) refers to various symbol systems within the culture, as forms of crystallized knowledge, and that various modes exist for transmission of knowledge, ranging from simple observation to complex forms of schooling. The final element related to cognitive growth that Bruner et al. (1966) describes is evolutionary history, particularly as this pertains to the evolution of brain development in humans and concomitant higher cortical functions. Thus, in explaining the relationship between culture and cognition, acquisition of competence may be attributed to (a) a genetically determined process, (b) learning, as influenced by cultural attributions, or (c) both, that is, an interaction of the two.

Gardner (1984, 1993) believes that developmental psychology and cultural psychology have contributed to models of culture in relationship to personality and affect, but less so to culture as regards cognition. Regarding neuropsychological assessments, a qualitative, holistic neuropsychological approach may, therefore, be helpful in this regard.

TYPES OF NEUROPSYCHOLOGICAL ASSESSMENT

Vanderploeg (1994) views the clinical assessment of brain–behavior relationships as having advanced from the use of single tests of "organicity" to a complex multifaceted process that consists of integrating test findings with the historical data, life situation and unique aspects of individual performance. Thus, in conducting neuropsychological assessments, a holistic model of human functioning is required to systematize such diverse information, resulting in evaluation techniques that are similarly diverse. These techniques may include the use of interview, case history, behavioral observations, and tests. Data can be interpreted quantitatively or qualitatively. According to Bauer (1994), what distinguishes the two approaches is that the former is concerned with the quantification and measurement of cognitive and mental abilities whereas the latter is more concerned with eliciting characteristic signs or symptoms of brain disease and linking behavioral syndromes to regional brain function through anatomical–clinical correlation.

Data can be interpreted quantitatively, that is, numerically, by standardized tests, experimental tasks, with standardized scoring and normative scores based on linear statistical models. Neuropsychological tests are comprised of homogeneous items that ideally involve interval-level measurement and meet appropriate standards of reliability and validity. Typically this approach adopts a priori test selection and yields numerical scores that are evaluated by comparing the subject's performance to normative standards. Thus, there is reliance on statistical predictions of brain damage from psychological tests. In contrast, a qualitative approach is based on behavioral observations and by assessments grounded in process analysis (for e.g., what is responsible for failure/success) rather than by providing an outcome score (level of achievement). A selective hypothesis-testing approach is adopted and examination of brain–behavior relationship takes place by for e.g., syndrome analysis, where emphasis is given to the nature or underlying cause of difficulties.

Halstead-Reitan's neuropsychological test battery is an example of a quantitative neuropsychological assessment (Reitan, 1986) ; whereas Luria's Neuropsychological Investigation (LNI; Christensen, 1975) and Kaplan's (1988) process are examples of qualitative neuropsychological assessments. The LNI is a pure example of such (i.e., it is a clinical investigation where qualitative aspects are described not quantified), whereas Kaplan's may be viewed as a compromise between quantitative and qualitative methods by making use of both methodologies: Here, standardized tests are neither scored nor necessarily administered in the standardized manner, whereas qualitative aspects are quantified and subjected to statistical analyses.

Luria's (1977) critique of the quantitative approach is that as psychometric tests measure specific cognitive functions to evaluate successful performance in relation to a normative sample, they, firstly, are based on preconceived classifications of functions related to contemporary psychological ideas, and secondly, they provide results without identifying how process could affect outcome. The cross-cultural applicability of psychometric tests may similarly be hampered by adopting such an approach. Furthermore, as regards brain injury, Goldstein (1952) has earlier argued against the use of quantitative methods in that the "concrete attitude" often displayed by brain injured patients could result in a quantitative approach being invalidated.

In contrast, a qualitative approach, according to Luria, should always (a) give a detailed analysis of how the observed performance comes about and be based on a hypothesis testing, so as to identify contributing factors (i.e., by process analysis), and (b) identify whether a symptom is due to an elementary level of dysfunction or due to the disorganization of a more complex level of activity. This, therefore, allows for a broad and flexible analysis of subjective variability inherent to the individual, potentially including cultural influences. The LNI has, for example, been used on Zulu (Tollman & Msengana, 1990) and Mexican subjects (Ostrosky-Solis et al., 1985) where cultural influences have been found to greatly impact the manner in which tasks can be completed. Regarding the Tollman study, however, Nell (2000) critiques the expectation that culturally mediated differences will be eliminated by providing, for example, accurate translation or substituting local content for that in the original, as this rests on the unspoken assumption that there are cognitive universals. Nonetheless, in contrast to a standardized quantitative approach, a qualitative approach offers the opportunity for process to be evaluated. Furthermore, flexibility in task administration aids in addressing variability.

Both quantitative and qualitative approaches can distort or misinterpret information, a concern that is of particular relevance to the cross-cultural application of neuropsychological assessments. According to Lezak (1995), quantitative data is limited due to its abstract representation of behavior, multidetermination of single test score responses, and the provision of limited response sets. These are obviously serious limitations in terms of cross-cultural applications. Alternatively, Lezak's critique of qualitative data is primarily viewed as a lack of objectivity, that is, relying on the subjective evaluation of an observer rather than on objective normative parameters. Arguably, in terms of neuropsychological assessment's cross-cultural application, certain subjective evaluations, such as those intended to identify cross-cultural diversity, for example, may be viewed as less misleading than using objective normative data not based on "culturally fair" measures. Furthermore, if qualitative data for neuropsychological assessments is theory driven (as is the LNI), subjectivity can be systematized by brain–behavior syndrome analysis, observation of ecologically valid tasks, and contextualized by a comprehensive interview/narrative analysis of contributing neuropsychological variables. The purpose of the interview is, thus, to constrain subjective interpretation by emphasizing culturally defined meanings.

DIFFICULTIES IN CROSS-CULTURAL QUANTITATIVE ASSESSMENT

The following examples aim to show how a quantitative approach in neuropsychological assessments has limited applicability when using westernized tests in a cross-cultural context: In western culture, cognitive assessment is historically rooted in the composite measure of intelligence. Current neuropsychology, however, does not support this view of cognitive assessment as sufficient. Luria (1977) described cognitive functioning in terms of functional systems, where complex cortical functions are viewed as consisting of the coordinated effect of several neural networks working together, but with specialization in functional activity. Luria states, " the material basis of the higher nervous processes is the brain as a whole, but ... the brain is a highly differentiated system, whose parts are responsible for different aspects of the unified whole" (p. 33). Functional systems are hierarchically identified in the LNI (Christensen, 1975). Basic areas of functioning such as simple motor, tactile-kinaesthetic, auditory and visual modalities, are viewed as elements integrated in complex functions such as memory, expressive and receptive language, problem solving, and so forth.

Lezak (1995) in providing a compendium of tests and assessment techniques for neuropsychological assessments states, "there is no general cognitive or intellectual function, but rather many discrete ones that work together so smoothly when the brain is intact, that cognition is experienced as a single, seamless attribute" (p. 23). Cognitive functions may be classified into four major classes, namely receptive functions (i.e., the selection, acquisition, classification, and integration of information), memory and learning (i.e., information storage and retrieval), thinking (i.e., mental organization/reorganization of information), and expressive functions (i.e., the means through which information is communicated or acted on). Modern neuropsychological assessments identify discrete cognitive functions not in isolation but in terms of functional systems where feedback and feedforward mechanisms emphasize their interconnectedness.

Historical difficulties in the cross-cultural applicability of cognitive assessment is provocatively illustrated by Gould's (1982) article, "A nation of morons," an early example of cross-cultural bias in intelligence testing. Gould described how, in America, Binet's scale was used in the early part of the 20th century for army recruiting. Later, in the 1920s, this data influenced the decision to restrict immigration, without recognizing that the tests were biased and that adherents held a purely hereditarian argument, that is, that test results only reflected innate differences in intelligence, nothing more. For purposes of illustration, this example is presented in some depth. Three types of tests were used; (a) literate recruits were given a written examination (entitled the Army Alpha) that was comprised of items such as analogies, filling the next number in a sequence, and so forth; (b) illiterates, that is, men who failed Alpha, were give a pictorial test (the Army Beta), which included tasks such as running a maze, counting the number of cubes, translating numerals into symbols, and so forth. Thus, although an attempt was made at being "culturally fair," and pictures, numbers, and symbols were used, two flaws remained, namely that pencil work was required and, a knowledge of numbers and how to write them was required (on three of the seven subparts of the test). Those who failed Army Beta were supposed to be recalled for an individual examination at a later date. Unfortunately, not only was the validity of the tests flawed but the procedures for ascribing the test types to the literate and illiterate groups were also inconsistent. In addition, the conditions under which the tests were taken were often inadequate.

Nonetheless, data was produced in the 1920s from 160,000 of these army cases, and a classification system was devised, where individuals with a mental age (MA) of less than 3 were classified as "idiots," individuals with an MA between 3–7 were "imbeciles," and those with an MA between 8–12 were "morons," that is, high-grade "defectives" who could be trained to function in society. Such classifications resulted in European immigrants, for example, being graded by their country of origin. As a result, the average person of many a nation was in the "moron" category, and where southern Europeans and Slavs of eastern Europe were classified as less intelligent than people of western and northern Europe.

These early findings naturally resulted in controversy that, to date unfortunately, has not fully been resolved. Nell (2000), in reviewing the ongoing debate as this pertains to cross-cultural applications of the quantitative approach, notes that the most appealing response, politically and intellectually, to the problems raised by test score variations across countries and cultures is radical environmentalism, which holds that culture makes mind. This is in sharp contrast to the nativist view that holds that intelligence is primarily genetically determined and therefore immutable. Nell (2000) cites the 1994 publication of *The Bell Curve* by Herrnstein and Murray, who countered critique of IQ testing as essentially useless (due to difficulties with cross-cultural applicability, construct validity, etc.) by arguing that IQ and what it measures are "real," that is, that IQ tests demonstrate no external bias (measured against the criteria of school and college success) and dutifully cited data showing that IQ scores vary substantially across ethnic and cultural groups. These findings were, in turn, counterargued as racially and culturally discriminatory due to internal bias. Coupled with these controversies in quantitative assessment is the fundamental distinction of the psychometric contra information-processing approach, where in the former view intelligence is perceived as structure whereas in the latter, process is emphasized. Thus, while not without flaws, psychometric tests are typically used because of their proven diagnostic utility, and because they can be supplemented by information-processing probes and qualitative test interpretation in neuropsychological assessments.

Finally, regarding the issue of whether western-based neuropsychological assessments have been adapted for minority groups within a dominant culture, Pérez-Arce (1999) for example, in describing the use of neuropsychological tests on a minority group (Hispanics) within a dominant culture (USA), argues that North American psychology is steeped in empiricism (positivism). This has resulted in the search for universals in cognitive operations across individuals by using a normative approach with simple demographic indices such as age, gender, educational level, and on occasion, ethnicity. The influence of social and cultural factors have not, however, been systematically studied. Thus, both culture-free and culture-fair tests have been proposed, where culture-free tests refer to those theoretically ideal tests where some inherent quality of human capacity could be equally well measured in all cultures. As Cole (1996) states, "the simple fact is, we know of no tests that are culture free, only tests for which we have no good theory of how culture variation affect performance" (p. 56). Culture-fair tests, on the other hand, refer to conditions where either a set of items equally unfamiliar to all possible persons in all possible cultures is used, or multiple sets of items are modified for use in each culture to ensure that each version of the test would contain the same amount of familiarity. Gould (1982) views the former condition as virtually impossible to achieve, whereas the latter is possible.

CULTURALLY VARIABLE CONCEPTS

Gould (1982) refers to the aforementioned debate in terms of the distinction that exists in understanding cognition from a hereditarian view, which argues for a universal, culture-free, unchanging, objectively measurable, biologically determined property, "g" (general intelligence) and a cultural psychology perspective that adheres to the view that culture influences (a) behaviors considered to be intelligent, (b) the processes underlying intelligent behavior, and (c) the direction of intellectual development, such that psychological theories of intelligence must offer generalizations that are relative to a particular time and context.

Further support for the cultural psychology view is found in examples of how cognitive concepts are culturally variable—not universal constants. A few examples are given for purposes of illustration: Regarding perception, cross-cultural studies show differences in the effect of the Müller-Lyer and horizontal/vertical illusions for industrialized and nonindustrialized groups (e.g., Segall, Cambell, & Herskovits, 1966). These and other findings were interpreted (and although disputed; see Cole, 1996) as perception being a process of construction, that is, learned, and therefore influenced by culture. Similarly, the concept of intelligence has been found to be culturally variable. Many languages have no word that corresponds to the western-based term. For example, the Baganda of East Africa use a word that refers instead to a combination of mental and social skills that make a person, steady, cautious, and friendly (Wober, 1974). In addition, many specific cognitive functions such as categorization, memory, and problem solving, when evaluated cross culturally, are found to be biased, for example, educational effect are found for sorting tasks (e.g., Evans &

Segall, 1969) and with the supposed maturational aspects of verbal problem-solving tasks (e.g., Luria, 1974/1976). Furthermore, as regards memory, cultures with oral traditions do better at remembering meaningful oral materials than do those from American culture that focus on written communication (e.g., Cole, Gay, Glick & Sharp, 1971). See also Nell (2000) for a more comprehensive discussion of these issues.

Cultural influences are also found, as regards cognitive development. Piaget's theory is used as an example, which suggests that the proposed stages of development occur in the same order in different cultures (Kuhn, 1988). However, cross-cultural findings suggest that there are age variations at which children in different societies typically reach, for example, the third (concrete operations) and fourth (formal operations) Piagetian stages, (e.g., Shayer, Demetriou, & Perez, 1988), and that there is considerable cultural variation to the order in which children acquire specific skills within Piaget's stages (e.g., Dasen,1975). Furthermore, cross-cultural research has indicated that nonwestern cultures do not necessarily regard scientific reasoning as the ultimate developmental end point, and that in some cultures, very few people are able to complete the fourth-stage (i.e., formal operations) Piagetian tasks (e.g., Shea 1985).

Similarly, definitions of emotion and experience of self vary cross culturally (e.g., Russell, 1991). For example, as regards the self, there appears to be independent (western culture) versus interdependent (nonwestern) construal of self and these self-construals have been found to influence self-perception, perception of others, and have consequences for emotional experience and motivational factors (Markus & Kitayama, 1991; Shweder & Bourne, 1984).

Thus, difficulties in neuropsychological assessments are related to (a) cognition not being a composite measure but consisting of discrete functions that coexist in a functional system; (b) cross-cultural definitions and processes of cognition being variable; (c) holistic neuropsychological assessments which includes cross culturally variable measures of emotions and self and (d) if assessment is quantitative in nature, data reflecting outcome, not process, which unless culturally fair, will misrepresent function. As a result of these difficulties, culturally and individually variable aspects of neuropsychological assessments are often neglected. However, as Cole (1996) points out, even when methodology is altered to take into account cultural variability, other difficulties arise. For example, if cognition is studied as context and activity dependent, then identifying sources of continuity are minimized. Thus, a tension will always exist in choosing one methodology over another, and the solution may lie in combining the strengths of both.

Furthermore, as Bruner (1990), notes "cultural psychology ... is what psychology looks like when it concerns itself centrally with meaning ... it must venture beyond the conventional aims of positivist science with its ideals of reductionism, casual explanation and prediction." (pp. xii–xiii). This suggests an alternate epistemology that is described in greater detail below.

A HOLISTIC, QUALITATIVE APPROACH

It will be argued that neuropsychological assessments are embedded and influenced by multiple domains. For example, a model of holistic human assessment offered by the World Health Organization (WHO, 2002) is the International Classification of Functioning, Disability, and Health (ICF), which provides a standard language and framework for the description of health and health-related states, based on a biopsychosocial model: Disability and functioning are viewed as outcomes of interactions between health conditions (diseases, disorders, and injuries) and contextual factors. Contextual factors include external environmental factors (for example, architectural characteristics, legal and social structures, etc.) and internal personal factors (e.g., gender, age, coping styles, education, overall behavior pattern, etc). Three levels of human functioning are identified, namely, (a) level of body or body part, (b) the whole person (individual) and (c) the whole person in a social context (societal perspectives). Both intact and disrupted functioning can be explored at all of these levels. Disability therefore involves dysfunctioning at one or more of these same levels and is described as (i) impairments, (ii) activity limitations, and (iii) participation restrictions. Thus, disruptions to body functions and structures (pathophysiology) result in losses or disorders of cognitive, emotional, or physiological functions (impairments). These impairments affect a person's ability to perform everyday life activities (activity/functional limitations) that in turn defines the nature and extent of a person's involvement in life situations (participation), contextualized by environmental and personal factors.

Another holistic model proposed by Trexler (1999), based on an earlier version of the aforementioned and the National Center for Medical Rehabilitation and Research (NCMRR) as adapted for holistic brain injury assessment and rehabilitation, includes the following: (a) individual factors (e.g., coping skills, family support) and pathophysiology; (b) level of impairment—motor and sensory functions (e.g., dexterity, praxis, speed), language and visuoperceptual functions, executive and cognitive functions (e.g., language, memory, problem solving) and neurobehavioral functions (e.g., awareness, disinhibiting, perseveration); (c) level of functional limitations—mobility, activities of daily living, communication and emotional reactions; (d) level of disability—productivity and quality of life; and finally, (e) level of social limitations. As regards treatment planning and outcome in brain injury rehabilitation, a similar array of variables is proposed by Sohlberg and Mateer (2004).

Thus, when neuropsychological assessment is viewed as holistic in nature, multiple domains are addressed, and as has been seen, cross-cultural variations are implicit in the expression of these domains. A qualitative method allows cultural variations to be considered by being based on (a) fundamentally different epistemological premises, operationalized by phenomenology and systems theory, and (b) by adopting multiple assessment methods. Thus, traditional psychometric tests are not the primary source of data collection, and if tests are used, their structure and function is fundamentally different in orientation. In addition, qualitative assessment measures may also include participant observation, observation via video, in-depth interviewing (including use of narrative or life histories), and questionnaires (Marshal & Rossman, 1995). Using a combination of measures arguably addresses concern regarding construct and ecological validity.

When considering a holistic approach to neuropsychological functioning, each of the aforementioned measures may be used. For example, at the level of impairment, LNI or other cognitive tasks may be administered, with interpretations based on brain–behavior syndrome and process analysis, whereas at the level of functional limitations, observational methods can be used. Furthermore, impairment, activity, and participation can be assessed using multisource (i.e., patient, significant others, health care professional versions) questionnaire-type measures (adapted as verbal rather than written versions if literacy, type of brain injury is an issue). In order to fully address cross-cultural issues, however, all levels of functioning should be considered from for e.g., a narrative approach that systematizes personal and cultural themes (e.g., McAdams, 1996).

Regardless of techniques used, an understanding of the epistemology of the qualitative approach is essential for the appropriate use, particularly as regards cross-cultural concerns. As such two of these premises is now presented in greater detail.

Epistemological Foundation 1: Phenomenology

This regards the fundamental human tendency as identifying experience and ascribing meaning. Spinelli (1989) indicated that historically, Kant argued for not knowing the thing itself, that is, "noumenon," but only the "phenomenon," that is, as it appears to us. Franz Brentano developed the notion of "intentionality," that is, a definition of the first, most basic, interpretative mental act. Edmund Husserl further developed transcendental phenomenology with its emphasis on essence, intentionality, and the distinction between "noema," that is, what is experienced and "noesis," that is, how it is experienced. He also operationalized the phenomenological method, which emphasized (a) defining the process of meaning construction, (b) bracketing, that is, acknowledging and thereby limiting bias in interpreting meaning, (c) description rather than explanation, and (d) treating all experience as having equal value.

Thus, briefly stated, the phenomenological view may be described as follows: As human beings, we attempt to make sense of all our experiences and through mental acts we strive to impose meaning upon the world. Reality is thus viewed as an interpretational process based on the interaction of the internal (our experience of self) with the external (i.e., the world around us) such that phenomena of the world is experienced rather than its reality. Phenomenology is concerned with the difference between the appearance of things (as determined by brain processing) and what those things actually are (external matter- objective reality). Thus, humans do not have access to an ultimate reality, but only hypothesis testing of what reality might be. Although interpretations of reality are relative, similar interpretations may be shared, as determined by biological mechanisms or sociocultural schemata. Meaningless experience is aversive, and, as such, attempts are always made to find meaning in experiences of "reality" and, as such, this is one of the constants of human experience. (Spinelli, 1989; Valle & King, 1978).

From a cultural perspective, Bruner (1990) reiterates the value of meaning as being central to psychology by arguing that the "cognitive revolution" (i.e., the attempt to bring "mind" back into the human sciences, starting in the 1950s) was diverted from this, its original purpose, to computational metaphors. Thus, Bruner (1990) argues for intentional states to be considered once more and that these can only be realized through participation in the symbolic systems of a culture. His view is based on three propositions, namely that (a) humans participate in culture and the develop of cognition through culture; (b) by participation in culture meaning-making, humans and culture are connected, therefore rendering meaning public and shared; and (c) due to the existence of folk psychology, that is, a culture's account of who humans are (providing "theories" of mind, motivation, etc.), culture and intentional states are linked. Thus, for Bruner, analysis of meaning is to recognize culture's intimate relationship to cognition and experience of self.

Epistemological Foundation 2: Systems Theory

Systems theory (see for e.g., Hansen, 1995; Von Bertalanffy, 1968) is centered on nonlinear causality and contextual analysis. It is a theory of patterns, concerning relational wholes and, as such, is an alternative to traditional epistemology that is linear and mechanistic. Systems theory may be viewed as a metatheory useful for purposes of description as it is not assumptive. The point of departure is nonsummativity, where the whole is viewed as greater than the sum of the parts. This is in direct contrast to classic views of linear cause and effect, where models of human behavior have been steeped in logical positivism and nomotheism.

5. QUALITATIVE ASSESSMENT

A system can be defined as any two or more parts that are related. Thus, nature is viewed as being ordered as a hierarchically arranged continuum, with its more complex larger units superordinate to the less complex smaller units. Thus, be it cell, organ, person, or family, each indicates a level of complex, integrated, organization and holds a high degree of consensus regarding existing characteristics. Furthermore, the designation "system" indicates the existence of a stable configuration in time and space and each level in the hierarchy represents an organized dynamic whole, its name reflecting many of its distinctive properties and characteristics. Stable configuration is maintained not only by the coordination of component parts in an internal dynamic network, but also by the characteristics of the larger system of which it is a component part. Thus, each level is a system with a particular level of organization, with distinctive properties and characteristics for that level of organization, requiring explanations unique for that level. Each system is, at the same time, a component of higher systems. As such, change in any one part of a system changes all parts. Systems theory is based on the principle of context. In addition, the following principles apply, namely, cybernetics and feedback, as elaborated by equifinality and multifinality is described below.

Cybernetics refers to the study of the self-regulating properties of a system where there is no preconception of what direction the self-regulation will take. In humans, an example of cybernetics is the ability to reflect on self. Cybernetics is studied by analyzing process such as action/inaction of interrelated parts over time where action and inaction are viewed as equally causal in a system. A systemic concept of change is in overall patterns, requiring time and process to determine what the relative patterns of alteration and continuity mean. Thus, process is emphasized rather than outcome.

Feedback refers to the ability of a system to reintroduce output as input. Feedback elaborates patterns of change and nonchange. It provides a language for looking for ongoing processes in systems. Causality is interactive and continuous rather than finite and linear. Systems are served by both positive and negative feedback. Positive feedback results in change, whereas negative feedback does not. Equifinality refers to the same result occurring from a variety of stimuli, whereas multifinality refers to a variety of results from the same stimuli; both, therefore, qualify the basic notion of feedback.

CONCLUSION

The qualitative approach adopts from phenomenology, (a) meaning construction as its premise for understanding human functioning; (b) the methodology by which meaning can be explored as a variable construct, that is, a description of process rather than explanations, avoiding a priori theoretical assumptions by treating all experience as equally important; and (c) the influence of culture as implicit to meaning. From systems theory, the qualitative method makes use of (a) a holistic model for understanding human functioning while acknowledging the distinct aspects of a system as integrally related to one another; (b) change as dynamic (i.e., as interrelated by the feedback process); and (c) viewing human functioning in terms of patterns, such that process rather than outcome analysis is possible

Thus, by definition, the qualitative approach implicitly recognizes cultural variations. It is based on process evaluation of brain–behavior relationships rather than evaluating outcome based on abstract constructs. In addition, use of a holistically based narrative interview provides a contextualized foundation for understanding task completion (while acknowledging that construct validity may remain problematic). Although the universal constants of human functioning should continue to be addressed, and if possible, be evaluated by using culturally fair methods, the qualitative approach remains highly relevant as it recognizes cultural and individual variability in the most fundamental of human activities, namely, construction of meaning.

REFERENCES

Bauer, R. M. (1994). The flexible battery approach to neuropsychological assessment. In R. D. Vanderploeg (Ed.), *Clinician's guide to neuropsychological assessment* (pp. 259–290). Hillsdale, NJ: Lawrence Erlbaum Associates.

Ben-Yishay, Y., & Larkin, P. (1989). Structured group treatment for brain injury survivors. In E. W. Ellis & A.-L. Christensen (Eds.), *Neurospychological treatment after brain injury* (pp. 271–296). Norwell, MA: Kluver Academic.

Bruner, J. S., Olver, R. R., & Greenfield, P. M. (1966). *Studies in cognitive growth*. New York: Wiley.

Bruner, J. (1990). *Acts of meaning*. Cambridge, England: Harvard University Press.

Christensen, A.-L. (1975). *Luria's Neurospychological Investigation: Manual and test materials* (1st ed.). New York: Spectrum.

Christensen, A.-L., & Caetano, C., (1999). Neuropsychological rehabilitation in the interdisciplinary team: The postacute stage. In D. T. Stuss, G. Wincour, & I. H. Robertson (Eds.), *Cognitive neurorehabilitation* (pp. 188–200). New York: Cambridge University Press.

Christensen, A.-L., & Danielsen, U. T. (1987). Neuropsychological rehabilitation in Denmark. In M. Meier, A. Benton, & L. Diller (Eds.), *Neuropsychological rehabilitation* (pp. 381–386). New York: Guildford.

Cole, M. (1996). *Cultural psychology: A once and future discipline*. London: Belknap/Harvard University Press.

Cole, M., Gay, J., Glick, J. A., & Wharp, E. W. (1971). *The cultural context of learning and thinking: An exploration in experimental anthropology*. New York: Basic Books.

Dasen, P. R. (1975). Concrete operational development in three cultures. *Journal of Cross-Cultural Psychology, 6*(2) 156–172.

Evans, J. L., & Segall, M. H. (1969). Learning to classify by color and function: A study of concept discovery by Ganda children. *Journal of Social Psychology, 77*, 35–55.

Gardner, H. (1984). The development of competence in culturally defined domains: A preliminary framework. In R.A. Shweder & R. A. LeVine (Eds.), *Culture theory: Essays on mind, self and emotion* (pp. 257–276). Cambridge, England: Cambridge University Press.
Gardner, H. (1993). *Frames of mind: The theory of multiple intelligences* (2nd ed.). London: Fontana Press.
Goldstein, K. (1952). Effects of brain damage on personality. *Psychiatry, 15,* 245–260.
Gould, S. J. (1999) A nation of morons. In Richard Gross (Ed.), *Key studies in psychology* (3rd ed., pp. 583–600). London: Hodder & Stoughton.
Hansen, B. G. (1995). *General systems theory: Beginning with wholes.* London: Taylor & Francis.
Kaplan, E. (1988). A process to neuropsychological assessment. In T. Boll & B. K. Bryand (Eds.), *Clinical neuropsychology and brain function: Research, measurement and practice* (pp. 129–167). Washington DC: American Psychological Association.
Kuhn, D. (1988). Cognitive development. In M. H. Bornstein & M. E. Lamb (Eds.), *Developmental psychology: An advanced textbook* (pp. 205–260). Hillsdale, NJ: Lawrence Erlbaum Associates.
LeVine, R. A. (1984). Properties of culture: An ethnographic view. In R. A. Shweder & R. A. LeVine (Eds.), *Culture theory: Essays on mind, self and emotion* (pp. 67–88). Cambridge, England: Cambridge University Press.
Lezak, M. D. (1995). *Neuropsychological assessment* (3rd ed.). New York: Oxford University Press.
Luria, A. R. (1976). *Cognitive development: Its cultural and social foundations* (M. Lopes & L. Soloatoff, Trans.). Cambridge, MA: Harvard University Press. (Original work published 1974)
Luria, A. R. (1977). *Higher cortical functions in man* (2nd ed.) (Basil Haigh, Trans.). New York: Consultants Bureau.
Markus, H., & Kitayam, S. (1991). Culture and the self: Implications for cognition, emotion, and motivation. *Psychological Review, 98*(2), 224–253.
Marshal, C., & Rossman, G. B. (1995). *Designing qualitative research* (2nd ed.). London: Sage.
McAdams, D. P. (1996). Personality, modernity and the storied self: A contemporary framework for studying persons. *Psychological Inquiry, 7,* 295–321.
McCarthy, R. A., & Warrington, E. K. (1990). *Cognitive neuropsychology: A clinical introduction.* San Diego, CA: Academic Press.
Nell, V. (2000). *Cross-cultural neuropsychological assessment: Theory and practice.* Mahwah, NJ: Lawrence Erlbaum Associates.
Ostrosky-Solis, F., Canesco, E., Quintanua, L., Navarro, E., Meneses, S., & Ardila, A. (1985). Sociocultural effects in neurospychological assessment. *International Journal of Neuroscience, 27*(1–2), 53–66.
Pérez-Arce, P. (1999). The influence of culture on cognition. *Archives of Clinical Neuropsychology, 14*(7), 581–592.
Prigatano, G. P., Fordyce, D. J., Zeiner, H. K., Roueche, J. R., Pepping, M., & Wood, B. (1986). *Neuropsychological rehabilitation after brain injury.* Baltimore, MD: Johns Hopkins University Press.
Reitan, R. M. (1986). The Halstead-Reitan Neuropsychological Test Battery. In D. Wedding, A. M. Horton, & J. Webster (Eds.), *The neuropsychology handbook* (pp. 134–160). New York: Springer.
Russell, J. A. (1991). Culture and the categorization of emotion. *Psychological Bulletin, 110,* 426–450.
Segall, M. H., Cambell, D. T., & Herskovits, J. (1966). *The influence of culture on visual perception.* Indianapolis: Bobbs-Merrill.

Shayer, M., Demetriou, A., & Pervez, M. (1988). The structure and scaling of concrete operational thought: Three studies in four countries. *Genetic, Social and General Psychology Monographs, 114*(3), 307–375.

Shea, J. D. (1985). Studies of cognitive development in Papua New Guinea. *International Journal of Psychology, 20*(1), 33–61.

Shweder, R. A., & Bourne, E. J. (1984). Does the concept of the person vary cross-culturally? In R. A. Shweder & R. A. LeVine (Eds.), *Culture theory: Essays on mind, self and emotion* (pp. 158–199). Cambridge, England: Cambridge University Press.

Sohlberg, M. M., & Mateer, C. A. (2004). *Cognitive rehabilitation: An integrative neuropsychological approach.* London: Guilford.

Spinelli, E. (1989). *The interpreted world: An introduction to phenomenological psychology.* London: Sage.

Tollman, S. G., & Msengagna, N. B. (1990). Neuropsychological assessment: Problems in evaluating the higher mental functioning of Zulu-speaking people using traditional western techniques. *South African Journal of Psychology, 20*, 20–24.

Trexler, L. E. (1999). Empirical support for neuropsychological rehabilitation. In A.-L. Christensen & B. P. Uzzell (Eds.), *International handbook of neuropsychological rehabilitation* (pp. 137–150). New York: Kluwer.

Valle, R. S., & King, M. (1978). *Existential-phenomenological alternatives for psychology.* New York: Oxford University Press.

Vanderploeg, R. D. (1994). Interview and testing: The data-collection phase of neuropsychological evaluations. In R. D. Vanderploeg (Ed.), *Clinician's guide to neuropsychological assessment* (pp. 1–42) Hillsdale, NJ: Lawrence Erlbaum Associates.

Von Bertalanffy, L. (1968). *General systems theory: Foundations, development, applications.* New York: George Brazziler.

World Health Organization. (2002). *Towards a common language for functioning, disability and health.* Retrieved January 31, 2005, from ICF.ww3.who.int/icf

Wober, M. (1974). Towards an understanding of the Kiganda concept of intelligence. In J. W. Berry & P. R. Dasen (Eds.), *Culture and cognition* (pp. 261–280). London: Methuen

Chapter **6**

Cognitive Abilities in Different Cultural Contexts

Alfredo Ardila
Florida International University

Kevin Keating
Broward Community College

Cognitive abilities usually measured in neuropsychological tests represent, at least in their contents, learned abilities whose scores correlate with the subject's learning opportunities and contextual experiences. Cultural variations are evident in test scores, as culture provides us with specific models for ways of thinking, acting, and feeling (Ardila, 1995; Berry, 1979). Findings of perceptual differences between cultures mark the role of culture as central in mediating and amplifying our cognitions, regarding that which is situationally relative and relevant.

Although basic cognitive processes are universal, cultural differences in cognition reside more in the situations to which particular cognitive processes are applied than in the existence of the process in one cultural group and its absence in the other (Cole, 1981). Culture prescribes what should be learned, at what age, and by which gender. Consequently, different cultural environments lead to the development of different patterns of abilities (Ferguson, 1956). Cultural and ecological factors play a role in developing different cognitive styles (Berry, 1979).

A general review of differences in abilities reported in different cultural groups is presented. Further, some cultural factors potentially affecting test performance are considered. Finally, some tentative conclusions are presented.

PERCEPTUAL ABILITIES

Rosselli and Ardila (2003) have emphasized that, when visuoperceptual test performance in different cultural groups is compared, significant differences are evident. Performance on nonverbal tests such as copying figures, drawing maps, or listening to tones can be significantly influence by the individual's culture.

Rosselli, Ardila, Bateman, and Guzman (2001) compared the performance of Colombian children (western, low-industrialized society) with the American normative sample (western, industrialized society) on several verbal and nonverbal measurements. In most of the tests, the performance of the two cultural groups was similar. However, in the Seashore Rhythm test, the Colombian group performed significantly better, two standard deviations above the mean for American normative data reported by Findelieis and Weight and cited by Nussbaum and Bigler (1997). It may be conjectured that musical learning represents a significant cultural value for Colombian children. Cultural differences in the Seashore Rhythm test have also been reported among the subcultures in the United States. African American males showed significantly higher scores in the Seashore Rhythm test as compared to European Americans and Hispanics (Bernard, 1989; Evans, Miller, Byrd, & Heaton, 2000). The Seashore Rhythm test was originally developed to assess musical ability (Mitrushina, Boone, & D'Elia, 1999) but the perceptual skills this test requires may be shaped by cultural influences. Arnold, Montgomery, Castaneda, and Longoria (1994) documented a significant effect of acculturation on the Seashore Rhythm test in a group of Mexican Americans with better performance in those that were better acculturated. Cultural effects on the Seashore Rhythm test, likely associated with familiarity and relevance of tone discrimination task, have been reported (Klove, 1974).

Significant differences in nonverbal test performance between western and nonwestern schoolchildren have been reported by Mulenga, Ahonen, Aro, and Mico (2001). They administered the NEPSY (Korkman, Kirk, & Kempt, 1998) to a small sample of Zambian children and compared their performance with the U.S. norms. They found that Zambian children performed poorer in the domain of language, attention, and executive functions but better in visuospatial tests (design copying). Mulenga et al. made the interesting observation that, although there were clear instructions to perform the task as fast as possible, most children tended to work slowly. Other authors have confirmed this finding that members of many cultures are frequently slower in speed of performance when compared with U.S. children. "Fast performance" is obviously an important culture value in the United States, but it is absent in many other cultural groups. Zairian children for example, are slower in the Tactual Performance Test than the American and Canadian children (Boivin, Giordani, & Bornefeld, 1995). The authors noticed that the difference between the African children and the North American children could be due to differences in experience with the test items. Whereas in the North American culture children have played with standard geometrical shapes at a very early age, many of the Zairian children could not name most of the shapes of the blocks. Obviously, each individual has to be compared with his or her own group, sharing the same cultural values, experiences, and environmental conditions. Spanish children are slower in the Trail Making Test as compared with U.S. children (Leon-Carrion, 1989). The fairness of timed tests in the assessment of cognitive abilities is challenged by these results. Or rather, there is a need for culture-specific norms in timed tests. Both speed and accuracy at performance are values in the U.S. culture, which also emphasizes competitiveness and success.

Sensory Discrimination

Some differences in sensory discriminations have been found when comparing different human groups. Three different sets of variables have been proposed to account for these differences: (1) environmental conditions, (b) genetic factors, and (c) enculturation practices.

As an example of environment-dependent differences, it has been pointed out that Kalahari Bushmen present a better auditory acuity for higher frequencies than western samples taken from the United States and Denmark (Reuning & Wortley, 1973). Differences are most striking in older subjects. It has been conjectured that in the Kalahari desert there is less hearing loss associated with age. Long-term exposure to higher levels of noise in western societies apparently correlate with a rapid decline in auditory acuity of high frequencies.

Color blindness (Daltonism) represents an X-linked chromosomal defect, consequently manifesting more commonly in males than in females. Interestingly, color blindness is less frequent among hunter and gatherer societies than in societies with an agricultural tradition. To account for this difference, it has been proposed that poor color discrimination would be disadvantageous when hunting and gathering (Post, 1971).

Cultural practices may account for many sensory preferences found worldwide. Anglo-American society has a very clear preference for sweet foods, whereas preference for hot foods is found in many Amerindian groups. The judgment about the loudness of a sound is different in Japan, Germany, and Great Britain (Kuwano, Namba, & Schick, 1986), probably related with the type of auditory environment that is considered most desirable. Cultural preferences in colors, shapes, sounds, tastes, odors, and so forth represent an evident observation. Houses are painted with different colors in Greece and England; food has a different taste in China and Brazil; and aesthetic preferences are highly variable in different societies.

Perceptual Constancy

Characteristics of perceptual abilities in different cultures can be illustrative. Perceptual constancy (stability of perception despite changes in the actual characteristics of the stimuli) represents the most fundamental ability in the interpretation of the surrounding spatial environment (Ardila, 1980).

Cross-cultural comparisons have in general demonstrated that perceptual constancy (size and shape constancy) is more accurate in low-schooled and nonwestern societies people than in literate and westernized subjects (Pick & Pick, 1978). Beveridge (1940) demonstrated a greater constancy of shape and size among West African adults than among British adults. Myambo (1972) observed almost perfect shape constancy in uneducated Malawi adults, whereas the educated Africans and Europeans did not perform so accurately. Size constancy can be crucial when recognizing and interpreting pictorial material, and has been demonstrated to be both a contextually and experientially rather than a developmentally acquired characteristic (Turnbull, 1961).

Visual Illusions

Cultural differences in the susceptibility to visual illusions have been well demonstrated. Segall, Campbell, and Herkovits (1966) compared 14 nonwestern and three western societies in the susceptibility to six visual illusions (Sander parallelogram, the Muller-Lyer illusion, two versions of the horizontal–vertical illusion, the Ponzo illusion and the Poggendorff illusion). Western samples were more illusion prone that nonwestern participants, particularly with the Muller-Lyer illusion and Sander Parallelogram. Subjects from regions with open vista were more susceptible to the horizontal–vertical illusion. Results were interpreted as supporting the hypotheses that: (a) There is a learned tendency among people raised in environment with geometrical shapes (houses, furniture, etc.) to interpret nonrectangular figures as representing rectangles in perspective; (b) people living in environments with wide vistas have learned that vertical lines can represent long distances; and (c) exposure to pictorial material facilitates a greater level of susceptibility to visual illusions. Bolton, Michelson, Wilde, and Bolton (1975) noted high altitude/broad vista cultures (versus low altitude/limited vista) display high levels of susceptibility to Muller-Lyer, Sander parallelogram, and horizontal–vertical illusions.

SPATIAL ABILITIES

Cross-cultural differences in spatial orientation strategies under normal and pathological conditions could be illustrative to understand how spatial information is processed. Brain organization of spatial abilities under pathological conditions has been extensively studied in contemporary schooled western (particularly European and North American) people. To our best knowledge, however, clinical observation about disturbances in spatial abilities associated with brain pathology in other (nonwestern) cultures has not been reported.

Reference Systems

People living in different environments develop different systems of spatial reference (rivers, mountains, sun position, streets, buildings, etc). Geographic features affect the terms of local reference systems, and differences in reference systems may, in turn, be related to differences in perception of spatial orientation (Pick & Pick, 1978). The analysis of different reference systems can be illustrative.

Gladwin (1970) analyzed the system used by Puluwat sailors to navigate among clusters of islands in the Western Pacific. He disclosed that many different features of the sea and sky comprise the information on which the navigation system is based. Knowledge of the habits of local sea birds provides cues for one's location. The sailors learn to detect changes in a coral reef's formation depending on the conditions of the weather, sea, and sky. Ability to detect change in the "feel" of the boat moving through the waves on a particular course is a skill used to maintain a course. There is a complex reference system based on the position and patterns of stars in the night sky, and the rules for navigating between specific islands are described in terms of the star patterns and islands. Parallax information is also explicitly included in the system as descriptions of the way in which the islands "move" as the boat passes on one or the other side of them (Pick & Pick, 1978).

Amazonian Indians simultaneously use a variety of different types of information to move around in the jungle. They use small rivers, orientation and color of trees, soil characteristics, sun position, animal routes, olfactory cues, and many other signals to move in the jungle. Vegetation is mildly different when closer to rivers, moss grows differently in trees according to the sun direction, and direction of river variation. Additionally, when moving in the jungle, they permanently break small bush branches to recognize later that they have already crossed (and approximately how long ago) that particular point. All these environmental signals are simultaneously interpreted for establishing orientation and moving around in the jungle (Ardila, 1993).

Evidently, members of different cultures and dwellers in different spatial environments operate in terms of complex spatial reference systems, depending on the particular demands of their geographic environments.

Cultural Differences in Visuospatial Abilities

Cross-cultural differences in perceptual abilities have been extensively studied (e.g., Brislin, 1983; Laboratory of Comparative Human Cognition, 1983; Segall, 1986). Illiterate African people do better than western literate subjects in perceptual constancy tasks with real objects. However, they perform worse when the external space is represented on paper (i.e., in a nonfamiliar contextual format).

Hudson (1960, 1962) studied depth perception using pictures that contained figures of an elephant, an antelope, and a man with a spear; the basic question referred to that the man was doing with the spear. There were four pictures differing with respect to the cues available for the interpretation of the picture. This set of pictures was used with different groups of people from Africa and Europe. It was observed that European children around 7–8 years have a great difficulty perceiving the picture as three dimensional. However, around 12 years, virtually all perceived the picture as three dimensional. Not so with Bantu or Guinean children. Nonliterate Bantu and European laborers responded to the picture as flat, not three dimensional. They were unable to interpret figures represented on a paper in three dimensions; this also holds true in general for illiterate people (Ardila, Rosselli, & Rosas, 1989). In general, people untrained to use maps cannot understand and cannot draw a map, even a simple map such as the map of the place where the subject is situated.

Significant cross-cultural differences in visuoperceptual abilities have been observed. Deregowski (1980) argued that in all societies children exhibit a preference for drawing in two dimensions, and that this persists if they do not have practice in three dimensional drawings. Dawson (1967) suggested that general exposure to pictorial material might not be enough for learning pictorial representation and some use of pictorial material is also required. Deregowski, Muldrow, and Muldrow (1972) found in a remote group in Ethiopia with little experience to pictures, a significant difficulty in identifying detailed and clear drawing of animals.

Berry (1971, 1979) proposed that hunting people with specific ecological demands usually present good visual discrimination and excellent spatial skills. For instance, the embedded figures test is better performed by cultural groups for whom hunting is important for survival. Ecological demands and cultural practices are significantly related to the development of perceptual and cognitive skills. A good example of a specific culture-dependent cognitive skill was that reported by Gay and Cole (1967). When Kpelle farmers were contrasted with a sample from the American working class, the former were considerably more accurate in estimating the amount of rice on several bowls of different sizes containing different amounts of rice. By the same token, any cattle farmer is able to calculate accurately the weight of a cow; or any dactilographist can easily and quickly distinguish two different fingerprints; or any neurologist can distinguish a Parkinsonian patient at one glance. Cultural demands and training history are strongly associated with visuoperceptual abilities.

MEMORY

An Amazonian jungle Indian joked with the poor memory of an anthropologist who needed to be writing down everything in order to remember. For the Amazonian jungle Indian, it was obvious that the tree names are not represented with letters and the way to follow a particular jungle route was not written down. This simple observation illustrates a tremendous difference in memory: Cultural differences in memory to a significant extent refer to the situations where memory is used and how memory is mediated. This Amazonian jungle Indian very likely was able to repeat long epic poems, myths, and ceremonial verbal rituals. Also, very likely, this individual failed in memorizing words or repeating digits. To memorize words out of context or to repeat digits simply following the instructions of an ununderstandable examiner is not really a situation where memory should be applied.

Lewis (1976) reported that Australian Aboriginals had a phenomenal memory for recalling virtually every topographical feature of any place that they had ever crossed. Nonetheless, performance in laboratory memory tests was not necessarily good. Ardila and Moreno (2001) found in a group of Aruaco Indians from Colombia that memory for the Rey-Osterrieth Complex Figure was extremely low, whereas spatial memory for everyday elements was notoriously higher (spatial memory was tested in the following way: Nine everyday elements with approximately the same size were used—bean, two different pebbles, corn, small wood, two different seeds, piece of coal, and chickpea. They were distributed in a 3 × 3 arrangement, three columns with three rows. The subject was instructed to carefully watch them for 10 s. The examiner then mixed the elements and the subject was asked to place them in their original positions. Each element placed in the correct position was scored 1. Total score was 9). Immediate memory for the Rey-Osterrieth Complex figure was on average 5.9/36 (about 16.4%), whereas spatial memory for everyday elements averaged 5.2/9 (about 57.8%).

Another significant difficulty in comparing memory across different cultural groups refers to the limitations in memory testing. Usually only declarative memory is tested in neuropsychology batteries, whereas procedural memory is ignored. Declarative memory is strongly related with school learnings, whereas procedural memory refers to learning how to perform different activities. A very significant school attendance effect is observed in declarative memory tests (e.g., Ardila et al., 1989), whereas procedural memory is more dependent on manual working activities.

In brief, findings of cross-cultural differences in memory refer to the situations in which memory is used. Culturally relevant and significant information is recalled at a higher rate, and performance is greater on those tasks that are considered important and relevant. It is understandable that individuals from psychometric-oriented societies and schooled subjects will perform higher in standard memory tests. The question when testing for memory is to find out what tasks are really relevant for a particular cultural group. This requires developing innovative techniques for studying cognitive processes in everyday activities across a variety of settings. A higher performance is expected on culturally significant tasks.

LANGUAGE

Phoneme Discrimination

The basic sound unit in language is called a phoneme. Each language possesses a rather limited amount of phonemes (some 14–50) combined in diverse ways to form all the language words. Phoneme discrimination is extremely easy for the language's native speakers. When pairs of artificially produced phonemes, corresponding to different phonemic categories are presented, discrimination is virtually perfect. However, when acoustically equally different sounds are presented that fall in the same phonemic category, discrimination is almost at the chance level (Strange & Jenkins, 1978). We perceive language in discrete sound categories.

Even though there are common phonemes found across different languages, there are also differences among languages in the set of phonemes that are used. When discriminating phonemes in a foreign language, and those phonemes are nonexisting in the native language, discrimination is extremely difficult. For example, English speakers can only discriminate two categories (d, t) for a series of sounds where Thai speakers use three (d, t, and an aspirated t; Abrahamson & Lisker, 1970). When phonemes are relatively coincidental between two languages (e.g., Spanish and Greek), phoneme discrimination in the second language is very easy.

Infants can differentiate phonemes before they can produce them. They can even distinguish phonemes that are not found in their environment (Eimas, 1975). Later on, the ability to make these nonexisting in the environment distinctions will disappear. Many second language speakers can learn to produce certain phonemes, but they cannot distinguish them when auditorily presented, even when their own language records are used. Similarly, the ability to differentiate tones for adult speakers of nontonal languages may be very low, and sometimes, virtually impossible.

Universals in Language

The search for universals in language has represented a major endeavor for linguistics. Lenneberg (1967) argued that the processes by which language is realized are innate. Humans possess certain basic biologic organizational and cognitive abilities that permits language development. Language universals can be characterized as occurring on different language levels: phonemic, semantic, and grammatical.

Some universal phonemes have been observed when comparing different human languages (Greenberg, 1963, 1978). Some soundless stop (e.g., /p/) and nasal (e.g., /m/) phonemes have been regarded as universals. Three vowels are supposed to represent the minimal vocalism (/a/, /i/, and /u/). These universal language sounds are the result of the specific characteristics of the human articulatory system. As a general rule, those phonemes appearing earlier during language development are more universal than those acquired later. They are also easier to articulate.

It has been assumed that when comparing word meanings, some words are observed universally across languages. Swadesh (1952, 1967) proposed that there is a minimal vocabulary found in every language, further known as "Swadesh word list." Every human, regardless of the environmental conditions, time, and cultural factors is exposed to some constant phenomena and conditions. Equivalent words to refer to these phenomena and conditions are found in every language. As a matter of fact, there are two major versions of this basic universal vocabulary, a shorter one including 100 words, and a longer one including 200 words. The shorter Swadesh word list includes: (1) grammatical words (e.g., I/me), (2) quantifiers (e.g., many), (3) adjectives (e.g., big), (4) human distinctions (e.g., woman, men), (5) animals (e.g., bird), (6) highly frequent elements (e.g., tree), (7) body-parts (e.g., head), (8) actions (e.g., eat), (9) natural phenomena (e.g., sun), and (10) colors (e.g., white). Departing from the Swadesh word list, Ardila (unpublished) proposed a cross-linguistic naming test, including, (a) body-parts (10 words), (b) natural phenomena (nontouchable; 5 words), (c) external objects (potentially known through the sight and the touch; 5 words); (d) animals (5 words), (e) colors (5 words), (f) actions (10 words).

Chomsky (1980) has suggested that there is a universal grammar that is innate and that determines the potential for human language. He made a basic distinction between the surface structure of a language and its deep structure. The expressed surface structure can vary, but it points to a deep structure of meaning. Whereas languages can differ in the way they express different events and ideas, a convergence can be found in the deep meaning of the sentences. By the same token, the distinction between things and actions (nouns and verbs) is also found in all languages (Greenberg, 1978), even though the opposition between nouns and verbs can be stronger in some languages and weaker in others. In many languages, the very same word can play the role of noun and verb. Adjectives are taken from nouns, and it is not unusual that in some adjectives, an explicit and overt relationship with the noun is observed (e.g., the orange is orange). Time and place adverbs, as well as verb tenses, are highly variable. They are correlated with a whole array of environmental conditions, linguistic idiosyncrasies and cultural interpretations. However, all languages distinguish spatial directions such as right and left, up and down, and in front and behind. A significant effort has been devoted to the cross-cultural analysis of time and place adverbs (e.g., Whorf, 1956). Present tense seems to be universal, but the future and past as well as the conditional forms can be expressed in rather different ways.

Classification Systems

The comparative study of language raises the question of how people in different societies name and classify aspects of their world. Conkin (1971) published a bibliography that contains 5,000 entries, all references to analyses of classification and to comparisons of systems. Topics included are kinship, colors, and ethnobiology. This bibliography has become a reference point to compare how different systems function, and how words are selected and assembled to name elements of the external world. Some examples are presented.

It has been observed that the number of words to name colors is quite variable. Some societies have as few as two color terms (black or dark and white or light) whereas some other societies have as many as 11 basic colors. Color names appear in a specific order. For example, if a language has a word for red, it would have ones for black and white. If it had a term for yellow, it would have a word for black, white, and red; and so on (Berlin & Kay, 1969). It may be argued that the color names reflect the relative importance that a culture places in the color spectrum. As a matter of fact, it is observed that when new color names are required (for instance, by painters) new names appear. Blue, for instance, can be subdivided in many hues: blue sky, baby blue, robin egg, and so forth.

Strategies used in classifying animals and plants have been a matter of significant analysis and discussion. Berlin (1992) proposed seven principles of categorization and five principles of nomenclature that characterize ethnobiological systems in different societies. Ethnobiological names appear to be due to salient morphological and behavioral features of plants and animals. Clustering usually is based in salience or perceptual proprieties. Similarities and differences in clustering occur across languages. Fish, for instance, is a relatively evident category, but the members included in the category are not totally coincidental. For example, the sting-ray can be or not included as a fish. Different high-level ranks can also exist. For example, in English, canary corresponds to birds (one level), whereas in Spanish, canary is *pájaro* (subtype of birds) and *pájaros* are *aves* (birds). For Spanish speakers, there are two levels whereas in English, there is only one.

Language Disturbances in Different Languages

Language disturbances associated with brain pathology have been studied in just a handful of Indo-European languages, primarily French, English, German, Russian, Italian, and Spanish. Our knowledge about language disturbances in other tonal and non-Indo-European languages (a nonneglectable percentage of human languages) is limited. We do not know yet if our current Indo-European languages aphasia model is applicable or not to tonal languages (Yu-Huan, Ving-Guan, & Gui-Qing, 1990). Or rather to say, to what extent it may be applicable. Recent evidence, however, seems to suggest that there are some universal principles in the brain organization of language and in the language pathology associated with brain damage (Paradis, 2001). Thus, for any language, language disturbances are associated with left-hemisphere pathology; phoneme discrimination defects are found in cases of temporal damage, whereas grammatical impairments result from left posterior frontal pathology. Right hemisphere damage, on the other hand, is associated with emotional language defects, regardless of the idiosyncrasies of the language (Gandour, 1998).

Differences can be observed also with regard to written language disturbances associated with brain pathology. Alexias and agraphias have been well studied in Indo-European language writing systems. Comparative research on alexias and agraphias in different languages, except for some studies on the Japanese Kana and Kanji writing system disturbances (e.g., Sasanuma & Fujimura, 1971; Sugishita, Otomo, Kabe, & Yunoki, 1992; Yamadori, 1975, 1988), has been relatively scarce. Alexias and agraphias are not completely equivalent in different writing systems (Karanth, 2003). Taking two relatively close languages such as English and Spanish, some differences in reading errors when using a graphophonemic reading system (Spanish), and a partially logographic reading system (English) have been pointed out (Ardila, 1991, 1998; Ardila, Rosselli, & Pinzón, 1989).

SOME FACTORS INFLUENCING COGNITIVE TEST PERFORMANCE

Some attempts are found in the history of psychological testing to develop measures that would be "culture-free" or rather "culture-fair" (Anastasi, 1988; Cattell, 1940). Initially, it was supposed that the effect of culture could be controlled if verbal items were eliminated, and only nonverbal, performance items were used. However, this assumption turned out to be wrong (Rosselli & Ardila, 2003). Researchers testing a wide variety of cultural groups in many countries have sometimes observed even larger group differences in performance and other nonverbal tests than in verbal tests (Anastasi, 1988; Ardila & Moreno, 2001; Vernon, 1969). Therefore, not only verbal, but also nonverbal tests may be culturally biased. The use of pictorial representations itself may be unsuitable in cultures unaccustomed to representative drawings, and marked differences in the perception of pictures by individuals of different cultures have been reported (Miller, 1973). Furthermore, nonverbal tests often require specific strategies and cognitive styles characteristic of middle-class western cultures (Cohen, 1969). Currently, it is accepted that culture-free cognitive tests are simply impossible (Greenfield, 1997).

Cultural factors such as familiarity, speed, and testing environment can affect neuropsychological test performance. It is not surprising that the members of the cultural group the test developer belongs to usually obtain the best results. Familiarity however, not only refers to the materials used in testing (figures, blocks, etc) and their contents (houses, bikes, etc.) but also to the strategies used to solve the problems, and the attitudes required for succeeding. Competitiveness, for example, in many societies is viewed with suspicion. Cooperation and social ability may be by far more important. Ardila (2005) proposed that at least eight different culture-dependent values underlie cognitive testing: (1) one-to-one relationship, (2) background authority, (3) best performance, (4) isolated environment, (5) special type of communication, (6) speed, (7) internal or subjective issues, and (8) the use of specific testing elements and strategies. He further emphasized that "the distance" (e.g., gender, age, ethnicity) between the examiner and the examinee may potentially impact the testing situation. Cognitive testing represents a social situation that is governed by implicit cultural rules.

Testing environment is a poorly analyzed question in psychometry. Usually testing requires a highly structured and rigid situation. Testing is carried out individually. As a matter of fact, a whole array of cultural values underlie the testing situation. These are the typical values observed in psychometric-oriented societies, but they are far from modal values in many cultural groups (Greenfield, 1997). Frequently, intellectual or cognitive testing may be perceived as aversive in some cultures. In Latin America, usually highly educated people dislike, and try to avoid testing. Intellectual testing may even be perceived as a kind of humiliating situation and disrespectful of privacy. People with little education, on the other hand, may be afraid and embarrassed when tested. In consequence, frequently testing can be much more effectively if performed in a flexible and informal way, than if using a rigid and highly standardized situation. In many worldwide societies (e.g., many Amerindian groups), it is absurd that other people cannot observe, collaborate with, and help the testee. Activities are socially carried out with the participation of several people and there is not any apparent reason for the privacy in testing. For Hispanics, to illustrate another type of attitude, the interpersonal relationship with the examiner may be most important (Geisinger, 1992).

All these factors significantly complicate cross-cultural comparisons in cognitive abilities. They represent, however, central issues to understanding cognitive abilities in other cultural contexts.

CONCLUSIONS

Some significant differences in cognitive abilities have been demonstrated. They include visuoperceptual, visuoconstructive, memory, and languages abilities. Results in cognitive tests are under the influence of a significant number of variables, such as ecological conditions, previous training, age, gender, linguistic and cultural values. Cross-cultural comparisons in cognitive abilities are particularly difficult. Psychometric testing has been developed departing from the cultural values of competitiveness, high productivity, literacy, speed, and so forth in the societies where the tests were developed. Instrumentation should link cognition to context and culture to avoid having our findings reflect an ethnocentric artifact of our methodology.

REFERENCES

Abrahamson, A. S., & Lisker, L. (1970). Discriminability along the voicing continuum: Cross-language tests. *Proceeding of the Sixth International Congress of Phonetic Science* (pp. 569–573). Prague: Academic.

Anastasi, A. (1988). *Psychological testing*. New York: Macmillan.

Ardila, A. (1980). *Psicologia de la percepción* [Psychology of perception]. Mexico: Editorial Trillas.
Ardila, A. (1991). Errors resembling semantic paralexias in Spanish-speaking aphasics. *Brain and Language, 41,* 437–455.
Ardila, A. (1993). Historical evolution of spatial abilities. *Behavioral Neurology, 6,* 83–88.
Ardila, A. (1995). Directions of research in cross-cultural neuropsychology. *Journal of Clinical and Experimental Neuropsychology, 17,* 143–150.
Ardila, A. (1998). Semantic paralexias in Spanish language. *Aphasiology, 12,* 885–900.
Ardila, A. (2006). *A cross-linguistic naming test.* Unpublished manuscript.
Ardila, A. (2005). Cultural values underlying cognitive testing. *Neuropsychology Review, 15,* 185–195.
Ardila, A., & Moreno, S. (2001). Neuropsychological evaluation in Aruaco Indians: An exploratory study. *Journal of the International Neuropsychological Society, 7,* 510–515.
Ardila, A., Rosselli, M., & Pinzón, O. (1989). Alexia and agraphia in Spanish speakers: CAT correlations and interlinguistic analysis. In A. Ardila & F. Ostrosky (Eds.), *Brain organization of language and cognitive processes* (pp. 147–175). New York: Plenum Press.
Ardila, A., Rosselli, M., & Rosas, P. (1989). Neuropsychological assessment in illiterates: Visuospatial and memory abilities. *Brain and Cognition, 11,* 147–166.
Arnold, B. R., Montgomery, G. T., Castaneda, I., & Longoria, R. (1994). Acculturation and performance of Hispanics on selected Halstead-Reitan neuropsychology tests. *Assessment, 1*(3), 239–248.
Berlin, B., & Kay, P. (1969). *Basic color terms: Their universality and evolution.* Berkeley: University of California Press.
Berlin, B. (1992). *Ethnobiological classification: Principles of categorization of plants and animals in traditional societies.* Princeton, NJ: Princeton University Press.
Bernard, L. C. (1989). Halstead-Reitan neuropsychological test performance of black, Hispanic, and white young adult males from poor academic backgrounds. *Archives of Clinical Neuropsychology, 4,* 267–274.
Berry, J. W. (1971). Ecological and cultural factors in spatial perceptual development. *Canadian Journal of Behavioral Sciences, 3,* 324–336.
Berry, J. W. (1979). Culture and cognition style. In A. Marsella, R. G. Tharp, & T. J. Ciborowski (Eds.), *Perspectives in cross-cultural psychology* (pp. 117–135). New York: Academic Press.
Beveridge, W. M. (1940). Some racial differences in perception. *British Journal of Psychology, 30,* 57–64.
Boivin, M. J., Giordani, B., & Bornefeld, B. (1995). Use of the Tactual Performance Test for cognitive ability testing with African children. *Neuropsychology, 9,* 409–417.
Bolton, M., Michelson, C., Wilde, J., & Bolton, C. (1975). The heights of illusion. *Ethos, 3,* 403–424.
Brislin, R. W. (1983). Cross-cultural research in psychology. *Annual Review of Psychology, 34,* 363–400.
Cattell, R. B. (1940). A culture free intelligence test. Part I. *Journal of Educational Psychology, 31,* 161–179.
Chomsky, N. (1980). *Rules and representations.* Oxford, England: Blackwell.
Cohen, R. A. (1969). Conceptual styles, culture conflict, and nonverbal tests. *American Anthropologist, 71,* 828–856.

Cole, M. (1981). Cross-cultural psychology: A combined review. *Contemporary Psychology, 26*(5), 330–334.

Conkin, H. C. (1971). *Folk classification: A topically arranged bibliography of contemporary and background references through 1971.* New Haven, CT: Department of Anthropology Yale University.

Dawson, J. L. M. (1967). Cultural and physiological influences upon spatial perceptual processes in West Africa (Parts 1 & 2). *International Journal of Psychology, 2,* 115–128.

Deregowski, J. B. (1980). Perception. In H. C. Triandis & W. Lonner (Eds.), *Handbook of cross-cultural psychology* (Vol. 3, pp. 21–115). Boston: Allyn & Bacon.

Deregowski, J. B., Muldrow, E. S. & Muldrow, W. F. (1972). Pictorial recognition in a remote Ethiopian population. *Perception, 1,* 315–323.

Eimas, P. D. (1975). Auditory and phonetic coding of the cues for speech. Discrimination of the [r-l] distinctions by young infants. *Perception and Psychophysics, 18,* 341–347.

Evans, J. D., Miller, S. W., Byrd, D. A., & Heaton, R. K. (2000). Cross-cultural applications of the Halstead-Reitan batteries. In E. Fletcher-Jenzen, T. L. Strickland, & C. R. Reynolds (Eds.), *Handbook of cross-cultural neuropsychology* (pp. 287–303). New York: Kluwer-Academic.

Ferguson, G. (1956). On transfer and the abilities of man. *Canadian Journal of Psychology, 10,* 121–131.

Gandour, J. (1998). Aphasia in tonal languages. In P. Coppens, Y. Lebrun, & A. Basso (Eds.), *Aphasia in atypical populations* (pp. 117–142). Mahwah, NJ: Lawrence Erlbaum Associates.

Gay, J., & Cole, M. (1967). *The new mathematics and an old culture.* New York: Holt, Rinehart & Winston.

Geisinger, K. (Ed). (1992). *Psychological testing of Hispanics.* Washington, DC: American Psychological Association.

Gladwin, T. (1970). *East is a big bird: Navigation and logic in Puluwatatoll.* Cambridge, MA: Harvard University Press.

Greenberg, J. H. (1963). *Universals of language.* Cambridge, MA: MIT Press.

Greenberg, J. H. (1978). *Universals of human language* (Vols. 1–4). Stanford, CA: Stanford University Press.

Greenfield, P. M. (1997). You can't take it with you: Why ability assessments don't cross cultures. *American Psychologist, 52,* 1115–1124.

Hudson, W. (1960). Pictorial depth perception in subcultural groups in Africa. *Journal of Social Psychology, 52,* 193–208.

Hudson, W. (1962). Cultural problems in pictorial perception. *South African Journal of Sciences, 58,* 189–195.

Karanth, P. (2003). *Cross-linguistic studies of acquired reading disturbances.* New York: Kluwer/Plenum.

Klove, H. (1974). Validation studies in adult clinical neuropsychology. In R. M. Reitan & L. A. Davison (Eds.), *Clinical Neuropsychology: Current status and application* (pp. 211–236). Washington, DC: Winston.

Korkman, M., Kirk, U., & Kempt, S. L. (1998). *NEPSY–A developmental neuropsychological assessment.* San Antonio, TX: Psychological Corporation.

Kuwano, S., Namba, S., & Schick, A. (1986). A cross-cultural study on noise problems. In A. Schick, H. Hoge, & G. Lazarus-Mainka (Eds.), *Contributions to psychological acoustics* (pp. 370–395). Oldenburg, Germany: Universitat Oldenburg.

Laboratory of Comparative Human Cognition. (1983). Culture and cognitive development. In P. Mussen (Ed.), *Handbook of child psychology: History, theory and methods* (Vol. 1., pp. 342–397). New York: Wiley.
Leon-Carrion, J. (1989). Trail Making Test scores for normal children : Normative data from Spain. *Perceptual and Motor Skills, 68,* 627–630.
Lenneberg, E. H. (1967). *Biological foundations of language.* New York: Wiley.
Lewis, D. (1976). Observations on route-finding and spatial orientation among the Aboriginal peoples of the Western desert region of Central Australia. *Oceania, 46,* 249–282.
Miller, R. J. (1973). Cross-cultural research in the perception of pictorial materials. *Psychological Bulletin, 80,* 135–150.
Mitrushina, M. N., Boone, K. B., & D'Elia, L. F. (1999). *Handbook of normative data for neuropsychological assessment.* New York: Oxford University Press.
Mulenga, K., Ahonen, T., & Aro, M. (2001). Performance of Zambian children on the NEPSY: A pilot study. *Developmental Neuropsychology, 20,* 375–384.
Myambo, K. (1972). Shape constancy as influenced by culture, Western education, and age. *Journal of Cross-Cultural Psychology, 3,* 221–232.
Nussbaum, N. L., & Bigler, E. (1997). Halstead-Reitan neuropsychological batteries for children. In C. R. Reynolds & E. Fletcher-Janzen (Eds.), *Handbook of Clinical Child Neuropsychology* (pp. 219–236). New York: Plenum.
Paradis, M. (Ed.). (2001). *Manifestations of aphasia symptoms in different languages.* Oxford, England: Pergamon Press.
Pick, A. D., & Pick, H. L. (1978). Culture and perception. In E. C. Carterette & M. P. Friedman (Eds.), *Handbook of perception: Vol. 10. Perceptual ecology* (pp. 19–39). New York: Academic Press.
Post, R. H. (1971). Possible cases of relaxed selection in civilized populations. *Human Genetics, 13,* 253–284.
Reuning, H., & Wortley, W. (1973). Psychological studies of Bushmen [Monograph]. *Psychologia Africana, 7,* 1–113.
Rosselli, M., & Ardila, A. (2003). The impact of culture and education on nonverbal neuropsychological measurements: A critical review. *Brain and Cognition, 52,* 226–233.
Rosselli, M., Ardila, A., Bateman, J. R., & Guzman, M. (2001). Neuropsychological test scores, academic performance and developmental disorders in Spanish-speaking children. *Developmental Neuropsychology, 20,* 355–374.
Sasanuma, S., & Fujimura, O. (1971). Kanji versus Kana processing in alexia with transient agraphia. *Cortex, 7,* 1–18.
Segall, M. H., Campbell, D. T., & Herkovits, M. J. (1966). *The influence of culture on visual perception.* Indianapolis, IN: Bobbs-Merrill.
Segall, M. H. (1986). Culture and behavior: Psychology in global perspective. *Annual Review of Psychology, 37,* 523–564.
Strange, W., & Jenkins, J. J. (1978). Role of linguistic experience in the perception of speech. In R. D. Walk & H. L. Pick (Eds.), *Perception and experience* (pp. 125–169). New York: Plenum.
Sugishita, M., Otomo, K., Kabe, S., & Yunoki, K. (1992). A critical appraisal of neuropsychological correlates of Japanese ideogram (kanji) and phonogram (kana) reading. *Brain, 115,* 1563–1586.
Swadesh, M. (1952). Lexicostatistic dating of prehistoric ethnic contacts. *Proceedings of the American Philosophical Society, 96,* 152–163.
Swadesh, M. (1967). *El lenguaje y la vida humana* [Language and human life]. Mexico: Fondo de Cultural Económica.

Turnbull, C. (1961). Notes and discussion: Some observations regarding the experiences and behavior of the Bambute pygmies. *American Journal of Psychology, 7,* 304–308.
Vernon, P. E. (1969). *Intelligence and cultural environment.* London: Methuen.
Whorf, B. L. (1956). *Language, thought and reality.* Cambridge, MA: MIT Press.
Yamadori, A. (1975). Ideogram reading in alexia. *Brain, 98,* 231–238.
Yamadori, A. (1988). Writing and hemispheric coordination. *Aphasiology, 2,* 427–432.
Yu-Huan, H., Ying-Guan, Q., & Gui-Qing, Z .(1990). Crossed aphasia in Chinese: A clinical survey. *Brain and Language, 39,* 347–356.

Chapter 7

Speech, Language, and Neuropsychological Testing: Implications for African Americans

Constance Dean Qualls
State University of New York College at Buffalo

Psychological testing of African Americans has been a longstanding point of controversy in the United States. The major dilemma deals with the disparate performance between African Americans and whites. While some African Americans perform comparably to their white counterparts on tests of cognitive functioning and intelligence, a significant proportion of African Americans score lower on these measures (Jencks & Phillips, 2000). The reasons for the black–white differences in performance on cognitive (includes measures of verbal abilities, vis-à-vis speech and language) and neuropsychological tests are many and complex, and the theoretical explanations posed are largely flawed and unsupported by scientific research. As a consequence, little progress has been made toward improving cognitive test performance in African Americans, and, thereby, increasing their chances for educational and economic success. Lowenstein, Arguelles, and Arguelles (1994) acknowledged that one of the greatest challenges facing neuropsychologists today is the assessment of individuals from culturally and linguistically diverse backgrounds.

This chapter presents the current state of affairs of the literature on speech, language, and neuropsychological testing of African Americans. To shed light on this topic, three areas of research are discussed, including (1) black–white test score gap, (2) African American English (AAE), and (3) testing older African Americans. The term "cognitive tests" in this chapter represents measures that assess cognitive ability/functioning (i.e., reasoning, memory, perceptual abilities, attention, language, and so forth), intelligence, aptitude, achievement, and neuropsychological functioning (e.g., identification of disorders of the brain such as dementia).

BLACK–WHITE TEST SCORE GAP

Individual differences in performance on cognitive tests are observed and should be considered paramount for assessment and intervention purposes. Individual differences notwithstanding, there continues to be a significant gap in the scores between African Americans and white Americans on tests assessing cognitive abilities and cognitive functioning. This "black–white test score gap" persists from kindergarten through adulthood, with the typical American black scoring more than 75% and 85% below that of the typical American white (Jencks & Phillips, 2000). Phillips (2000) and her colleagues concluded that more than half of the gap in reading comprehension seen at the end of the 12th grade is attributable to the gap that existed at the beginning of the first grade. From elementary to middle to high school, black–white math and vocabulary gaps widen by a little less than 2 points per year, or 18–23 SAT points (Phillips, 2000).

Throughout the 20th century, the gap has narrowed considerably, indicating some progress has been made. However, the gap continues to fuel debates about whether cognitive equality can be achieved, particularly between African Americans and whites in the United States (Jencks & Phillips, 2000). Educational achievement is the driving force behind occupational and economic success and has remained a major campaign issue for politicians at all levels of government. For example, the No Child Left Behind (NCLB) Act of 2001 (see Anderson, 2005) was an outcome of the 2000 presidential election. Designed to improve student achievement and to change the culture of America's schools, NCLB has a specific focus on improving the academic achievement of "disadvantaged" children. The effectiveness of NCLB in improving test scores among poor and nonmajority populations remains to be seen and will likely be inconclusive, at least in the near future, because research investigating effective measures for improving education and achievement is yet to be firmly established (Ferguson & Brown, 2000).

Theoretical explanations for the black–white test gap are largely unsupported and highly controversial. Three are discussed, including genetic, methodological, and environmental. The genetic theory, advanced by Hernstein and Murray in 1994, suggested that the black–white test score gap is explained by genetic inequality. A great deal of discussion has fueled this debate, but, in the final analysis, no evidence has ever been presented in support of this view.

A widely held view among many blacks and some whites is that all cognitive tests are racially biased (Jencks & Phillips, 2000). A reasonable question then is do those African Americans who hold this view perform differently than those who do not? The answer to this question assumes the possibility of a "racial bias effect" for some African Americans that would negatively affect their performance on tests. For example, one might speculate that those persons who, prior to taking the test, have determined that the test is racially biased may feel ambivalent regarding the outcome and not put forth the necessary effort to adequately prepare for it. People are naturally inclined to spend more time and effort preparing for competitive contexts in which they feel success is possible than contexts where success is unlikely. Five types of test bias have been identified, including labeling bias, content bias, methodological bias, prediction bias, and selection system bias (Jencks, 2000). Each of these is now summarized below.

Labeling bias occurs when a test claims to measure one thing but really measures something else; thus, labeling bias violates internal validity. The terms "intelligence" and "aptitude" are widely used to describe innate potential as well as developed abilities. After many years of debate, it is agreed that intelligence tests measure developed rather than innate abilities; developed abilities represent the interaction between one's environment and their innate abilities (Jencks, 2000). The notion of intelligence testing, therefore, presents a racially biased estimate of innate ability that cannot simply be changed by changing the content of the test (Jencks & Phillips, 2000). The logical remediation, according to Jencks, is to accurately represent the test as measuring developed abilities. This has implications for test development, test standardization, and test interpretation. Content bias occurs when a test contains items that favor one group over another. The language of the test (e.g., formal English and grammar vs. a dialect of American English such as Appalachian English or African American English), as well as familiarity with other aspects of majority American culture, could possibly underestimate the abilities of individuals from nonmajority groups. Jencks suggested that test score differences between blacks and whites may reflect differences in "the way blacks and whites are taught to deal with what they do not know and the emphasis they put on learning new cognitive skills" (p. 14). Methodological bias in a test measures mastery of some skill or body of information in such a way that underestimates the competence of one group over another. Although the research is sparse, methodological bias, as defined here, implies the possibility of an interaction between the person administering the test and the person taking the test. For instance, the way in which the test is described may differ depending on a person's group membership. Prediction bias and selection bias have to do with prediction of outcome, for example, using the scores of a test (i.e., SAT or GRE; PRAXIS or General Aptitude Test Battery) to estimate future academic and occupational outcomes (Jencks & Phillips). At best, these tests show moderate correlations with performance, thus, the fairness of using these tests for enrolling students and hiring personnel continues to be questionable (Jencks, 2000). Globalization has increased the stakes to the extent that high achievement on cognitive tests is now a priority in the United States. A survey of reading achievement of fourth-grade students in 35 countries, including the United States, showed that in 2001, U.S. fourth-graders scored well above the international mean of 500 (Martin, Mullis, Gonzalez, & Kennedy, 2003). However, some reading subtopics showed a declining trend: From 1991 to 2001, U.S. fourth graders' narrative reading literacy scores by dropped 20 points. Despite the fact that the information is from a restricted population and the scores reflect ability in a single area—narrative reading literacy, the implications of Martin et al.'s findings are far reaching. This means that test/cognitive performance is even more important than in past years. Further, until such time that bias in testing is accounted for, some African Americans will continue to be disadvantaged on cognitive tests.

Environmental explanations for the black–white test score gap range from family and school to societal effects (Jencks & Phillips, 2000). To date, a limited number of family variables have been studied relative to their influence on the black–white test score gap. These include parental schooling, socioeconomic level, single-parent status, parenting strategies, and extended family involvement. Of these, and the many other family characteristics that correlate with a child's test scores, a mother's socioeconomic status while growing up and her current parenting practices explain considerably more (Phillips, Brooks-Gunn, Duncan, Klebanov, & Crane, 2000). When African American and white mothers have similar schooling experiences, their children's scores will tend to look more alike than different. Even more salient is parenting practices, a factor that appears to significantly influence children's test scores (Jencks & Phillips).

Regarding school effects, teacher expectations have been widely studied. After reviewing the literature, Ferguson and Brown (2000) concluded that: a) Teachers have lower expectations for African Americans than for whites; b) teacher's expectations influence to a greater extent African American students' performance as compared to white students' performance; c) teachers expect less of African Americans than whites because African American students' past performance and behavior have been worse; d) teachers perpetuate disparities in academic achievement, some of which is attributable to their experiences with low-achieving African American students; and e) exhorting teachers to have more faith in African American children's potential is unlikely to change their expectations, although experience with high achieving African American students can make [somewhat of] a difference. Reducing class size positively affects test scores; this is especially the case for reading scores, but not math scores (Ferguson & Brown, 2000). Other school variables that have a positive impact on test scores for African Americans are high-scoring teachers (e.g., on competency tests such as the PRAXIS) and school desegregation (Jencks & Phillips, 2000).

Much of the literature on the societal influence on test performance in African Americans deals with two phenomena: fear of "acting white" and stereotype threat. For some African American students, working hard and getting good grades imply racial disloyalty (Fordham & Ogbu, 1986); thus, the social costs for academic success is higher for African Americans than for whites (Jencks & Phillips, 2000). Jencks and Phillips suggested that the "acting white" hypothesis does not explain why African Americans do more poorly on achievement tests than whites, but it might explain why African American students are less motivated to work toward better performance. Stereotype threat deals with the anxiety of confirming a negative stereotype (Steele & Aronson, 1995). These authors believe that African Americans who are affected by the stereotype threat score lower on achievement tests because their attention is diverted from the test content to thinking that, if they perform poorly, they will confirm the stereotype that all African Americans do poorly on cognitive and achievement tests. It might be that the level of difficulty of the test as well as how the results will be used will determine the relative strength of the stereotype threat. Sackett, Hardison, and Cullen's (2004) reinterpretation of Steele and Anderson's data showed that elimination of the stereotype threat did not eliminate the gap in performance. Thus, Sackett et al. cautioned against attributing primary causation of African American's depressed performance on cognitive tests to stereotype threat.

Disentangling the many factors that exert influence on the test performance of African Americans is an ongoing challenge. However, there are emerging areas of research that quite possibly will provide better and more complete explanations for the black–white test score gap and, thus, provide direction with regard to reducing/eliminating this disparity. These include parent–child interactions, intra and interracial student–teacher relations and their impact on expectations, and the psychological and cultural differences that have yet to be accurately described and empirically tested (Jencks & Phillips, 2000).

AFRICAN AMERICAN ENGLISH (AAE)

Linguistic variation is a highly systematic social practice that is often linked to race or ethnicity. African American English is a variety or dialect of general English that is defined as a systematic, highly regular language system that has its own set of phonologic, semantic, syntactic, and pragmatic rules (American Speech-Language-Hearing Association, 2003; see also Green, 2002). Many terms have been used when referring to this language system, including Black English, Black English Vernacular, African American English Vernacular, and Ebonics. In this chapter, the term African American English (AAE) is used. The use of AAE is motivated by a number of factors; three important ones are situational context (e.g., home, community vs. school, workplace), speaker relations (e.g., parent–child, boss–worker, friends/age-peers, shared experiences, and so forth), and the goal of the interaction (e.g., socialization vs. educational or occupational pursuit). Further, the level at which a person has acculturated or assimilated will determine whether or not they will use AAE, how often they use it, and in what context they will use it. Hence, there are large within-group differences in the use of AAE among African Americans, and AAE use is largely determined by one's level of acculturation. Acculturation, as cited in Battle (2002), is the level at which one assumes mainstream cultural attributes, including the language, cultural norms, behaviors, and values, in relation to those of their own culture; assimilation is the adoption of mainstream cultural attributes into one's social and cultural networks (i.e., work, residence, leisure activities, family).

It is presumed that individuals who speak AAE are a homogeneous group who are African Americans only. Horton-Ikard and Miller (2004) found that African American children in low and middle SES (socioeconomic status) groups had similar rates of dialect use. However, research is needed to examine frequency and patterns of use of AAE in African Americans at high SES levels. One might speculate that there will be lower rates of use because of higher rates of acculturation. On the other hand, because SES is largely based on occupation, income, and wealth, the latter two cannot necessarily assume high levels of education. This last scenario suggests that AAE use in high SES African Americans might be comparable to that of low and middle SES African Americans. If this is the case, level of acculturation/assimilation would be a better predictor of AAE use than SES. A notable example is Sweetland's (2002) sole study participant, Delilah, a 23-year-old white female, who exemplified what Rampton (1995a) termed as *code-crossing*. Code-crossing occurs when people who "shouldn't" (e.g., whites) speak a code (in this case, AAE) because they are not members of the group associated with the code (e.g., African Americans) they employ (Rampton, 1995a; Sweetland, 2002). A detailed analysis of Delilah's everyday speech revealed that she consistently used the distinctive features associated with AAE, although, in certain contexts, she chose to and was able to proficiently use "standard" American English (SAE; Sweetland, 2002). Delilah's successful use of AAE was a result of her ability to assimilate into the African American culture.

Similar to psychological testing of African Americans, AAE, the language system used by some African Americans, has generated a great deal of debate in the United States. Following is a brief historical account of the controversies surrounding AAE (see Green, 2002 for a complete discussion). In the 1960s, there was controversy as to whether AAE was a deficit in language or a variation of mainstream English. Over the next 20 years, the AAE debate culminated in the idea that AAE was, in fact, a rule-governed dialect of American English. In 1979, the judge in the *Ann Arbor School District* case ruled that the speech patterns of African American elementary school-aged children served as a barrier to their education if teachers fail to take it into account. Some years later, in 1996, the *Ebonics* controversy once again erupted, only this time in Northern California. The Oakland Unified School District Board of Education approved a policy mandating that all students be provided instruction that was necessary for them to achieve proficiency in SAE. Before the policy was officially disclosed to the public, false claims in the media stated that the Oakland school children would be taught AAE in the classroom. The reality was that the Oakland School Board resolved to recognize Ebonics as the "primary language of African American children" that should be considered in their language arts lessons (Rickford, 2005). Yet, the confusion displayed among the populous was related to negative attitudes toward AAE and the lack of adequate knowledge about the linguistic features of AAE (Green, 2002; Seymour, Abdulkarim, & Johnson, 1999). Of note is that the negative attitudes emanated from both African Americans and whites. Charity, Scarborough, and Griffin (2004) suggested that recognition of AAE as a systematic variety of English should reduce negative attitudes associated with its use, a naïve statement at best. AAE continues to be highly stigmatized and the use of AAE continues to disadvantage its speakers both academically and economically.

Speech-language pathologists, educators, and neuropsychologists who are responsible for testing and assessing the speech, language, and cognitive abilities of African Americans should have adequate knowledge about AAE. This is crucial for differentiating one's dialect from disordered speech (Rodekohr & Haynes, 2001). However, understanding the rules of AAE does not mean becoming fluent in the dialect, or that one has to become a specialist before working with speakers of AAE (e.g., Green, 2002). Rather, it is sufficient to understand some of the ways in which AAE differs systematically from SAE (Oetting & McDonald, 2002). In her paper, Green (2002) presented a detailed description of the linguistic features of AAE with the intent that such descriptions could be used to determine whether their presence interferes with reading and other education achievement. Some key points are discussed here.

- Words in AAE are generally identical in pronunciation to words in mainstream English, although some may have different meanings.

- AAE speakers use the same inventory of sounds (phonological system) that is used in mainstream and other varieties of English; however, in some cases, the rules governing the occurrence of the sounds differ. For example, *consonant cluster reduction* (e.g., list → lis, desk → des, etc.) exists in AAE. This feature follows the Voicing Generalization Rule to omit the final consonant of a cluster formed by two consonants with the same voicing value. On the other hand, depending on the phonetic environment, some mainstream consonant clusters are produced by AAE speakers (e.g., *nt, nk*). Words ending in voiced *th* in mainstream English are produced with a final *v* in AAE; final voiceless *th* → *f* in AAE.
- Many of the features that distinguish AAE from other varieties of English are in the syntactic and semantic components of the language system. For examples, *aspectual be* indicates habituality or iterativity not tense, it always occurs in its basic form, and is never conjugated or inflected. AAE speakers use *aspectual be* to indicate that something recurs or happens from time to time (e.g., "Dee be running" means that Dee usually runs in AAE speakers; "Dee running" means that Dee is running now). For *marking the past,* AAE makes at least six distinctions; some are constrastive with SAE and some are not. For example, AAE speakers employ the form "he drunk the milk" to mark the simple past where the event culminates before now. To mark the remote past (whole event or some part of it is in the remote past), they may say "he bin drink the milk."
- AAE speakers use *multiple negative* constructions to indicate a single negative meaning. The particular feature used implies a specific meaning and is considered to be an existential construction in that it expresses something about existence or nonexistence. Some exemplars are "Nobody don't be at the library," meaning nobody is usually at the library; "Don't nobody be at the library," meaning not a single person is usually at the library; and "It don't be nobody at the library," meaning usually, there isn't anybody at the library.
- When AAE speakers produce constructions that approximate those of SAE, they are not simply attempting to speak mainstream English and missing the mark, these are well-formed AAE constructions (Green, 2002).

Studies of AAE have historically focused on identifying and describing dialect features. A contemporary view is that linguistic theory should explain the unique linguistic features of AAE (Coles-White, 2004). Coles-White studied one of the grammatical features of AAE, negative concord, to determine its merit for assessing the development of comprehension skills in young AAE speakers. Negative concord, as defined by Martin (1992), is the expression of two negative elements in a syntactic environment or sentence where they are *in* agreement [as opposed to double negation, denoting independent negatives]. An example of negative concord in AAE is "He *don't* have *no* friends"; an example of double negation is "He *don't* like going there with *no* friends." Coles-White explained that the meanings of these two sentences differ as a result of the differential use of negatives and concluded that that "... negative concord is represented and interpreted in the grammar similarly to *wh-* questions, so that if a child has difficulty in comprehending questions, the child may also have difficulty comprehending negative concord" (pp. 219–220).

Linguistic descriptions of the features of AAE will inform ways of examining patterns of influence of AAE for reading development. In SAE speakers, performance on measures of phonological processing, for example, a phoneme deletion task (e.g., *Say* "tink"; *Now say* "tink" without the *t*), is highly correlated with reading; this was not the case for AAE speakers in one study (Sligh & Conners, 2003). However, Sligh and Connors' findings must be interpreted with caution because they failed to account for at least two factors that may have impacted their results. There was no formal, systematic assessment of AAE features and use among the African American students, and students from all SES levels were included, thus not accounting for the association between SES and AAE use by the African American students (i.e., increased ability to code-switch with higher SES). As acknowledged by the researchers, their findings raise the possibility that speakers of AAE who have been identified as at-risk for reading difficulty may be missed and those who are not truly at-risk might be falsely identified as such (Sligh & Connors).

Thompson, Craig, and Washington (2004) suggested that, because the school curriculum is based on SAE vocabulary, entering African American students who speak AAE may be disadvantaged. In their elementary-grade African American students, Thompson et al. found that those children who were more successful at shifting between AAE and SAE performed better on achievement tests as compared to those who were unsuccessful dialect shifters. Many African American students enter school speaking AAE, but quickly decrease use of it in school contexts, particularly seen at grade 3 and higher (Thompson et al.). Similarly, Charity et al. (2004) studied the nature of the association between AAE and SAE use and academic literacy. These researchers hypothesized that AAE speakers entering school and who are more familiar with SAE should be advantaged on reading tasks. Their tasks included reading aloud, sentence imitation (used as the measure of familiarity with SAE), and story recall for kindergarten through second graders. Charity et al. found moderate to high correlations between early reading and dialect knowledge in the African American children, although the reason(s) for such an association remain unclear and warrant further investigation.

Other relevant considerations when assessing the cognitive abilities of AAE speakers include experimenter/clinician characteristics, teacher training, and linguistic inventories. Experimenter characteristics have been shown to exert some influence on the outcome of behavioral studies (Rosenthal, 1976). For example, researchers have studied the effects of race of the interviewer when collecting language samples of AAE speakers (Cukor-Avila & Bailey, 2001; Rickford & McNair-Knox, 1994). Rickford and McNair-Knox found that the use of AAE features are strongly conditioned by the interviewer's race, so that, all other things being equal (e.g., subject matter; interview forms, and so forth), the interviewee used a significantly greater percentage of AAE features in the interview with the African American interviewer. Cukor-Avila and Bailey's results failed to replicate Rickford and McNair-Knox's interviewer race effect on AAE use; however, they did show that different interviewers can produce significantly different results. Thus, factors such as personality (e.g., friendliness, level of comfort with strangers), interviewer use of dialectal forms, and/or interviewee perceptions of the interviewer must be considered during the interview or assessment process.

Inadequate teacher training contributes significantly to the problems faced by linguistic minority students (i.e., speakers of AAE) in the United States. A first step toward increasing teacher competence in working with nonstandard English speakers is ascertaining information about their attitudes and perceptions of these individuals. In a small sample of 88 self-selected informants from five secondary schools in New York City, Blake and Culter (2003) reported several findings. Among their findings, the majority of the teachers did not support bidialectal education and felt that federal funds should not be allocated for such programs (this is in contrast to their overwhelming support for bilingual education). Similarly, the majority of the respondents felt that AAE would not be useful as a tool for mastering SAE, although about half felt AAE would be useful for teaching social studies and math. The participants were roughly equally divided in their view of whether it is educationally sound to use the students' first (or home) language as a way of mastering SAE or school language.

Some researchers claim that inventories are useful in assisting educators, diagnosticians, and researchers with making decisions about the distinctive features of behaviors such as language. For example, Bland-Stewart (2003) identified the dialect-based phonological patterns that AAE-speaking 2-year-olds frequently use, although her results could not reliably distinguish typical phonological development from emergent dialect features. Craig, Thompson, Washington, and Potter (2003) developed a taxonomy of characteristic phonological features of child AAE speakers in elementary grades. Pollock and Meredith (2001) discussed the dynamic nature of AAE phonological forms, citing time-linked change and substantial regional variations that lead to a complete understanding of the full range of phonological features of AAE. AAE inventories should also include the semantic, grammatical, and pragmatic features associated with this dialect of English.

TESTING OLDER AFRICAN AMERICANS

Given the history of lower test score performance among school-aged and college-aged African Americans, it is not a surprise that older African Americans, as a group, show a similar pattern of performance on tests of cognition. Because of their unique history and life course, the term *double jeopardy* has been used to characterize older African Americans (Dowd & Bengston, 1978). Double jeopardy refers to the simultaneous membership in two or more devalued social groups, for example, old and African American, but most often, old, poor, and African American. Many older African Americans have endured racism, poverty, and poor health, and these factors have had a deleterious effect on psychological well-being and health (Utsey, Payne, Jackson, & Jones, 2002), and, ultimately, cognitive functioning.

Data from the Indianapolis Study of Health and Aging showed that cognitive impairment short of dementia [also referred to as mild cognitive impairment (MCI), cognitive impairment no dementia (CIND), or age-associate cognitive decline (AACD)] is common in older African Americans, affecting nearly 1 in 4 persons in this population (Unverzagt et al., 2001). Clinical diagnosis of MCI is determined by (1) informant-reported clinically significant decline in cognition, (2) physician-detected clinically significant impairment in cognition, (3) cognitive test scores(s) below approximately the 7th percentile, and (4) no clinically important impairment in performance of daily living tasks (Unverzagt et al., 2001; Wolf et al., 2004). The presence of MCI is a significant risk factor for the development of dementia (Alzheimer's Association, 2004). As a consequence, there is a significantly higher prevalence of Alzheimer's disease (AD; and other dementias) among African Americans, with estimates of as much as 100% higher than whites (Alzheimer's Association, 2002; Gurland et al., 1999).

Generally, older African Americans score lower than whites on cognitive tests. Health issues notwithstanding, the integrity of their performance and the interpretation of the scores must be tempered by potential sources of measurement bias and increased "false positive" rates (Fillenbaum, Heyman, Williams, Prosnitz, & Burchett, 1995; Froelich et al., 2001). Froehlich et al. cited education and cultural bias in self-report and informant measures as potential sources of measurement bias. African Americans have a lower mean education level that can significantly disadvantage them, particularly because many cognitive tests are biased toward high education levels. In addition to education level, the nature or quality of one's educational experiences must be taken into consideration when assessing the cognitive abilities of older African Americans (Allaire & Whitfield, 2004). For example, when tested on the identical battery (inductive reasoning, verbal meaning, processing speed, declarative memory, and everyday memory), African Americans who attended a segregated school differed in their pattern of performance compared to those who attended a desegregated school (Allaire & Whitfield). Nevertheless, some studies have found that race independently predicted performance on the Mini-Mental State Exam (MMSE; Folstein, Folstein, & McHugh, 1975) even when age, gender, education, income, occupation, and duration of dementia symptoms were controlled (e.g., Bohnstedt, Fox, & Kohatsu, 1994). In contrast, Murden, McRae, Kaner, and Bucknam (1991) reported no statistically significant differences in performance between African Americans and whites who had similar levels of education.

Even with education controlled, unusually high rates of the diagnosis of dementia on the MMSE have been seen for African Americans. Using a cut-off score of 23 (out of a possible 30) on the MMSE, a greater percentage of Bohnstedt et al.'s (1994) African Americans than whites were classified as demented, suggesting that the MMSE may overestimate cognitive decline in African Americans. Both Fillenbaum et al. (1990) and Gurland, Wilder, Cross, Teresi, and Barrett (1992) reported high rates of false positives for older African Americans on the MMSE; these findings show that the MMSE demonstrates poor specificity for detecting individuals who do not have dementia. In their African American-only sample, Albert and Teresi (1999) found that education and reading ability independently predicted cognitive impairment, as measured by the MMSE, and suggested that taking into account one's reading ability may improve the specificity of cognitive tests.

Other cognitive tests show results similar to the MMSE. The Consortium to Establish a Registry for Alzheimer's Disease (CERAD) neuropsychological battery evaluated cognitive performance in African American and white patients with AD (Welsh et al., 1995). Tests of verbal fluency, naming, mental status (MMSE), constructional praxis, word list memory, word list recall, and word list recognition were completed by the patients. The results showed that, after controlling for age, education level, estimated duration of disease, and dementia severity, Welsh et al.'s African American patients performed worse than the white patients on the MMSE, constructional drawings, and naming of line drawings. The Stroop Color and Word, a commonly used test in neuropsychological assessment, measures executive functioning. This test examines the interference effect, defined by Stroop (1935) as an increase in reaction time resulting from the introduction of task-irrelevant stimulus characteristics (Moering, Schinka, Mortimer, & Graves, 2004). Moering et al. produced the only normative data established to date for older African Americans on the Stroop test. Similar to whites, performance was a function of age, education, and gender; however, when these data were compared to normative data on whites, the African Americans performed at lower levels across age groups and education levels. Adjusting for education eliminated only a portion of the differences. Moering et al. provided some possible explanations for the discrepant scores between African Americans and whites, including health (e.g., hypertension has an association with cognitive decline).

Differential item functioning (DIF) has been identified as a potential source of test bias on tests of normal cognitive functioning (Jones, 2003) and dementia (Woodard, Auchus, Goodsall, & Green, 1998). Jones analyzed the cognitive status data from 15,257 African American and white adults, aged 50 and older, who were surveyed in two national databases, the Study of Asset and Health Dynamics of the Oldest Old (AHEAD) and the Health and Retirement Study (HRS), and found that 89% of the differences between the groups were attributable to measurement or structural differences. These findings were confirmed when DIF was controlled, which showed that much of the variance was due to DIF. The remaining group difference was then explained by background variables, for example, Jones reported that low education significantly depressed performance in the African American group, whereas high income advantaged the whites only. African Americans also showed lower performance compared to whites on immediate and delayed recall during parallel versions of the telephone interview of cognitive status (TICS; Hogervorts Bandelow, Hart, & Henderson, 2004). This was the case for individuals with educational levels higher and lower than 12th grade.

There is a general consensus that culture-free or culture-fair assessments should be developed and rigorously tested (Froehlich et al., 2001; Jones, 2003; Whitfield, Baker-Thomas, Heyward, Gatto, & Williams, 1999). Until such time that happens, some researchers are investigating whether existing cognitive measures are appropriate for older African Americans. Whitfield et al. concluded that the Everyday Problems Test (Willis, Jay, Diehl, & Marsiske, 1992) is appropriate for studying within-group variability in cognitive functioning among African Americans, and suggested that the next step would be to examine the African Americans' performance relative to whites to determine cultural influences on performance. Woodard et al. (1998) concluded that the Mattis Dementia Rating Scale (MDRS; Mattis, 1973) showed no evidence of overall test bias in their African American and white patients with dementia, although the African Americans showed greater dementia severity than the whites. DIF was demonstrated on 4 of the 36 MDRS items, showing a slight advantage for the African Americans. These results, however, should be interpreted with caution because of the small numbers of participants and possible differences in the quality of education between the groups (Woodard et al., 1998).

CONCLUSIONS

This chapter discussed three areas of research that provide insight about assessment of the speech, language, and neuropsychological abilities in African Americans across the life span; black–white test score gap, AAE, and testing older African Americans. Cognitive assessment of African Americans calls for a thorough appreciation of the copious and complex variables that operate within and externally to this cultural group. Of import is the legacy of forbidden literacy and poor educational opportunities for African Americans that may underlie the lack of progress of some African Americans (Qualls, 2001). On the other hand, many African American children and adults perform as well as individuals from other racial-ethnic groups on cognitive tests and health care assessments. Therefore, an individual differences approach is warranted to ensure unbiased interactions, expectations, and interpretations of behaviors. Too, as language is integral to culture, assessment that does not consider AAE as a rule-governed language that is used in specific ways and for specific purposes will grossly misrepresent the language and cognitive abilities of many African Americans. A life-span developmental paradigm should be adopted for the study of cognitive testing of African Americans. By studying the various age groups in isolation, the interaction between variables is much less clear. In contrast, when researchers take into account an individual's life experiences from early development to senescence, a more complete picture of the influence of the different variables discussed in this chapter may emerge. Finally, more research is needed to investigate and address the flaws inherent in existing tests of cognitive ability, intelligence, and achievement so that there will be the opportunity for equivalent, yet competitive, performance among individuals from all racial-ethnic backgrounds.

REFERENCES

Albert, S. M., & Teresi, J. A. (1999). Reading ability, education, and cognitive status assessment among older adults in Harlem, New York City. *American Journal of Public Health, 89,* 95–97.

Allaire, J. C., & Whitfield, K. E. (2004). Relationships among education, age, and cognitive functioning in older African Americans: The impact of desegregation. *Aging Neuropsychology and Cognition, 11,* 443–449.

Alzheimer's Association. (2002, February 12). *African Americans and Alzheimer's disease: The silent epidemic.* Retrieved June 6, 2005, from http://www.alz.org/Media/newsreleases/2003/AA_ALZ.pdf

Alzheimer's Association. (2004, July 18). *Studies detail prevalence and risk factors for MCI.* Retrieved May 17, 2005, from http://www.alz.org/news/03q4/102003mci.asp

American Speech-Language-Hearing Association. (2003). Technical report: American English dialects. *ASHA Supplement, 23,* 1–3.

Anderson, L. W. (2005, April 4). The No Child Left Behind Act and the legacy of federal aid to education. *Education Policy Analysis Archives, 13*. Retrieved May 30, 2005, from http://epa.asa.edu/epa/v13n2/
Battle, D. E. (2002). *Communication disorders in multicultural populations* (3rd ed.). Boston, MA: Butterworth-Heinemann.
Bland-Stewart, L. (2003). Phonetic inventories and phonological patterns of African American two-year-olds. *Communication Disorders Quarterly, 24*, 109–120.
Blake, R., & Cutler, C. (2003). AAE and variation in teachers' attitudes: A question of school philosophy? *Linguistics and Education, 14*, 163–194.
Bohnstedt, M., Fox, P. J., & Kohatsu, N. D. (1994). Correlation of Mini-Mental Status Examination scores among elderly demented patients: The influence of race-ethnicity. *Journal of Clinical Epidemiology, 47*, 1381–1387.
Charity, A. H., Scarborough, H. S., & Griffin, D. M. (2004). Familiarity with school English in African American children and its relation to early reading achievement. *Child Development, 75*, 1340–1356.
Coles-White, D. (2004). Negative concord in child African American English: Implications for specific language impairment. *Journal of Speech, Language, and Hearing Research, 47*, 212–222.
Craig, H., Thompson, C. A., Washington, J., & Potter, S. L. (2003). Phonological features of child African American English. *Journal of Speech, Language, and Hearing Research, 46*, 623–635.
Cukor-Avila, P., & Bailey, G. (2001). The effects of the race of the interviewer on sociolinguistic fieldwork. *Journal of Sociolinguistics, 5*, 254–270.
Dowd, J. J., & Bengston, V. L. (1978). Aging in minority populations: An examination of the double jeopardy hypotheses. *Journal of Gerontological Social Work, 5*, 127–145.
Ferguson, R. F., & Brown, J. (2000). Certification test scores: Teacher quality, and student achievement. In D. W. Grissmer & J. M. Ross (Eds.), *Analytic issues in the assessment of student achievement* (NCES 2000-050; pp. 133–156). Washington, DC: U.S. Department of Education National Center for Education Statistics.
Fillenbaum, G., Heyman, A., Williams, K., Prosnitz, B., & Burchett, B. (1990). Sensitivity and specificity of standardized screens of cognitive impairment and dementia among elderly Black and White community residents. *Journal of Clinical Epidemiology, 43*, 651–660.
Folstein, M. F., Folstein, S. E., & McHugh, P. R. (1975). "Mini-Mental State." A practical method for grading the cognitive state of patients for the clinician. *Journal of Psychiatric Research, 12*, 189–198.
Ford, G. R., Haley, W. E., Thrower, S. L., West, C. A. C., & Harrell, L. E. (1996). Utility of Mini-Mental State Exam scores in predicting functional impairment among white and African American dementia patients. *Journal of Gerontology, 51*(A), M185–M188.
Fordham, S., & Ogbu, J. U. (1986). Black student's school success: Coping with the burden of acting white. *Urban Review, 18*, 176–206.
Froehlich, T. E., Bogardus, S. T., & Inouye, S. K. (2001). Dementia and race: Are there differences between African Americans and Caucasians? *Journal of the American Geriatric Society, 49*, 477–484.
Green, L. (2002). A descriptive study of African American English: Research in linguistics and education. *Qualitative Studies in Education, 15*, 673–690.
Gurland, B. J., Wilder, D. E., Cross, P., Teresi, J., & Barrett, V. W. (1992). Screening scales for dementia: Toward reconciliation of conflicting cross-cultural findings. *International Journal of Geriatric Psychiatry, 7*, 105–113.

Gurland, B. J., Wilder, D. E., Lantigua, R., Ster, Y., Chen, J., Killerfer, E. H. P., & Mayeux, R. (1999). Rates of dementia in three enthnoracial groups. *International Journal of Geriatric Psychiatry, 14,* 481–493.
Hernstein, R., & Murray, C. (1994). *The bell curve: Intelligence and class structure in American life.* New York: Free Press.
Hogervorst, E., Bandelow, S., Hart, J., & Henderson, V. W. (2004). Telephone word-list recall tested in the Rural Aging and Memory Study: two parallel versions for the TICS-M. *International Journal of Geriatric Psychiatry, 19,* 875–880.
Horton-Ikard, R., & Miller, J. F. (2004). It is not just the poor kids: The use of AAE forms by African-American school-aged children from middle SES communities. *Journal of Communication Disorders, 37,* 467–487.
Jencks, C. (2000). Racial bias in testing. In C. Jencks & M. Phillips (Eds.), *The black-white test score gap* (pp. 55–85). Washington, DC: Brookings Institution Press.
Jencks, C., & Phillips, M. (Eds.). (2000). *The black-white test score gap.* Washington, DC: Brookings Institution Press.
Jones, R. N. (2003). Racial bias in the assessment of cognitive functioning of older adults. *Aging & Mental Health, 7,* 83–102.
Lowenstein, D. A., Arguelles, T., & Arguelles, S. (1994). Potential cultural bias in the neuropsychological assessment of the older adult. *Journal of Clinical and Experimental Neuropsychology, 16,* 623–629.
Martin, M. O., Mullis, I. V. S., Gonzalez, E. J., & Kennedy, A. M. (2003). *Trends in children's reading literacy achievement 1991–2001: IEA's repeat in nine countries of the 1991 reading literacy study.* Chestnut Hill, MA: Boston College. Retrieved June 2, 2005, from http://isc.bc.edu/pirls2001i/PIRLS2001_Pubs_TrR.html
Martin, S. (1992). *Topics in the syntax of nonstandard English.* Unpublished doctoral dissertation, University of Maryland, College Park.
Mattis, S. (1973). *Dementia Rating Scale professional manual.* Odessa, FL: Psychological Assessment Resources, Inc.
Moering, R. G., Schinka, J. A., Mortimer, J. A., & Graves, A. B. (2004). Normative data for elderly African Americans for the Stroop Color and Word Test. *Archives of Clinical Neuropsychology, 19,* 61–71.
Murden, R. A., McRae, T. D., Kaner, S., & Bucknam, M. E. (1991). Mini-Mental State Exam scores vary with education in blacks and whites. *Journal of the American Geriatric Society, 39,* 149–155.
Oetting, J. B., & McDonald, J. (2002). Methods for characterizing participants' nonmainstream dialect use in child language research. *Journal of Speech, Language, and Hearing Research, 45,* 505–518.
Phillips, M. (2000). Understanding ethnic differences in academic achievement: Empirical lessons from national data. In D. W. Grissmer & J. M. Ross (Eds.), *Analytic issues in the assessment of student achievement* (NCES 2000-050; pp. 103–132). Washington, DC: U.S. Department of Education National Center for Education Statistics.
Phillips, M., Brooks-Gunn, J., Duncan, G., Klebanov, P., & Crane, J. (2000). Family background, parenting practices, and the black-white test score gap. In C. Jencks & M. Phillips (Eds.), *The black-white test score gap* (pp. 103–148). Washington, DC: Brookings Institution Press.
Pollock, K. E., & Meredith, L. H. (2001). Phonetic transcription of African American Vernacular English. *Communication Disorders Quarterly, 23,* 47–53.
Qualls, C. D. (2001). Public and personal meanings of literacy. In J. L. Harris, A. G. Kamhi, & K. E. Pollock (Eds.), *Literacy in African American communities* (pp. 1–19). Mahwah, NJ: Lawrence Erlbaum Associates.

Rampton, B. (1995a). Language crossing and the problematisation of ethnicity and socialization. *Pragmatics: Quarterly Publication of the International Pragmatics Association, 5*, 485–513.

Rickford, J. R. (2005). *The ebonics controversy in my backyard: A sociolinguist's experiences and reflections.* Retrieved April 13, 2005, from http://www.stanford.edu/~rickford/ebonics/

Rickford, J. R., & McNair-Know, F. (1994). Addressee- and topic-influence style shift. A quantitative sociolinguistic study. In D. Biber & E. Finegar (Eds.), *Sociolinguistic Perspectives on Register* (pp. 235–276). New York: Oxford University Press.

Rodekohr, R. K. & Haynes, W. O. (2001). Differentiating dialect from disorder: A comparison of two processing tasks and a standardized language test. *Journal of Communication Disorders, 34*, 255–272.

Rosenthal, R. (1976). *Experimenter effects in behavioral research* (enlarged ed.). New York: Irvington.

Sackett, P. R., Hardison, C. M., & Cullen, M. J. (2004). On interpreting stereotype threat as accounting for African American-white differences on cognitive tests. *American Psychologist, 59*, 7–13

Seymour, H. N., Abdulkarim, L., & Johnson, V. (1999). The ebonics controversy: An education and clinical dilemma. *Topics in Language Disorders, 19*, 66–77.

Sligh, A. C., & Conners, F. A. (2003). Relation of dialect to phonological processing: African American Vernacular English vs. Standard American English. *Contemporary Educational Psychology, 28*, 205–228.

Steele, C. M., & Aronson, J. (1995). Stereotype threat and the intellectual test performance of African Americans. *Journal of Personality and Social Psychology, 69*, 797–811.

Stroop, J. R. (1935). Studies of interference in serial verbal reactions. *Journal of Experimental Psychology, 18*, 643–661.

Sweetland, J. (2002). Unexpected but authentic use of an ethnically-marked dialect. *Journal of Sociolinguistics, 6/4*, 514–536.

Thompson, C. A., Craig, H. K., & Washington, J. A. (2004). Variable production of African American English across oracy and literacy contexts. *Language, Speech, and Hearing Services in Schools, 35*, 269–282.

Unverzagt, F. W., Gao, S., Baiyewu, O., Ogunniyi, A. O., Gureje, O., Perkins, A., et al. (2001). Prevalence of cognitive impairment: data from the Indianapolis Study of Health and Aging. *Neurology, 57*, 1655 62.

Utsey, S. O., Payne, Y. A., Jackson, E. S., & Jones, A. M. (2002). Race-related stress, quality of life indicators, and life satisfaction among elderly African Americans. *Cultural Diversity and Ethnic Minority Psychology, 8*, 224–233.

Welsh, K. A., Fillenbaum, G., Wilkinson, W., Heyman, A., Mohs, R. C., Stern, et al. (1995). Neuropsychological test performance in African-American and white patients with Alzheimer's disease. *Neurology, 45*, 2207–2211.

Whitfield, K. E., Baker-Thomas, T., Heyward, K, Giatto, M., & Williams, Y. (1999). Evaluating a measure of everyday problem solving for use in African Americans. *Experimental Aging Research, 25*, 209–221.

Willis, S. L., Jay, G., Diehl, M., & Marsiske, M. (1992). Longitudinal change and prediction of everyday task competence in the elderly. *Research on Aging, 14*, 68–91.

Wolf, H., Hensel, A., Kruggel, F., Riedel-Heller, S. G., Arendt, T., Wahlund, L., & Gertz, H. (2004). Structural correlates of mild cognitive impairment. *Neurology of Aging, 25*, 913–924.

Woodard, J. L., Auchus, A. P, Goodsall, R. E., & Green, R. C. (1998). An analysis of test bias and differential item functioning due to race on the Mattis Dementia Rating Scale. *The Journals of Gerontology, 53*(B), P370–P374.

Chapter 8

Developmental Perspectives: Culture and Neuropsychological Development During Childhood

Lúcia Willadino Braga
The SARAH Network of Hospitals for the Locomotor System

Our knowledge of the anatomical development and neuroplasticity of the child's brain has expanded significantly over the years (Parker, 1990; Anderson, Catroppa, Morse, Haritou, & Rosenfeld, 2005). Growth of anatomical structures, the branching out of neuroprocesses, production of glial cells, and the myelination process are common to all human beings, independent of their cultural contexts. However, recent Pet Scan and functional magnetic resonance imaging (fMRI) studies reveal that, although the anatomical substratum of the central nervous system (CNS) is very similar in everyone, individuals of different cultures or even educational levels activate partially distinct neural networks when performing the same tasks in neuropsychological tests (Braga & Campas de Paz, 2000; Castro-Caldas, Petersson, Rei, Stone-Elander, & Ingvar, 1998; Peterson, Reis, Askelöt, Castro-Caldas, & Ingvar, 2000).

The issue of what is common and universal among all human beings and what varies depending on each culture has prompted much discussion in psychology (Berry, Poortinga, Marshall, & Dasen, 2000; Piaget & Inhelder, 1963; Vygotsky, 1978). In neuropsychology, the debate concerning the biological and the cultural is becoming increasingly significant. On the one hand neuropsychological tests aim toward establishing a relation between performance in various tasks and the location of the lesion, whereas on the other we have evidence that these tests are rarely independent of culture and educational level, that is to say, there is a need for adaptations in neuropsychological tests that heed cultural differences and varying levels of education in different cultures (Ardila, Rosselli, & Ostrosky,1992; Ardila, Rosselli, & Rosas, 1989; Castro-Caldas et al.,1997; Ostrosky, Canseco, Quintanar, Navarro, & Ardila,1985).

In this chapter, we address these issues within the scope of the child's development, in addition to briefly reviewing Jean Piaget and Lev Semanovith Vygotsky's theories on the subject.

CONSTRUCTIVIST THEORIES OF DEVELOPMENT

Piaget: Cross-Cultural Studies and the Search for the Epistemic Subject

In the 1920s, the Swiss biologist Jean Piaget began his studies on the cognitive development of the child, searching for aspects common to all human beings during the various stages of childhood and adolescence, independent of cultural influences. His aim was to describe the epistemic subject (Piaget,1926,1932).

Piaget established a parallel between intelligence and biological functions, defining intellectual function as part of the individual's physiological totality. He proposed the existence of one same mode of cognitive operation shared by all humans throughout the various stages of life. Thus, cognitive functioning tendencies would be present in all ages, despite variations related to the maturity level and experience of each person. Piaget called this mode of operating functional invariants and defined as invariant the organization and adaptation functions in the cognitive development process of the human being. Through interaction with the environment, these invariants would permit the emergence and transformation of the cognitive structures for the whole human race (Piaget, 1932, 1937, 1952).

In addition to the mode of cognitive function, Piaget also defined four great sequential stages of development (divided into substages) experienced by all individuals during neurodevelopment (Piaget & Inhelder, 1963, 1966). These stages would, theoretically, appear in every culture, with possible variations related to the age at which each stage commenced. They were termed sensorimotor (0 to approximately 24 months of age), preoperational (2 to 7 years old), concrete operational (seven to 11 or 12 years old) and formal operational (from age 12 onward).

In the Piagetian model, organic growth, neurological maturation, and overall physiology are elements fundamental to psychological development. However, the model has a constructivist focus that maintains that children construct their own development through interaction with the en-

8. DEVELOPMENTAL PERSPECTIVES

vironment; in other words, children are the primary agents of their own development (Piaget, 1945).

Studies about the biology of human cognition began to expand in 1955, with the founding of the International Center for Genetic Epistemology in Geneva. Piaget, together with a team of collaborators and students, became dedicated to researching more profoundly the epistemic subject in the various stages of development. Some of his collaborators began studying the repercussions of the theoretical model on the child's scholastic learning, whereas others concentrated on analyzing the model's applicability in other cultural contexts.

The stages and main principles of piagetian theory were soon carried over to educational models and to the teacher's approach in the classroom. Although Piaget did not specifically write about education, his pupils and collaborators conducted studies in this area based on the theoretical construct that development precedes learning; in other words, it is necessary to await the child's development process, which emerges as a consequence of the relation between biological maturation and interaction with the environment, before initiating formal instruction of new contents. The repercussions on education spread throughout the world and were henceforth applied in schools (regular as well as special education programs) that naturally included children with brain injury as well.

Piaget's theoretical bases were also widely used in the early years of pediatric neuropsychology. Because the child with brain injury, either congenital or acquired, presents developmental problems and Piaget's model is basically a theory of development, it started to be used in establishing parameters for evaluation; the constructivist focus was transformed into a reference for post-brain injury reeducation (Young, 1991).

Another area of research developed at the International Center for Genetic Epistemology, which is also a central point in neuropsychology, was devoted to research in different cultural settings. The main goals of this group's studies were discovering the importance of social interaction on the child's cognitive development and the influence of culture on development, as well as testing the universality of piagetian theory, because Jean Piaget had not investigated the social context in cognitive development (Doise, 1985; Forman & Kraker, 1985). Various studies derived from Piaget's theory began to demonstrate, for example, that interaction with other children is an important facilitator of cognitive development for all involved children, that is to say, social interaction in the performance of group tasks contributed to cognitive development (Doise & Mackie, 1981; Mugny & Doise, 1978; Perret-Clermont & Nicolet, 1988).

Dasen (1977) conducted extensive research about the relation between culture and development and studied the difference between competence and performance in relation to Piaget's stages. He defined competence as a logical representation that the individual recognizes or could implement within a real environment (i.e., language is a universal competence, even for the deaf) whereas performance requires a real device that can implement, in true-life situations, the skill embodied in the competence. In this work, published in 1977 about the cultural aspects of Piaget's theory, Dasen compared children from Swiss urban regions with Canadian Eskimos using piagetian tests and demonstrated that competence in concrete operational structures is apparently universal, but the way in which these competencies are translated into spontaneous behavior is determined by culture. In 1979, Dasen, Lavallée, and Retschitzki tested this hypothesis on Baoulé children from the Ivory Coast. They studied children aged 7 to 14 years old using three quantity conservation tests, one compensation test, and a class inclusion test; the results showed that, in general, competence was present but performance was not. The structures necessary for performance were forged by training, which could be used to reduce the development gap, frequently demonstrated between children from technologically advanced countries and those from other countries. The authors concluded that the gap in performance did not represent an absence of competence: Some competencies are stimulated in certain cultures whereas in others, they are neglected. In a later study, Dasen (1981) discussed why the Baoulé children had better results than the Eskimos in the quantity conservation task and suggested that it was likely due to the fact that those African children lived on farms and rural areas and thus participated in the planting, harvesting, stocking, and selling of agricultural products. Conversely, the Eskimos had better performance in the horizontality conservation task because spatial abilities are more valued in nomadic than in stationary populations. Nell (2000), after analyzing several studies based on piagetian theory in different cultural contexts proposed that "there is persuasive evidence in this series of piagetian tasks studies that the fundamental operations of intellect are invariant across cultures, but that—to use a Vygotsky`s metaphor—culture powerfully determines which cognitive buds will come into flower, and which will lie dormant until they are triggered by situational press" (p. 77).

Vygotsky: A Sociocultural Approach to Development

Lev Semonovitch Vygotsky (1978), who was born in the same year as Jean Piaget, developed a theory based on Karl Marx's material dialectic and Friederich Engels's thinking. Vygotsky demonstrated the importance of culture, society, and education on the cognitive development of the child. He conducted in-depth studies of the relationship between thought and language (Vygotsky, 1987) and proposed the concept of unified analysis in the study of human psychology. Within his concept, language development has a social origin since birth. Vygotsky transposed the notion of mediation, through the use of instruments created by Engels, to the field of psychology. The development of higher mental functions would be mediated by a system of signs that are, together with the instruments, created by society throughout history and are elements that transform culture. Therefore, cognitive development would have a sociocultural genesis.

Vygotsky had access to various publications by Piaget; however, Piaget only became acquainted with his work after his death (Vygotsky died at a young age in 1936). Vygotsky's (1978) view about the relationship between learning and development was opposite to that of Piaget. For Vygotsky, these processes were interrelated from the child's first day of life. Although he acknowledged that learning should in some way be compatible with the child's level of maturity, Vygotsky affirmed that the emphasis should be on the premise that learning results in mental development. In the Vygotskian model, learning is a universal aspect of the process of developing culturally organized psychological functions. Learning presupposes that human development is social in nature and thus constitutes a process whereby children gain entry into the intellectual life of the society and culture to which they belong. In contrast to Piaget's theory that development permits learning, Vygotsky postulated that sociocultural learning promotes development.

A very important aspect of Vygotsky's theory was the establishment of the zone of proximal development (ZPD) concept, which defines functions that have not yet matured; in other words, problems that the child is unable to solve independently, but can do so with the assistance of a qualified peer or an adult partner. As Vygotsky stated, "these functions could be termed the buds of development rather than the fruits of development" (Vygotsky, 1978, p.86). The zone of proximal development represented the space between real development (that which the child is able to do unassisted) and potential development (that which the child can do with assistance).

The zone of proximal development concept had repercussions on pediatric neuropsychology because today's zone of proximal development is tomorrow's real development, and therefore the evaluation of children with brain injury should, in principle, consider not only what they can do unaided but also what they are able to do when assisted. Within this prism, the process of neuropsychological reeducation should also not be limited to working with the functions that the child has already developed but rather, and primarily, should stimulate the child to transcend these limits.

Many professionals, when performing cognitive assessments of the child with brain injury, have incorporated Vygotsky's (1978) zone of proximal development theory. The conventional use of psychometric tests permits the observation of only real development; however, if, after exhausting all the tasks that the child could resolve alone, the examiners started to work with the child, observing the responses, they could uncover the potential development as well.

Vygotsky (1978) questioned the use of conventional psychometric tests, "this procedure oriented learning toward yesterday's development" (p. 88) and argued that the conventional approach could lead the examiner to underestimate the child's capacities. He illustrated this by comparing two children with the chronological age of 10 and mental age of 8 and then, in one way or another, proposing that the children solve the problems with his assistance. Under these circumstances, he observed that the first child could deal with problems up to a 12-year-old's level and the second up to a 9-year-old's level. Vygotsky then queried, "can I say that they are the same age mentally?" (p. 86). In the case of children with cerebral palsy (CP) and traumatic brain injury (TBI), this observation is of particular relevance for two reasons: (1) Neuropsychological evaluation also has the function of orienting the reeducation program; and (2) due to movement disorders or language disturbances often present after brain injury, the children's expression may become limited and, consequently, the assessment of their real and potential development may be hindered (adaptations that facilitate communication or the manipulation of objects could be elaborated for the application of the test). A cooperative approach of coconstruction permits the expression of capacities, thus enabling a true assessment of the brain injured child's real and potential development that in turn generates elements for the creation of an efficient rehabilitation program. It is important to stress that this does not invalidate the use of standardized identification tests in neuropsychological evaluation of the functions affected by the brain injury; rather, this approach simply contributes new elements of reflection that can be incorporated into the examiner's approach to the cognitive evaluation process.

Vygotsky (1993) wrote a book based on his research specifically directed toward children with some type of disability, called *Problems of Abnormal Psychology and Learning Disabilities: The Fundaments of Defectology*. In this book, he proposed that the fundamental laws of development are the same for both normal and handicapped children; in other words, culture is fundamental to development. The only possible differentiation would lie in the fact that handicapped children may create their own pathways to cognitively process the society in which they live. Vygotsky (1993) maintained that the development of the handicapped child is hampered. Consequently, this may occasion creative processes (physical and psychological) that imply in both the creation and recreation of the child's personality due to the restructuring of all adaptive functions and the formation of new processes generated by the handicap, thus permitting the creation of new roundabout paths for development with a basis in culture. Stated succinctly: The physical or mental deficiency could cause limitations and obstacles to the development of the child, but also stimulate creative compensatory processes. Vygotsky affirmed that much of what is inherent to normal develop-

8. DEVELOPMENTAL PERSPECTIVES

ment vanishes or is curtailed due to a defect, and subsequently results in a new and special type of development generated in part by social and cultural interaction.

Vygotsky (1993) admitted that there exists limits in the compensatory processes produced by the handicapped child. He argued, however, that when a defect destroys the existing balance between adaptive functions, the adaptive system is completely restructured on new bases. The entire system moves in the direction of a new balance.

The most relevant point in the theoretical model created by Vygotsky is the principle of the social formation of the mind, which states that the entire development of children with or without deficiency is, since birth, mediated by culture and the social context in which they live. Thus, within Vygotsky's perspective, despite the fact that the child has an analogous neurological substratum and experiences similar phases of maturation, there exist in each society differences in relation to what is or is not valued by culture, and this has a direct influence on the abilities that will develop in the child.

NEUROPSYCHOLOGICAL PROBLEMS IN DEVELOPMENT

The problems that hamper the development of the higher mental functions comprise a very broad spectrum and could occur due to a variety of etiologies. Genetic diseases, cerebral palsy, traumatic brain injury, and stroke, as well as developmental problems such as learning disabilities, dyslexia, attention deficit hyperactivity disorder (ADHD), dyscalculia, and are very frequent. The relevance of each of these problems in the child's development and social insertion depends not only on how much the central nervous system was affected, but also on the significance, within the cultural context that the child lives, of the abilities that were impaired or preserved.

Cerebral Palsy

Cerebral palsy is a syndrome resulting from a nonprogressive lesion to the developing brain that leads to a movement and posture disorder. It is frequently accompanied by associated disorders such as mental retardation, language difficulties, convulsions, and neuropsychological disturbances related to the executive functions, communication, perception, and attention (Braga, 1996).

In CP, the motor difficulties range from severe spastic tetraplegia to mild forms of hemiplegia and monoplegia. There is a group of children that, despite having severe motor involvement, maintain the cognitive functions intact. Conversely, others are able to attain a good level of motor development but present mental retardation or neuropsychological problems that impair scholastic performance. Some children have severe motor and cognitive states whereas others present intact cognitive functions and only mild states with barely perceptible alterations of muscular tonus.

With this wide range of variations, the prognosis of the dimension of CP-related problems for the family and for the social insertion of these children is extremely dependent on the culture and the community in which they live. Illiterate societies or parents with little or no schooling, who earn their living with professional activities centered around physical labor, often have great difficulties accepting the motor deficiencies of the child with CP because they are unable to see a way to make them part of the productive community. In these cases, the fact that the cognitive functions are preserved is sometimes not of great value.

On the other hand, in cultures where schooling and academic competency is important, or in which parents have professions linked to intellectual activity or that are minimally dependent on manual labor, it is more difficult to accept the child who has CP associated with mental retardation than a child with CP who has good cognitive development but is confined to a wheelchair. In technologically advanced cultures, academic opportunities and a job market with chances for gainful employment through intellectual activity, motor deficiencies are of lesser importance whereas neuropsychological disturbances, such as attention deficit, take on immense significance to the family and community (Braga, 1996).

Traumatic Brain Injury

Contrary to CP and genetic diseases such as fragile X syndrome or trisomy 21, which lead to differentiated development from birth, severe TBI and stroke abruptly alter a development that has been taking place within what are considered "normal" patterns. However, these problems also have varying repercussions from culture to culture.

TBI, when severe, could affect various functions and bring significant repercussions to the child's daily life. Depending on the location of the injury, changes in muscular tonus could lead to hemiplegia or tetraplegia. The child may suffer alterations in gait, become unable to walk, or become dependent on support aids such as walkers or crutches. When not correctly evaluated, motor deficits could lead to the impression that the child has cognitive or sensorial deficits that may not be present at all.

Mild trauma does not always have consequences that are evaluated right away. Oftentimes, immediately following the trauma, the physicians give emphasis to aspects of physiological functioning and may ignore cognitive problems that will become more accentuated in the future. Head injury might affect the acquisition of new skills. An evaluation conducted at a given age often fails to take into account those functions that are not ordinarily developed at that specific age. Abilities that are still being evolved, such as

8. DEVELOPMENTAL PERSPECTIVES 153

reading, could suffer greater damage than those that had already been consolidated. Many of the neuropsychological deficits resulting from mild injuries are only perceived later in the development, when poor performance in school signals that something is wrong.

Children with mild brain injury are generally slower in reacting to visuomotor, visuospatial, spatial dexterity, and tasks involving the processing of visual and verbal information. They can also experience difficulties in dealing with information of greater complexity; consequently, as the children advance from one school grade to the next and the quantity of information and breadth of learning stimuli increases, a decline in performance in relation to their peers is often observed. The integration of these children is easier in rural societies than in urban areas with great technological infrastructures. In cultures more geared toward activities such as planting and harvesting, fishing, or livestock raising, neuropsychological deficits have a lesser influence on the child's daily life. However, in urban areas, scholastic performance is greatly valued and technological devices are sometimes not able to overcome or bypass the difficulties that surface during the process of learning to read and write.

Learning Disabilities

Another category of childhood neuropsychological disturbances involves developmental problems such as learning disabilities, dyslexia, and dyscalculia.

Children with learning disabilities do not have mental retardation, nor do they have any disabling physical problem. In sum, a child with learning disabilities is one who has at least average potential and yet has some problem that interferes with learning.

The causes of developmental learning problems are still little known. Children with learning disabilities do not appear to have a high incidence of trauma at birth; some authors have verified that there may exist genetic factors with greater frequency of learning difficulties in children with sex chromosome disorders such as Turner's syndrome (Hier, Atkins, & Perlo, 1980).

Various studies that have attempted to locate the areas in the brain that were affected in children with learning disabilities revealed that the areas more involved in language and syntax, that is, the parietal lobe, seem to present abnormality in these children (Dean,1980; Galaburda & Eidelberg,1982; Levine, Hier, & Calvanio,1981;). Several authors began to associate a number of learning problems with neurochemical deficiencies (Keogh, 2000).

It has been noted that, in societies in which reading and writing are taught early, children present some type of learning problem while they are still in preschool. The child may demonstrate difficulties in recognizing forms and sizes and later, in identifying letters of the alphabet and the sounds of different letters. As far as society is concerned, in contrast to children with attention deficit disorder, those with learning disabilities exhibit good interpersonal relationships with their classmates. In societies where reading and writing is taught at 6 or 7 years of age, learning disabilities are diagnosed later, when the children are 8 or older; they may still consistently interchange the letters "d" and "b" and have trouble determining right from left (Accardo, 1980).

Learning disabilities include a wide gamut of problems that could appear isolated or associated with other developmental neuropsychological difficulties. Nevertheless, these children present normal intelligence and do not have attention deficits. According to Geschwind (1983), the concept of learning disability is less absolute than normally assumed. In illiterate societies, the advantages of the dyslexic may be more evident that the disadvantages. In literate societies, however, the dyslexic may be discriminated against because of a reduced aptitude at reading and writing. On the other hand, children with dysmusia (specific difficulties with music) pass through the entire educational system of literate societies without any great difficulties. Geschwind described the case of a child with dysmusia who did not have any problems with grammar, handwriting, or calculation. He pointed out that, when evaluating learning disabilities, we cannot focus only on changes in the central nervous system; we need also to understand that the advantages or disadvantages are deeply rooted in local or cultural circumstances.

The same concept seems applicable to other specific learning disabilities and to children with attention deficit disorders. The latter exhibit problems with concentration, impulsiveness, clumsiness, or hyperactivity. These children would most probably have better chances of participating actively in an illiterate society.

In sum, we could conclude that, in relation to all the problems that occur during development, children are considered more or less "deficient" because of the daily life, and the cultural and social contexts in which they live.

NEUROPSYCHOLOGICAL EVALUATION OF THE DEVELOPING CHILD: BRAIN INJURY, CULTURE, AND SCHOOLING

Until very recently, the bases of neuropsychological evaluations of children were psychological tests aimed at assessing general cognitive ability. These tests were, and continue to be, associated with neurological exams such as cranial nerves examination motor and praxis examination (Baron, Fennel, & Voeller, 1995). Research into aspects directly linked to neuropsychology frequently involves adapting tasks developed for adults and then applying them to children. This approach often fails to take into account the vast differences between the adult brain and the child's developing one. Only recently have we seen the emergence of neuropsychological evaluations specifically designed and standardized for children with brain injury or learning disabilities. Nevertheless, even with the creation of new tests, we are still faced with basic questions about the relation between lesion and function, and the issue of cultural and educational influence on the child's performance in neuropsychological testing.

The nature of a neuropsychological test implies that it is correlated with the function of a particular network or region of the brain. Brain injury in a particular region would, therefore, result in the loss of the skill assessed by the test. Presently, however, many researchers are defending the theory that performance in neuropsychological tests depends on the cultural level of each individual (Ardila et al, 1989, 1992; Castro-Caldas et al., 1997; Ostrosky, 1985). Several test batteries that have been adapted for use in populations with low socioeconomic levels, or in different cultures, assume that they are assessing equivalent skills (Ostrosky, Ardila, Rosselli, Lopez-Arango, & Uriel Mendoza, 1998).

Levav, Mirky, French, and Bartko (1999) compared results of neuropsychological evaluations of children between 8 and 12 years old in five countries: United States, Ecuador, Canada, Israel, and Ireland. The results of a multivariate analysis revealed that the reaction time measures obtained in tests of sustained attention are minimally affected by country and level of education; in contrast, tests assessing the ability to focus attention and solve a problem, to shift strategies, and to inhibit an automatic response tendency differ significantly by country and level of education.

Several studies demonstrate that babies in different countries obtain number perception before language acquisition (Antell & Keating, 1983; Geary, 1994; Wynn, 1992). By having contact with their bodies and their first toys, babies acquire a natural representation of numbers; between 12 and 18 months of age, when children achieve their first words, they are already capable of deciding which of two collections is more numerous, regardless of their cultural context (Starkey, 1992).

Nell (2000) cited a case study conducted in South Africa in 1988 in which Richter and Griesel compared 722 Black South African children between 2 and 30 months old with a group that served as the reference for standardization of the Bayley Scales of Mental and Motor Development. According to the authors, the South African children significantly outperformed the Americans at ages 2, 3, 4, 5, 6, 8, 10, and 15 months on the mental scale scores and American children obtained better results at other ages, whereas no significant differences between the two groups were found at other months. Nell (2000) also referred to a study conducted by Verster and Prinsloo (1988) that showed that in the 3 to 5 year age bracket, no significant differences were revealed in cognitive tests when South African children who spoke English were compared with those who spoke Afrikaans; however, from the age of 6 onward, with the initiation of reading and writing skills, these differences started to become significant. The aforementioned studies may lead to the hypothesis that in early infancy the influence of culture does not in fact seem to be so important.

It has been verified that social and cultural factors generate more significant repercussions on the neuropsychological evaluation process during the phases in which the acquisition of reading and writing skills become increasingly influential on the child's development, from age 6 or 7 onward (Fuson & Kwon, 1992; Miura, Okamoto, Kim, & Steere, 1993).

Kendall, Verster, and von Mollendorf (1988) asserted that a number of elements from the classroom help testing performance, for example, practice using a pencil, facility with symbols (such as letters and numbers), familiarity with the use of booklets, perception of the importance of paying attention, the habit of following instructions, the custom of preparing for an exam situation, and sitting still as contributors to speed and quality of work. Nevertheless, studies developed with children who do not yet know how to read and write or with restricted skills in these tasks reveal that the capacity for dealing with simple informal mathematics is universal and independent of culture and social class (Klein & Starkey, 1988; Saxe & Posner, 1983). A study conducted with Brazilian children who do not attend school but sell goods on the street in order to survive, demonstrates that the capacity for handling money, performing addition and subtraction, understanding cost, and executing adjustment of prices proportional to current inflation develop despite the absence of scholastic training (Saxe, 1991).

Another aspect important to the discussion of scholastic influence on the child's performance during neuropsychological assessment is the importance that cultures confer on each type of learning as well as the value that it imprints on the schooling process. For example, various studies have shown that Asiatic children have better scholastic performance than American children (Fuson & Kwon,1992; Miura et al., 1993). Research has also demonstrated the influence of socioeconomic class on certain aspects of the learning process in children who know how to read and write; those from lower socioeconomic backgrounds, in the same country, yield inferior scores in most of the evaluated abilities (Jordan, Huttenlocher, & Levine,1994).

We developed a cross-cultural study using the Nucalc calculation evaluation battery for children (Dellatolas et al., 2000). Four hundred and sixty school children aged 7 to 10 years from Brasilia, Brazil (n = 141), Paris, France (n = 160), and Zurich, Switzerland (n = 159) were asked to perform number processing and calculation tasks. The working hypothesis of this investigation was that cultural, educational, and linguistic factors might differentially affect the different components of mathematical development. The same battery of number processing and calculation tests (von Aster, Deloche, Dellatolas, & Meier, 1997) was applied to four groups of children aged 7 to 10 years old from Brazil, France, and Zurich. The battery includes 11 subtests. The four groups differed according to cultural factors, linguistic factors (e.g., different structure of number names in German, French and Portuguese), socioeconomic background and educational systems.

The results of this study demonstrate that counting dots was the only task showing no significant age or group effect. Children performed at a remarkably high level in all groups and age classes, which demonstrates that most children master all the "counting principles" (Gelman & Gallistel, 1978). Counting backwards showed a significant age effect but only a slight marginally significant group effect and no interaction between age and group; this pattern suggests that this task depends more on age than on schooling or culture. Perceptive estimation was characterized by a strong age-by-group interaction, with an increasing level of performance with age in the two European groups, but a decreasing (even if not significant) level of performance with age in the Brazilian group. Such a pattern suggests that European and Brazilian children use different strategies in this task, the former possibly more related to number knowledge, the latter more related to quantities sense. The results led to the division of the Brazilian group into two: Brazil1, consisting of children from middle-class backgrounds and Brazil2, with children from low socioeconomic backgrounds. Among children aged 7 to 8 years, there was a striking difference between the Zurich group (30% correct), and the Brazil2 group (97% correct). The low performance in perceptive estimation of the young children from Zurich may be related to their low performance in tasks involving transcription and comparison of numbers. The very high-level performance of the younger children of Brazil2 clearly suggests that perceptive estimation is independent of schooling (it may be acquired by observing street activities) and furthermore that the acquisition of formal mathematical skills might interfere with the perceptive estimation ability.

In summary, despite its limitations, this transcultural comparison of normally developing young school children provides evidence that linguistic, cultural, and pedagogical factors have varying effects on different components of number processing and calculation, such as counting, literal number knowledge, calculation, or estimation. Therefore, the batteries with neuropsychological calculation tests should consider possible variations in relation to these elements.

There is also overwhelming evidence for important differences in development across national boundaries (Towse & Saxton, 1997), which have been attributed, among other factors, to pedagogical influences such as different teaching methods (Fuson, 1992; Perry, van der Stoep, & Yu, 1993), different attitudes toward learning (Geary, 1994; Stevenson et al., 1990; Stevenson, Chen, & Lee, 1993), preschool experience (Towse & Saxton, 1997; Stein, 1999) and linguistic influences (Miller & Stigler, 1987; Miura et al., 1993; Towse & Saxton, 1997). These cultural or linguistic factors may have a strong effect on some components of development but no effect on others (Carraher, Carraher, & Schliemann, 1985; Nunes, Schliemann, & Carraher, 1993; Shalev, Manor, Amir, & Gross-Tsur, 1993).

The various studies analyzed here lead us to conclude that in the neuropsychological evaluation of the child, several of the functions studied are more susceptible to the influence of culture, schooling, socioeconomic background, and language whereas others appear to be unaffected by these variables. The child's age is also a fundamental aspect in relation to the permeability of culture, that is to say, as we have mentioned before, the neuropsychological development of babies is less dependent on cultural influences.

It is important to bear in mind that the child is in constant development and has a central nervous system that is still being formed; thus, neuropsychological evaluation should seek to provide data that correlate higher mental functions with the injury. However, we cannot lose sight of the cultural influences exerted by the context in which the child lives.

In other words, analysis of this data suggests that it is not feasible to have a single instrument for the neuropsychological assessment of a child in different cultures without first making the necessary adaptations. Tests that evaluate the various neuropsychological functions for each stage of development must be created. Furthermore, when an evaluation instrument developed in one culture is transposed to another, it needs to undergo adaptation and standardization that takes into account age, developmental stage, level of schooling, and culture.

Finally, with this chapter our aim was to highlight the importance that culture and society have on the neuropsychological development of the child. Although anatomically, most children have similar brain structures in common throughout the various states of development, culture and society neverthele4ss have a significant impact on their ability to use and create problem-solving strategies; their overall neuropsychological development; which neural networks they will use in solving cognitive tasks (these may be partially different due to social interaction); and on the nature and quality of social interaction that they will have with the world around them.

REFERENCES

Accardo, P. J. (1980). *A neurodevelopmental perspective on specific learning disabilities*. Baltimore: University Park Press.

Anderson, V., Catroppa, C., Morse, S., Haritou, F., & Rosenfeld, J. (2005). Functional plasticity or vulnerability after early brain injury. *Pediatrics, 116*(6), 1374–1382.

Antell, S. E., & Keating, D. P. (1983). Perception of numerical invariance in neonates. *Child Development, 54,* 695–701.
Ardila, A., Rosselli, M., & Ostrosky, F. (1992). Cultural factors in neuropsychological assessment. In A. E. Puente & R. J. Mcffrey (Eds.), *Handbook of neuropsychological assessment: A biopsychosocial perspective* (pp. 181–192). New York: Academic Press.
Ardila, A., Rosselli, M., & Rosas, P. (1989). Neuropsychological assessment in illiterates: Visuospatial and memory abilities. *Brain and Cognition, 11,* 147–166.
Baron, I. S., Fennel, E. B., & Voeller, K. (1995). *Pediatric neuropsychology in the medical setting.* New York: Oxford University Press.
Berry, J. W., Poortinga, Y. H., Marshall, H., & Dasen, P. (2000). *Cross-cultural psychology: Research and application.* Cambridge, England: Cambridge University Press.
Braga, L. W. (1996). *Cognição e paralisia cerebral: Piaget e Vygotsky em questão* [Cognition and cerebral palsy: Piaget and Vygotsky] (2nd ed.). Salvador, Brazil: Sarah Letras.
Braga, L. W., & Campos da Paz, A., Jr. (2000, September). *Number processing in the brain: A preliminary study using fMRI.* Paper presented at The Year 2000 Conference of Brain Injury, Brasilia, D.F.
Carraher, T. N., Carraher, D. W., & Schliemann, A. D. (1985). Mathematics in the streets and in the schools. *British Journal of Developmental Psychology, 3,* 21–29.
Castro-Caldas, A., Petersson, K. M., Reis, A., Stone-Elander, S., & Ingvar, M. (1998). The illiterate brain: Learning to read and write during childhood influences the functional organization of the adult brain. *Brain, 121,* 1053–1063.
Castro-Caldas, A., Reis, A., Guerreiro, M., Leal, M. G., Ferrajota, L., & Fonseca, J. (1997). Literacy and aphasia revisited. *Journal of Neurology, 244,* 5–47.
Dasen, P. R. (1977). Cross-cultural cognitive development: The cultural aspects of Piaget's theory. *Annals of the New York Academy of Sciences, 285,* 332–337.
Dasen, P. R. (1981). "Strong"and "weak"universals: Sensori-motor intelligences and concrete operations. In B. Lloyd & J. Gay (Eds.), *Universals of human thought* (pp. 137–156). Cambridge, England: Cambridge University Press.
Dasen, P. R., Lavallée, M., & Retschzki, J. (1979). Training conservation of quantity (liquids) in West African (Baoulé) children. *International Journal of Psychology, 14,* 576–568.
Dean, R. S. (1980). Cerebral localization and reading dysfunction. *Journal of School Psychology, 18,* 324–332.
Dellatolas, G., von Aster, M., Braga, L. W., & Deloche, G. (2000). Number processing and mental calculation in school children aged 7 to 10 years: A transcultural comparison. *European Child & Adolescent Psychiatry, 9* (Suppl. 2), I/1–I/9.
Doise, W. (1985). Social regulations in cognitive development. In R. A. Hinde (Ed.), *Social relationships and cognitive development* (pp. 294–308). Oxford: Clarendon Press.
Doise, W., & Mackie, D. (1981). On the social nature of cognition. In P. Forgas (Ed.), *Social cognition: Perspectives on everyday understanding* (pp. 53–83). London: Academic Press.
Forman, E. A., & Kraker, M. J. (1985). The social origins of logic. In M. W. Berkowisk (Ed.), *Peer conflict and psychological growth* (pp. 23–39). San Francisco: Jossey-Bass.
Fuson, K. C. (1992). Research on teaching and learning addition and subtraction of whole numbers. In G. Leinhardt, R. Putman & R. A. Hattrup (Eds.), *Analysis of arithmetic for mathematics teaching* (pp. 39–63). Hillsdale, NJ: Lawrence Erlbaum Associates.
Fuson, K. C., & Kwon, Y. (1992). Korean children's understanding of multidigit addition and subtraction. *Child Development, 63*(2), 491–506.
Galaburda, A. M., & Eidelberg, D. (1982). Symmetry and asymmetry in the human posterior thalamus. *Archives of Neurology, 39,* 333–336.

Geary, D. C. (1994). *Children's mathematical development*. Washington, DC: American Psychological Association.
Gelman, R., & Gallistel, C. R. (1978). *The child's understanding of number*. Cambridge, MA: Harvard University Press.
Geschwind, N. (1983, November). Dysmusia and dyslexia. Paper presented at the Annals of the 33rd Orton Dyslexia Society Meeting, San Diego, CA.
Hier, D. B., Atkins, L., & Perlo, V. P. (1980). Learning disorders and sex chromosome aberrations. *Journal of Mental Deficiency Research, 24,* 183–186.
Jordan, N. C, Huttenlocher, J., & Levine, S. C. (1994). Assessing early arithmetic abilities: Effects of verbal and nonverbal response types on the calculation performance of middle- and low-income children. *Learning and Individual Differences, 6*(4), 413–432.
Kendall, I., Verster, M. A., & von Mollendorf, J. W. (1988). Tests performance. In S. H. Irvine & J. W Berry (Eds.), *Human habilities in cultural context* (pp. 239–299). Cambridge, England: Cambridge University Press.
Keogh, R. (2000) Learning disabilities and neurochemical deficiencies. *Children Learning, 3,* 39–45.
Klein, A., & Starkey, P. (1988). Universals in the development of early arithmetic cognition. *New Directions for Child Development, 41,* 5–26.
Levav, M., Mirky, A. F., French, L. M., & Bartko, J. J. (1999). Multinational neuropsychological testing: Performance of children and adults. *Journal of Clinical and Experimental Neuropsychology, 20,* 658–672.
Levine, D. N., Hier, D. B., & Calvanio, R. (1981). Acquired learning disabilities for reading after left temporal lobe damage in childhood. *Neurology, 31,* 257–264.
Miller, K. F., & Stigler, J. W. (1987). Counting in Taiwanese: Cultural variation in a basic cognitive skill. *Cognitive Development, 2,* 279–305.
Miura, I. T., Okamoto Y., Kim C. C., Chang C. M., Steere, M., & Fayol, M. (1993). Comparisons of children's cognitive representation of number: China, France, Japan, Korea, Sweden, and the United States. *International Journal of Behavioral Development, 17,* 401–411.
Mugny, G., & Doise, W. (1978). Socio-cognitive conflict and structure of individual and collective performance. *European Journal of Social Psychology, 8,* 181–192.
Nell, V. (2000). *Cross-cultural neuropsychological assessment: Theory and practice*. Hillsdale, NJ: Lawrence Erlbaum Associates.
Nunes, T., Schliemann A. D., & Carraher, D. W. (1993). *Street mathematics and school mathematics*. Cambridge, England: Cambridge University Press.
Ostrosky, F., Ardila, A., Rosselli, M., Lopez-Arango, G., & Uriel Mendonza, V. (1998). Neuropsychological test performance in illiterates. *Archives of Clinical Neuropsychology, 13,* 645–660
Ostrosky, F., Canseco, E., Quintanar, L., Navarro, E., & Ardila, A. (1985). A sociocultural effects in neuropsychological assessment. *International Journal of Neuroscience, 27,* 53–66.
Parker, R. S. (1990). *Traumatic brain injury and neuropsychological impairment*. New York: Springer-Verlag.
Perret-Clermont, A. N., & Nicolet, M. (1988). *Interagir et connaitre* [To interact and to know]. Cousset, Switzerland: DelVal.
Perry, M., Van der Stoep, S. W., & Yu, S. L. (1993). Asking questions in first grade mathematics classes: Potential influence on mathematical thought. *Journal of Educational Psychology, 85,* 31–40.
Petersson, K. M., Reis, A., Askelöf, S., Castro-Caldas, A., & Ingvar, M. (2000). Language processing modulated by literacy: A network analysis of verbal repetition in literate and illiterate subjects. *Journal of Cognitive Neuroscience, 12*(3), 364–382

Piaget, J. (1926). *The language and thought of the child*. New York: Harcourt Brace.
Piaget, J. (1932). *Le jugement moral chez l'enfant* [Moral judgment of the child]. Paris: Presses Universitaires de France.
Piaget, J. (1937). *La construction du réel chez l'enfant* [The construction of reality in the child]. Neuchâtel: Delachaux et Niestlé.
Piaget, J. (1945). *La formation du symbole chez l'enfant* [Formation of symbols in the child]. Neuchâtel: Delachaux et Niestlé.
Piaget, J. (1952). *The origins of intelligence in children*. New York: Norton.
Piaget, J., & Inhelder, B. (1963). *La psychologie de l'enfant* [The psychology of the child]. Paris: Presses Universitaires de France.
Piaget, J., & Inhelder, B. (1966). *L'image mentale chez l'enfant* [Mental Imagery in the child: A study of the development of imaginal representation]. Paris: Presses Universitaires de France.
Saxe, G. B. (1991). *Culture and cognitive development: Studies in mathematical understanding*. Hillsdale, NJ: Lawrence Erlbaum Associates.
Saxe, G., & Posner, J. (1983). The development of numerical cognition: Cross cultural perspectives. In H. P. Ginsburg (Ed.), *Development of mathematical thinking* (pp. 23–54). New York: Academic Press.
Shalev, R. S., Manor, O., Amir, N., & Gross-Tsur, V. (1993). The acquisition of arithmetic in normal children: Assessment by a cognitive model of acalculia. *Developmental Medicine Child Neurology, 35*, 593–601.
Starkey, P. (1992). The early development of numerical reasoning. *Cognition, 43*, 93–126.
Stevenson, H. W., Chen, C., & Lee, S. (1993). Mathematics achievement of Taiwanese, Japanese, and American children: Ten years later. *Science, 259*, 53–58.
Stevenson, H. W., Lee, S., Chen, C., Stigler, J. W., Hsu, C., & Kitamura, S. (1990). Contexts of achievement. *Monographs of the Society for Research in Child Development, 55*(1–2, Serial No. 221).
Towse, J. N., & Saxton, M. (1997). Linguistic influences on children's number concept: Methodological and theoretical considerations. *Journal of Experimental Child Psychology, 66*, 362–375.
Verster, J. M., & Prinsloo, R. J. (1988). The diminishing test performance gap between English speakers and Afrikaans speakers in South Africa. In S. H. Irvine & J. W. Berry (Eds.), *Human abilities in cultural context* (pp. 534–559). Cambridge, England: Cambridge University Press.
Von Aster, M., Deloche, G., Dellatolas, G., & Meier, M. (1997). Number processing and calculation in 2nd and 3rd grade school children. *Zeitschrift für Entwicklungspsychologie und Päedagogische Psychology, 24*, 151–166.
Vygotsky, L. S. (1978). *Mind in society: The development of higher psychological process*. Cambridge, MA: Harvard University Press.
Vygotsky, L. S. (1987). Thinking and speech. In R. W. Rieber & A. S. Carton (Eds.), *The collected works of L. S. Vygotsky* (pp. 37–285). New York: Plenum.
Vygotsky, L. S. (1993). *Problems of abnormal psychology and learning disabilities: The fundaments of defectology*. New York: Plenum.
Wynn, K. (1992). Addition and subtraction by human infants. *Nature, 358*, 749–750.
Young, M. M. (1991). *Cognitive development in cerebral palsy children*. New York: Bell & Howell Company.

Chapter 9

Executive Functions in Hispanics: Toward an Ecological Neuropsychology

Carmen G. Armengol
Northeastern University

> *Every culture has its myths. One of our most persistent is that nonliterate people in less developed countries possess something we like to call a "primitive mentality" that is both different from, and inferior to our own. This myth has it that the "primitive mind" is highly concrete, whereas the "Western mind" is highly abstract; the "primitive mind" connects its concrete ideas by rote association, whereas the "Western mind" connects its abstract ideas by general relations; the "primitive mind" is illogical and insensitive to contradictions, whereas the "Western mind" is logical and strives to attain consistency; the "primitive mind" is childish and emotional, whereas the "Western mind" is mature and rational; and so on and on.*
>
> —George Miller (1971, p. vii)

Among neuropsychologists, the notion of executive functions has prompted much discussion and debate. Central to this debate is whether emotional and volitional factors should be incorporated into the definition. The purpose of this chapter is to argue for the necessity of incorporating sociocultural, historical, and emotional factors, as well as a developmental perspective, into any definition of executive functions that is offered. The application of such a definition to cross-cultural neuropsychological studies, and to Hispanics in particular, is also discussed.

Although this argument is not new, and follows the work of Vygotsky and Luria (both highly influential in neuropsychological circles worldwide), it is not universally acknowledged or even accepted (e.g., Denckla, 1996). Furthermore, although the vast majority of neuropsychological research in Latin American countries has followed the general theory and principles expounded by Luria and Vygotsky (Ardila, 1999; Facultad de Psicología, Universidad Autónoma de Morelos, 1998), very little systematic research has been done to examine the impact of different cultural environments on brain organization. The research that does exist describes differences between large cultural groups and the impact of sociodemographic variables (e.g., years of education and socioeconomic status) on batteries of neuropsychological measures. A cross-cultural perspective, which provides methodological approaches to operationalizing the overly vague and broad term *sociocultural factors*, has, however, been lacking (Gasquoine, 1999).

It is well established that education impacts neuropsychological performance on most, if not all, tests of executive functioning (Heaton, Grant, & Mathews, 1986, 1991), although more specific underlying factors responsible for this effect have not been elucidated. There is accumulating evidence that the acquisition of specific skills (e.g., literacy and bilingualism) result in differences in functional organization of the human brain (Kim, Relkin, Lee, & Hirsch, 1997; Castro-Caldas, Petersson, Reis, Stone-Erlander, & Ingvar, 1998; Perani et al., 1998). In a fascinating study comparing six literate with six illiterate right-handed women from the same social and cultural background in southern Portugal, Castro-Caldas et al. (1998) demonstrated, with the use of PET scans, that illiterates had difficulty repeating pseudowords and failed to activate the anterior cingulate cortex and basal ganglia during this task. Eviatar (2000) discusses related issues on the relationship between cultural/linguistic habits and brain organization, citing his own and others' work, and mentioning also that of Vaid and Singh (1989), who reportedly found that scanning habits due to reading from right to left do not show the left preference in the chimeric faces task usually interpreted as reflecting right hemisphere specialization for the processing of faces and emotions.

It seems reasonable to speculate on the extent to which growing up in different cultures, with differential reinforcement of behaviors and acquired skills, language, and values, produces differences in functional brain organization, particularly as they affect executive functions. That is, cultures may differ in the degree to which they emphasize and explicitly train individuals in "executive skills." This in turn may, or may not, affect functional brain organization and development.

From a personal perspective, as a Cuban Mexican graduate student coming to live in the United States, adapting to time-management habits in the

United States required considerable adjustment. I was not used to taking out an agenda to write down a dinner invitation for 2 months hence (specifically, between the hours of 7 p.m. and 10 p.m.). As another example, the Dutch take pride in their pragmatic and efficient approach to life. Indeed, the technological, cultural, and social achievements of a country occupying such a small expanse of land are truly remarkable. A conversation with an artist on Cape Cod, Massachusetts, who himself had been married to a Dutch national, drove the point home. He told of his first arrival at Schiphol Airport in Amsterdam. Coming to a set of escalators, he found them standing still. Taken aback by this, he thought to himself: "So much for the touted efficiency of the Dutch," only to discover that upon placing a foot above the escalator, it started moving! Levine (1998), in his book *A Geography of Time*, provides many fascinating and amusing anecdotes in his studies of differences in time management and the tempo of life across cultures.

To what extent might differences of this nature be reflected, for example, in tasks purporting to measure efficiency in planning and other "executive" tasks, especially when the dependent measure is reaction time- or completion time-based (e.g., Trailmaking A and B)? Cross-cultural differences, in this case, would not merely be a potentially confounding factor in interpreting test results, but would also provide a marvelous opportunity for examining the relationship between learned styles of responding and their impact on brain–behavior relationships. That is the focus of the following discussion.

In this chapter, a model of executive functions that incorporates the role of emotional learning and the contextual significance of acquired values is outlined. After describing the few studies that have examined the performance of Hispanic subjects on tests believed to measure executive functions, an approach that operationalizes specific cognitive and affective functions that are predictive of differences in neuropsychological measures is introduced. This approach is currently being pursued in research conducted by the author in Mexico City, and will be described briefly.

EXECUTIVE FUNCTIONS: AN EVOLVING CONSTRUCT

Planning, anticipation, goal selection, working memory, flexibility, inhibition, and self-monitoring are higher cortical functions considered prime examples of executive functions (Lezak, 1995; Stuss & Benson, 1986). Although there is consensus about the general meaning of these terms, it has proven surprisingly difficult to operationalize these constructs in a manner that fully captures the clinical presentation of patients who demonstrate deficits in these domains (Stuss & Alexander, 2000). In an attempt to bring some consensus to the field, and based on an informal survey of researchers in this area at a national conference, Eslinger (1996) proposed that executive functions be defined as:

> psychological processes that have the purpose of controlling implementation of activation-inhibition response sequences ... that is guided by diverse neural representations (verbal rules, biological needs, somatic states, emotions, goals, mental models) ... for the purpose of meeting a balance of immediate situational, short term, and long-term future goals ... that span physical–environmental, cognitive, behavioral, emotional, and social spheres. (p. 381)

Eslinger's attempt has, so far, not been successful. At least two difficulties have been identified in reaching a consensus regarding the definition of executive functions. One is the tendency among neuroscientists to equate executive functions with the frontal lobes. Another is the difficulty in operationalizing and measuring these functions, which are by nature multifactorial (Stuss & Alexander, 2000). I would argue that a third problem has been the tendency to ignore the differential real-life significance of various tasks, and the context in which goals are initiated and determined.

The prefrontal cortex has traditionally been credited with mediating executive functions (Stuss & Benson, 1986). Yet, nonlocalizationist perspectives on the subject have long brought to the fore the complex neural networks that underlie individual executive functions, along with the important role and contribution of subcortical structures (e.g., caudate, globus pallidus, nucleus accumbens, and thalamus; cf. Denckla & Reis, 1997; Lezak, 1995; Luria, 1966).

Furthermore, there has been an implicit, and at times explicit, tendency to limit executive functions to the realm of "cold cognition" (Denckla, 1996, p. 264). Denckla's definition equates executive functions with "control processes," and she maintains that "the constructs more readily susceptible to the status of central control processes are those of inhibition, delayed responding, maintenance of anticipatory set/preparedness to act, and planning of sequences of selected actions. *Efficiency* and *productivity* [italics added] are observable outcomes of these constructs" (p. 266). Inhibition of emotional responding, which she sees as "the salient EF [executive function] achievement of the preschool age group" allows for "more seemingly rational, objective behavior such as conformity to the task demands [never mind the content] of school or school-like group settings"(p. 267).

Barkley (1996), whom Denckla cites, also refers to Bronkowski's "separation of affect." He claims that the capacity for imposing a delay between stimulus and response enables the individual to "separate the instruction from its affective charge" (p. 315), and thereby attain a response that is "less emotionally charged, better informed, and more likely to be successful or adaptive that a more immediate, passionate, and thoughtless reaction would be."

9. EXECUTIVE FUNCTIONS IN HISPANICS

This emphasis on "separation of affect" finds an echo in earlier writings of Luria. Vygotsky and Luria undertook a seminal study in the early 1900s in the remote regions of Uzbekistan, where the Bolshevik revolution was transforming the area's way of life. Of particular interest to Luria and Vygotsky was the impact of the widespread introduction of literacy into an agrarian society that hitherto had not been exposed to it (Luria, 1976). Luria (1979) and Vygotsky conducted a number of studies specifically geared to analyzing "problem-solving and reasoning, imagination and fantasy, and the ways in which informants evaluated their own personalities" (p. 80). They referred to the latter as "anti-Cartesian experiments," as, contrary to the famous dictum *cogito ergo sum* (I think therefore I am), they found "critical self-awareness to be the final product of socially determined psychological development, rather than its starting primary point, as Descartes' ideas would have us believe" (p. 80). Luria (1979) summarized their findings with nonliterate subjects as follows:

> These people made excellent judgments about facts of direct concern to them, and they could draw all the implied conclusions according to the rules of logic revealing much worldly intelligence. However, as soon as they had to change to a system of theoretical thinking, three factors substantially limited their capability. The first was a mistrust of initial premises that did not arise out of their personal experience. This made it impossible for them to use such premises as a point of departure. Second, they failed to accept such premises as universal. Rather, they treated them as a particular statement reflecting a particular phenomenon. Third, as a result of these two factors, the syllogisms disintegrated into three isolated, particular propositions with no unified logic, and they had no way in which to channel thought into the system. In the absence of such a logical structure, the subjects had to answer the problems by guessing or referring to their own experience. Although our nonliterate peasant groups could use logical relations objectively if they could rely on their won experience, we can conclude that they had not acquired the syllogism as a device for making logical inferences. (p. 80)

In contrast, the educated subjects "immediately drew the correct, and to us obvious, conclusion from each of the syllogisms presented, *regardless of the factual correctness of the premises* [italics added] or their application to a subject's immediate experience" (Luria, 1979, p. 80).

Almost identical conclusions were reached by Cole and his collaborators (Cole, Gay, Glick, & Sharp, 1971) who studied the Kpelle children and young adults in Liberia. Comparisons were made between literate and nonliterate individuals, to gauge the impact of the American style of education that was being introduced into the area. Functions investigated included classification, learning and memory, and several aspects of reasoning, using procedures that presented problems that occurred in the subjects' natural environment and everyday experiences. The authors indicate:

It is *not* the case that the noneducated African is incapable of concept-based thinking nor that he never combines substances to obtain a general solution to a problem. Instead, we have to conclude that the situations in which he applies general, concept-based modes of solution are different and perhaps more restricted than the situations in which his educated age mate will apply such solutions. (p. 225)

One conclusion that might be drawn from these studies is that education promotes the ability to apply logical processes to abstract situations that have no immediate consequence (and therefore emotional charge) for the individual. In real life, as illustrated by situations like those that occur in Northern Ireland and the Middle East, it is clear that educated individuals who are perfectly capable of rational and abstract thought refuse to accept premises that are at odds with their experience or values. Even academicians, if sufficiently invested in a specific point of view, are unlikely to repudiate that viewpoint on the basis of counterevidence or even the logical arguments of others alone (Kuhn, 1970).

Barkley (1996), in his discussion of the relationship between attention and executive functions, comments that "For almost all animals, attending behaviors function to produce a change in the probability of an immediately subsequent consequence (environmental event) for that animal" (p. 309). For him, one of the major distinctions between attention and executive functioning is simply the temporal proximity of what he refers to as the [environmental event]–[response]–[consequence] chain. That is, executive control processes allow the individual to change the probability of a response by inhibiting prepotent responses in order to problem-solve using alternative and potentially more effective strategies. Similarly, Welsh and Pennington (1988) define executive function as "the ability to maintain an appropriate problem-solving set for attainment of a future goal" (p. 201).

What gets lost in these definitions is that the final value of these "more effective strategies" is determined by the degree to which they allow the individual to accomplish goals that are, in essence, *pre-selected on the basis of values shaped by the person's history of interactions with the environment* (i.e., on the basis of anticipated reward and avoidance of punishment). In essence, a critical component of executive functioning, the ability to determine and initiate behavior in pursuit of specific goals, is taken for granted or excluded from analysis.

To illustrate, on testing a teenage girl with the Wisconsin Card Sorting Test (WCST), the examiner observed that rather than simply placing a card under one of the stimulus cards, she would tentatively put it on or near a response pile, while continuing to hold onto the card. She would then quickly glance at the examiner, searching for nonverbal cues to solve what was for her clearly a game (rather than a "test"), and then remove the card at the last moment with a laugh to try again in hopes of better success the next time. Her "goal" was to have fun and use all available cues, rather than to try and solve the task in a serious and supposedly "goal-directed" and logical manner. A more familiar example of where perceived goals conflict with the actual goal would be the situation where the employee deliberately fails at golf, tennis, or whatever, so that the boss can win.

In some cultures, acquiescence and trying to please the examiner may take precedence over performing the task *per se* (see also Perez-Arce, 1999). Along these lines, Díaz-Guerrero (1994) and his collaborators have specifically addressed the impact in Mexican versus American culture that predominant attitudes and values have on an individual's approach to work, academic attainment, and cognitive development. He speaks, for example, of the relative emphasis placed on a person being considered *simpatico* (charming, friendly, caring) versus being efficient. Levav, Mirsky, French, and Bartko (1998) have documented differences between countries on reaction time on an auditory continuous performance task and on the Trailmaking test. Although many variables may account for such findings, it is reasonable to speculate that attitudes toward the testing situation may affect performance on certain (more sensitive) tests and not others.

The critical significance of these goal selection and initiation abilities becomes readily apparent in individuals who have lost the capacity to engage in these activities as a result of damage to orbital prefrontal cortex. Shallice and Burgess (1991) provide an excellent example of this. They describe a study of three head-injured patients with WAIS IQs between 120 and 130 who were given a battery of 13 tests "held to have a frontal component." Two of the patients were well within the normal range on all 13 tests, while the third was below normal on 3 tests (tests on which they did well, including the Cognitive Estimation Test, Bilateral Hand Movements, the Stroop Test, the Tower of London, word fluency, the Modified WCST, the Rey figure, and Proverb Interpretation). On the other hand, "All three patients showed little spontaneous organization in everyday life" (p. 135). When two tests were developed of "their ability to schedule a number of relatively straightforward activities in a restricted period of time," they failed dismally on both. "In addition, they performed in a qualitatively inappropriate fashion. Thus A started the test by making notes for 4 minutes, which he never subsequently used, and B spent 10 minutes on one task and did not even tackle a second that was very similar" (p. 135).

There are numerous other single case examples of individuals reported in the literature who perform well on standard psychometric tests but who are severely incapacitated in real life (e.g., Benton, 1991; Damasio, 1994; Eslinger & Damasio, 1985; Walsh, 1991). I recall one patient, described by a colleague, who was failing the WCST. When he was asked, after a long string of unsuccessful responses, what he could learn from the fact that the last three responses were wrong, he answered, with his usual pleasant smile,

"Beats me." When asked, again, if he could try to figure it out, he responded (again with his unruffled demeanor and pleasant smile), "Oh, I don't think that's my job." In other words, he had completely failed to establish set on the task, which was to infer the rules in order to respond correctly, and was therefore also quite undisturbed by his repeated failures.

Although acknowledging that the neuroanatomical basis for many of the specific aspects of executive functioning remains to be elucidated, there is a body of literature that describes at least two functional divisions of prefrontal cortex (e.g., Benton, 1991; Pribram, 1990; Walsh, 1991). Thus, the dorsolateral prefrontal cortex is associated with planning, organization, working memory, error utilization (the so-called *knowing–doing* disconnection described by Teuber, 1964), or the inability to let verbalization guide behavior), learning, and reasoning. The orbital prefrontal cortex is highly connected with limbic structures and is seen as mediating prioritizing, grasping the nature of the task (establishing set), and initiating goals and action. Inhibition and response selection are also critical functions thought to be mediated by this brain region.

Dias, Robbins, and Roberts (1996) have demonstrated that impairment of orbitofrontal cortex in monkeys results in "a sort of defect that makes impossible to change behavior when changing the emotional content of the stimuli," whereas damage to lateral prefrontal cortex produces "a loss of inhibitory control in attentional selection." Bechara, Tranel, and Damasio (2000) measured the galvanic skin response (GSR) of patients with bilateral lesions of the ventromedial cortex during two versions of a card game. Results indicated that these patients preferred the task with low immediate punishment but much lower future reward to that with high immediate punishment but even higher future reward. They interpreted this as inability to foresee the future myopia for the future, or an insensitivity to future consequences, while being primarily guided by immediate prospects. They refer to it as a "decision-making deficit." Interestingly the GSR in response to reward or punishment did not differ between controls and patients, but in an earlier study (Bechara, Tranel, Damasio, & Damasio, 1996) patients with prefrontal lesions (in contrast to normal controls) failed to generate anticipatory GSRs prior to selecting a given card. This was interpreted as their failing "to activate biasing signals that would serve as value markers in the distinction between choices with good or bad future outcomes" (p. 215). Bechara, Damasio, & Damasio (2000) review studies of the relationship between emotion, decision-making, and other cognitive functions such as working memory. Damasio's 1994 book, *Descartes' Error,* is an attack on the belief that mind and body can be separated, and that subjective feeling states can be dissociated from executive functions such as reasoning.

Rolls, Hornak, Wade, and McGrath (1994) describe the difficulties of patients with damage to the ventral part of the frontal lobes who perseverated on responses to previously rewarded stimuli, even though they were able to report verbally that the contingencies had changed. Such perseveration correlated with scores on a questionnaire reflecting the degree of disinhibited and socially inappropriate behavior demonstrated by these patients. Walsh (1991) describes a young woman with an IQ of 135 who consistently failed to succeed in jobs. For example, she excelled in the theoretical orientation to nursing provided by the hospital to new trainees but was dismissed within a few days of starting her work on the wards. On testing, she persisted in her errors even while verbalizing an awareness of the fact that "I always go wrong here." "She was unable to modify her behavior not only on successive trials, but even within the same trial, making repeated errors at the same choice point. She was mildly perplexed by her inability to learn but was quite happy to continue trying. Not once did she show any obvious frustration" (p. 187).

In summary, critical capabilities such as establishing set-on tasks, initiating, setting, and prioritizing goals that have *purpose* and *value* to the individual, and sensitivity to future consequences, must all be included in any ecologically sound definition of executive functions. Priorities cannot be established in a vacuum. The presumed ecological purpose of neocortical development (i.e., improved ability to respond to a complex and increasingly socially determined environment) should not be dismissed in favor of a reductionistic analysis of executive functioning as *process* without *content* ("cold cognition"). Although the ability to reason abstractly through the use of acquired symbolic forms may be highly adaptive to certain situations, in real life thinking without purpose (i.e., with the goal of action) may represent good reasoning but hardly, most would agree, intelligent (adaptive) behavior.

Values are derived and shaped largely from experience and through social instruction. In this sense, executive functions (knowing what to inhibit when and how to prioritize) must reflect the social and cultural environment of the individual. Where this is not so, psychopathology is deemed present (as a failure to learn from social and emotionally driven experiences), and there is a growing body of literature precisely examining the (presumed prefrontal) executive mechanisms underlying such failures in social learning (e.g., Hornak, Rolls, & Wade, 1996; Siegel, 1999). The importance of social and emotional intelligence has also been emphasized in the writings of Goleman (1994) and LeDoux (1996).

Acknowledging the critical contribution of social factors to executive functions does not deny the existence of a developmental process in the maturation of executive capabilities. Diamond (1991) has demonstrated that preschoolers before the age of approximately 3½ years demonstrate many of the behaviors (e.g., poor error utilization and failure to inhibit prepotent responses) that are characteristic of adults with acquired lesions to the frontal lobes. Importantly, in order to determine that the underlying "deficit" could not be accounted for by other cognitive factors (e.g., restricted working memory), Diamond employed well-designed control tasks, and adapted her tasks to those familiar to children. Thus, she was not content to simply describe differences on tasks between children of different ages, but was determined to analyze the underlying developmental processes. This is a methodology that cross-cultural neuropsychologists (i.e., those interested in the impact of culture on brain organization) should also employ, using culturally appropriate, familiar activities and objects, and going beyond a simple description of level of performance on tasks.

STUDIES OF EXECUTIVE FUNCTIONS IN HISPANICS

The few studies that have looked at executive functions in Hispanics to date are primarily descriptive in nature, form part of a more comprehensive protocol, and are driven by a concern to provide suitable tests for clinical use and normative data for interpretation (e.g., Ardila, Rosselli, & Puente, 1994; Artiola i Fortuni, Heaton, & Hermosillo, 1998; Ostrosky-Solís, Ardila, & Rosselli, 1999; Pontón et al., 1996; Rey, Feldman, Rivas-Vázquez, Levin, & Benton, 1999). For the interested reader, Ardila (1995, 1999) provides an overview of the history of neuropsychology in Latin America, and the various centers where tests have been developed and standardized.

In their study of Colombians of different age groups and educational levels, Ardila et al. (1994) included, as measures that traditionally might be thought of as reflecting "frontal" or executive contributions, digit span (forward and backward), visual cancellation, a verbal fluency measure, a verbal list learning task, and the Rey figure. In this and their previous studies, the impact of education as well as age is apparent on tasks across the board, including those deemed primarily motoric or visuospatial in nature. There is no explicit discussion of executive functions such as planning or inhibition, and the Rey figure was not analyzed in terms of any planning or organizational score.

Pontón and collaborators (Pontón et al., 1996; Pontón, González, Hernández, Herrera, & Higareda, 2000) adapted a number of tests from the World Health Organization Battery and administered them to 342 Spanish-speaking volunteers in the greater Los Angeles area, stratified by age and education. Other predictors included gender, scores on an acculturation scale, bilingualism, and duration of residence in the United States. Other than verbal fluency, digit span forward and backward, a verbal list learning test, a Color Trails test, and the Rey figure, there were no other traditional measures of executive ability. Once again, education was highly correlated with all measures, including visuospatial ability (e.g., Digit Symbol, Rey figure copy). Age was negatively correlated with test performance, and age and education interacted on digits backward such that older, less educated subjects scored the lowest.

In a comparison of older, predominantly Spanish-speaking and primarily English-speaking adults matched on age and years of education, Jacobs et al. (1997) found that English-speaking participants did better in 5 out of 14 measures. These included the Benton Visual Retention Test (matching and recognition memory), category verbal fluency, Boston Diagnostic Aphasia Examination complex ideation, and the Identities and Oddities of the Mattis Dementia Rating Scale (DRS). There were no differences on the Buschke Selective Reminding Test, Orientation on the Mini-Mental, Similarities on the Mattis DRS, phonemic word list generation, short version of the Boston Naming Test, auditory comprehension and repetition from the BDAE, and the Rosen Drawing test. Level of acculturation (measured as self-rated English proficiency) and years of immigration did not predict differences on those five tasks. When the Spanish-speaking group was divided into two subgroups, including those with the highest self-ratings of English proficiency versus those with the lowest self-rating, statistical differences emerged between the low proficiency Hispanics and the primarily English speakers, whereas the high proficiency English-speaking Hispanics did not differ from either group.

Artiola i Fortuni et al. (1998) conducted a normative study of 400 Spanish speakers from Spain and Mexico and reported significant effects of education and duration of residence in the United States on performance of the WCST. They comment on the clinical implications of these findings.

The study by Rey et al. (1999) is important in documenting that after controlling for age, gender, and education, no significant differences were observed across a range of tasks from the Multilingual Aphasia Examination presented to 75 predominantly Spanish-speaking Hispanics in Dade County, Florida., compared to the original standardization sample of English speakers on the same instruments. When the WCST was administered, almost identical findings emerged for the Hispanics when demographics were comparable to the original Heaton normative groups. These findings again emphasize the importance of education and age relative to first language. Degree of acculturation as a possible predictor of differences was not addressed in this study, which is unfortunate in the context of prior findings from other studies that such factors can and do make a difference (see earlier).

Ostrosky-Solís et al. (1999) constructed a brief neuropsychological (25 to 30 minutes administration time) test battery in Spanish, which measures a wide range of functions. The instrument was standardized with Mexican volunteers from five regions of the country. A factor analysis yielded seven major groups. Of interest is Factor 1, which the authors labeled the Executive Function Factor and which accounted for most of the variance (28.6%

out of a total of 61.7%). It correlated best with tasks such as Digits Backwards (.64), Copy of a Semicomplex Figure (.74), Calculation Abilities (.64), Language Comprehension (.70), and Sequences (.66). Other tasks with high loadings in this factor include Orientation to time (.58), Phonologic Verbal Fluency (.58), Similarities (.58), Twenty Minus Three (.54), and Recall of a Semicomplex Figure (.52). Years of education significantly affected performance on the majority of subtests, with the greatest effect evident on visuoconstructional, phonological verbal fluency and conceptual functions (similarities, calculation, and motor sequences). A ceiling effect at higher levels of education (10 to 24 years) was observed. Although the aim of the authors was not to investigate any specific function in depth but to provide a quick comprehensive screening instrument normed in a Spanish-speaking population, it is noteworthy that factors associated with executive functions showed the greatest differentiation among educational groups in their normative sample.

These studies clearly document that literacy and level of education have an impact on most tasks, but most particularly on those related to "executive functioning." This finding holds no surprise, and the importance of providing age and education corrections to normative data is undeniable, as attested to trends in presentation of normative data over the last 20 years (e.g., Heaton, Grant, & Adams, 1986, 1991; Leckliter & Matarazzo, 1989). Perhaps more interesting, however, is the impact of acculturation on performance on tasks tapping into executive functions (Artiola i Fortuni, et al., 1998; Jacobs et al., 1997). Further investigation into cultural factors that underlie these differences is needed.

Others have noted that socioeconomic status is often confounded with culture (Ardila, 1995; Pérez-Arce, 1999). This variable was rarely considered in the previously mentioned studies. The influence of socioeconomic status (SES) was illustrated in developmental studies of the ability to inhibit prepotent responses, using a Spanish version of the Stroop (Armengol, 2002; Armengol & Méndez, 1999). In a study comparing children from Grades 1 through 6 in a private versus public school in Mexico City, where SES was assessed by asking parents to fill out questionnaires regarding occupation and education, significant differences were found such that children from low SES backgrounds were significantly worse than students of high SES (Armengol, 2002). The study also found that the performance of bilingual children in Massachusetts from predominantly lower SES backgrounds was closer to that of low SES children in Mexico City. Values obtained on higher SES Mexican children were equivalent to the early normative data from Comalli, Wapner, and Werner (1962) in American children, although, unfortunately, SES data on the latter were not reported.

Interestingly, in the Mexico City sample, parental education was correlated with the child's degree of self-monitoring on the Stroop, as measured by the number of self-corrections made in the interference condition. This, and other relationships between parental education and child's performance (Armengol, 2002) raises important questions about the possible impact of the parents' executive abilities on their children's approach to tasks and how these might be transmitted.

Further studies are currently under way in Mexico City to investigate executive and attentional functions in elementary school children in relation to parental factors and to academic performance. In addition, parent and teacher ratings of each child's real life executive abilities were obtained, using a Spanish adaptation of the Behavioral Rating Inventory of Executive Functions or BRIEF (Gioia, Isquith, Guy, & Kenworthy, 2000). The BRIEF was developed as a screening instrument that samples several aspects of executive functioning through ratings by parents and teachers of behaviors described in 86 statements, which yield 8 clinical and 2 validity scales. The statements, which refer to eight areas of executive function (working memory, initiation [or *initiate*], planning and organization [or *plan/organize*], organization of materials, monitoring [or *monitor*], inhibition [or *inhibit*], shifting [or *shift*], and emotional control), are rated on a 3-point scale *(never, sometimes, frequently)*. For the U.S. normative sample, parents and teachers filled out protocols on children of various ages (5–18) from different areas of the United States. Factor analysis of the original standardization sample was carried out for teachers and parents separately. For the data obtained from teachers the analysis yielded two factors: one termed *meta-cognition*, and the other *behavioral regulation*. Scales comprising the first factor (meta-cognition) were *working memory, initiate, plan/organize,* and *inhibit* for the teacher samples. The behavioral regulation factor included *inhibit, shift,* and *emotional control* for the teacher samples. The parent data resulted in the *inhibit* scale loading only on the second factor, but for the rest, the scales' loading on the two factors were similar.

The BRIEF was translated into Spanish. A pilot study ($N = 15$) was conducted in Mexico by this author to ensure that the terminology and meaning of the statements was clear. Specific items were also screened for cultural appropriateness. This resulted in the modification of some items (e.g., one item in English refers to the child's ability to keep his or her locker at school tidy; in Mexico children do not have lockers at school). Preliminary analysis on ratings by parents and teachers of 242 children in Mexico City revealed interesting differences in the factor structure between a subset of the American normative sample matched by age and SES to the Mexican samples (Isquith, Gioia, & Armengol, 2000).

Most surprising were data from the Mexican parent sample, which resulted in a three-factor solution. Thus, for the Mexican parent sample, *Plan/Organize, Working Memory,* and *Initiate* yielded a first factor (*meta-cognition*); the second factor was comprised of the *Inhibit, Shift,* and *Emotional*

Control factors; the third factor resulted from the *Organization of Materials* scale. Interestingly, the *Monitor* scale failed to load on any factors for the Mexican parents. Items that comprise this scale include: (a) doesn't ask for help when needed, (b) doesn't check work for mistakes, (c) makes careless errors, (d) poor handwriting, (e) unaware of how behavior affects others, and (f) leaves work incomplete. It is interesting to note that these observations are viewed by parents as unconnected with each other, whereas for the teachers the relationship between these items holds. Further exploration of these issues is currently under way, and these ratings will be correlated with the children's actual performance on various measures of executive ability (e.g., a computerized sustained attention task, an adaptation of the California Card Sorting Test, the Stroop, and other measures of problem-solving and linguistic ability).

CONCLUSION

There is a reasonable amount of data documenting the impact of demographic variables such as education, socioeconomic status, and, to a lesser extent, degree of acculturation on a wide range of cognitive functions. A cross-cultural approach to neuropsychology depends on the ability of researchers to operationalize these broad constructs to allow for a more in-depth analysis of mediating variables. Executive functions, insofar that they play an important role in determining the individual's approach to tasks, present a natural area of study to focus on. These functions include: setting and prioritizing goals (based on learned values), awareness of environmental (and specifically social) contingencies, and the ability to determine which syllogistic premises are correct and which are not while problem solving.

Rather than defining executive functions in terms of nonmodality specific processes that are divorced from contingencies and affect, as some have argued, an ecological perspective requires that the *content*, and not just the *process* of executive functioning be considered. Thus parents from certain social strata may be more inclined to *value, model, and teach* specific behaviors that translate into higher scores on neuropsychological measures of executive ability (e.g., showing initiative, structuring one's own activities, approaching new situations with confidence, neatness, asking for help when needed, checking for mistakes, etc.). The author is currently collecting data relevant to these issues.

Much tacit knowledge that is embedded in cultures needs to be made explicit. The very fact that some theorists insist on a decontextualized definition of executive functions that excludes affect, all in the name of efficiency, may speak to a specific cultural bias. Latinos may well cringe at the thought of a highly "efficient" (to what end, one might ask) but joyless society. The

Kingdom of Bhutan may be on to something in insisting on Gross National Happiness as the measure of success, rather than Gross National Product!

ACKNOWLEDGMENT

The author wishes to acknowledge the invaluable assistance of Dr. Elisabeth Moes in the various stages of the preparation of this chapter.

REFERENCES

Ardila, A. (1995). Directions of research in cross-cultural neuropsychology. *Journal of Clinical and Experimental Neuropsychology, 17,* 143–150.
Ardila, A. (1999). Spanish applications of Luria's assessment methods. *Neuropsychology Review, 9,* 63–70.
Ardila, A., Rosselli, M., & Puente, A. E. (1994). *Neuropsychological evaluation of the Spanish speaker.* New York: Plenum Press.
Armengol, C. G. (2002). The Stroop test in Spanish: Children's norms. *Neuropsychologist, 16,* 67–80.
Armengol, C. G., & Méndez, M. (1999). Lectura y Stroop en bilingües. La prueba de interferencia Stroop y la eficacia en la lectura: Estudio normativo en escolares bilingües de cuarto grado [The Stroop test in bilinguals: The Stroop test of interference and language proficiency]. *Revista Española de Neuropsicología, 1,* 21–27.
Artiola i Fortuni, L., Heaton, R. K., & Hermosillo, D. (1998). Neuropsychological comparison of Spanish-speaking subjects from U.S.–Mexico border region versus Spain: The Wisconsin Card Sorting Test. *Journal of the International Neuropsychological Society, 4,* 77.
Barkley, R. A. (1996). Linkages between attention and executive functions. In G. R. Lyon & N. A. Krasnegor (Eds.), *Attention, memory, and executive function* (pp. 307–326). Baltimore. MD: Paul H. Brookes.
Bechara, A., Damasio, H., & Damasio, A. R. (2000). Emotion, decision making and the orbitofrontal cortex. *Cerebral Cortex, 10,* 295–307.
Bechara, A., Tranel, D., & Damasio, H. (2000). Characterization of the decision-making deficit of patients with ventromedial prefrontal cortex lesions. *Brain, 123,* 2189–2202.
Bechara, A., Tranel, D., Damasio, H, & Damasio, A. R. (1996). Failure to respond automatically to anticipated future outcomes following damage to prefrontal cortex. *Cerebral Cortex, 6,* 215–225.
Benton, A. L. (1991). The prefrontal region: Its early history. In H. S. Levin, H. M. Eisenberg, & A. L. Benton (Eds.), *Frontal lobe function and dysfunction* (pp. 3–34). Oxford, England: Oxford University Press.
Castro-Caldas, A., Peterson, K. M., Reis, A., Stone-Erlander, S., & Ingvar, M. (1998). The illiterate brain: Learning to read and write during childhood influences the functional organization of the adult brain. *Brain, 121,* 1053–1063.
Cole, M., Gay, J., Glick, J. A., & Sharp, D. W. (1967). *The cultural context of learning and thinking.* New York: Basic Books.
Comalli, P. E., Wapner, S., & Werner, H. (1962). Interference effects of Stroop color-word test in childhood, adulthood, and aging. *Journal of Genetic Psychology, 100,* 47–53.
Damasio, A. R. (1994). *Descartes' error: Emotion, reason, and the human brain.* New York: Grosset/Putnam.

Denckla, M. B.(1996). A theory and model of executive function: A neuropsychological perspective. In G. R. Lyon & N. A. Krasnegor (Eds.), *Attention, memory, and executive function* (pp. 263–278). Baltimore: Paul H. Brookes.
Denckla, M. B., & Reis, A. L. (1997). Prefrontal–subcortical circuits in developmental disorders. In N. A. Krasnegor, G. R. Lyon, & P. S. Goldman-Rakic (Eds.), *Development of the prefrontal cortex: Evolution, neurobiology, and behavior* (pp. 283–294). Baltimore: Paul H. Brookes.
Diamond, A. (1991). Guidelines for the study of brain–behavior relationships during development. In H. S. Levin, H. M. Eisenberg, & A. L. Benton (Eds.), *Frontal lobe function and dysfunction* (pp. 339–380). New York: Oxford University Press.
Dias, R., Robbins, T. W., & Roberts, A. C. (1996). Dissociation in prefrontal cortex of affective and attentional shifts. *Nature, 380,* 69–72.
Díaz-Guerrero, R. (1994). *Psicología del mexicano: Descubrimiento de la etnopsicología* [Psychology of the Mexican: Discovering ethnopsychology]. México, Mexico City: Trillas.
Eslinger, P. J. (1996). Conceptualizing, describing, and measuring components of executive functions: A summary. In G. R. Lyon & N. A. Krasnegor (Eds.), *Attention, memory, and executive functions* (pp. 367–395). Baltimore: Paul H. Brookes.
Eslinger, P. J., & Damasio, A. R. (1985). Severe disturbances of higher cognition after bilateral frontal lobe ablation. *Neurology, 35,* 1731–1741.
Eviatar, Z. (2000). Culture and brain organization. *Brain and Cognition, 42,* 50–52.
Facultad de Psicología, Universidad Autónoma de Morelos. (1998). *Vigotsky en la Psicología y la educación* [Vygotsky in education and psychology]. Cuernavaca, Morelos, México: Universidad Autónoma del Estado de Morelos.
Gasquoine, P. G. (1999). Variables moderating cultural and ethnic differences in neuropsychological assessment: The case of Hispanic Americans. *The Clinical Neuropsychologist, 13,* 376–383.
Gioia, G. A., Isquith, P. K., Guy, S. C., & Kenworthy, L. (2000). *Behavioral Rating Inventory of executive function*. Odessa, FL: Psychological Assessment Resources.
Goleman, D. (1994). *Emotional intelligence*. New York: Bantam Books.
Heaton, R. H., Grant, I., & Mathews, C. G. (1986). Differences in neuropsychological test performance associated with age, education, and sex. In I. Grant & K. M. Adams (Eds.), *Neuropsychological assessment of neuropsychiatric disorders* (pp. 100–120). New York: Oxford University Press.
Heaton, R. H., Grant, I., & Mathews, C. G. (1991). *Comprehensive norms for an extended Halstead-Reitan battery: Demographic corrections, research findings, and clinical applications*. Odessa, FL: Psychological Assessment Resources.
Hornak, J., Rolls, E. T., & Wade, D. (1996). Face and voice expression identification in patients with emotional and behavioral changes following ventral frontal lobe damage. *Neuropsychologia, 34,* 247–261.
Isquith, P., Gioia, G. A, & Armengol, C. G. (2000, July). *Executive control functions in children: Concepts and assessment methods*. Workshop delivered at the XXIII Annual Colloquium of the International School Psychology Association: School Psychology Around the World: Many Languages, One Voice for Children. Durham, NH.
Jacobs, D. N., Sano, M., Albert, S., Shofield, P., Dooneief, G., & Yaakov, S. (1997). Cross-cultural neuropsychological assessment: A comparison of randomly selected, demographically matched cohorts of English- and Spanish-speaking older adults. *Journal of Clinical and Experimental Neuropsychology, 19,* 331–339.
Kim, K. H., Relkin, N. R., Lee, K. M., & Hirsch, J. (1997). Distinct cortical areas associated with native and second languages. *Nature, 388,* 171–174.
Kuhn, T. S. (1970). *The structure of scientific revolutions*. Chicago: University of Chicago Press.

Leckliter, I. N., & Matarazzo, J. D. (1989). The influence of age, education, IQ, gender, and alcohol abuse on Halstead Reitan neuropsychological test battery performance. *Journal of Clinical Psychology, 45,* 484–512.
LeDoux, J. (1996). *The emotional brain.* New York: Simon & Shuster.
Levav, M., Mirsky, A. F., French, L. M., & Bartko, J. J. (1998). Multinational neuropsychological testing: Performance of children and adults. *Journal of Clinical and Experimental Neuropsychology, 20,* 658–672.
Levine, R. V. (1998). *A geography of time: The temporal misadventures of a social psychologist, or how every culture keeps time just a little bit differently.* New York: Basic Books.
Lezak, M. D. (1995). *Neuropsychological assessment* (3rd ed.). New York: Oxford University Press.
Luria, A. R. (1966). *Higher cortical functions in man.* New York: Basic Books.
Luria, A. R. (1976). *Cognitive development: Its cultural and social foundations.* M. López-Morrillas and L. Solotaroff (Trans). Cambridge, MA: Harvard University Press.
Luria, A. R. (1979). *The making of mind: A personal account of Soviet psychology* (M. C. Cole & S. Cole, Eds.). Cambridge, MA: Harvard University Press.
Miller, G. A. (1971). Foreword. In M. Cole, J. Gray, J. A. Glick, & D. W. Sharp (Eds.), *The cultural context of learning and thinking.* New York: Basic Books.
Ostrosky-Solís, F., Ardila, A., & Rosselli, M. (1999). NEUROPSI: A brief neuropsychological test battery in Spanish with norms by age and educational level. *Journal of the International Neuropsychological Society, 5,* 413–433.
Perani, D., Paulesu, E., Galles, N. S., Dupoux, E., Dehaene, S., Dettinardi, V., et al. (1998). The bilingual brain. Proficiency and age of acquisition of the second language. *Brain, 121,* 1841–1842.
Peréz-Arce, P. (1999). The influence of culture on cognition. *Archives of Clinical Neuropsychology, 14,* 581–592.
Pontón, M. O., Gonzalez, J. J., Hernandez, I., Herrera, L., & Higareda, I. (2000). Factor analysis of the Neuropsychological Screening Battery for Hispanics (NeSBHIS). *Applied Neuropsychology, 7,* 32–39.
Pontón, M. O., Satz, P., Herrera, L., Urrutia, C. P., Ortiz, F., Young, et al. (1996). The neuropsychological screening battery for Hispanics: A preliminary report. *Journal of the International Neuropsychological Society, 2,* 94–104.
Pribram, K. (1990). The frontal cortex-A Luria/Pribram rapprochement. In. E. Goldberg (Ed.), *Contemporary neuropsychology and the legacy of Luria* (pp. 77–98). Hillsdale, NJ: Lawrence Erlbaum Associates.
Rey, G. J., Feldman, E., Rivas-Vázquez, R. A., Levin, B. E., & Benton, A. (1999). Neuropsychological test development and normative data on Hispanics. *Archives of Clinical Neuropsychology, 14,* 593–602.
Rolls, E. T., Hornak, J., Wade, D., & McGrath, J. (1994). Emotion-related learning in patients with social and emotional changes associated with frontal lobe damage. *Journal of Neurology, Neurosurgery and Psychiatry, 57,* 1518–1524.
Shallice, T., & Burgess, P. (1991). Higher-order cognitive impairments and frontal lobe lesions in man. In H. S. Levin, H. M. Eisenberg, & A. L. Benton (Eds.), *Frontal lobe function and dysfunction* (pp. 125–138). New York: Oxford University Press.
Siegel, L. J. (1999). Executive functioning characteristics associated with psychopathy in incarcerated females (women inmates). *Dissertation Abstracts International, 59*(11-B), 6112.
Stuss, D. T., & Alexander, M. P. (2000). Executive functions and the frontal lobes: A conceptual view. *Psychological Research, 63,* 289–298.
Stuss, D. T., & Benson, D. F. (1986). *The frontal lobes.* New York: Raven Press.

Teuber, H. L. (1964). The riddle of frontal lobe function in man. In J. M. Warren & K. Akert (Eds.), *The frontal granular cortex and behavior* (pp. 410–444). New York: McGraw Hill.

Vaid, J., & Singh, M. (1989). Asymmetries in the perception of facial affect: Is there an influence of reading habits? *Neuropsychologia, 27,* 1277–1287.

Walsh, K. (1991). *Understanding brain damage* (2nd ed.). Edinburgh, Scotland: Churchill Livingstone.

Welsh, M. C., & Pennington, B. F. (1988). Assessing frontal lobe functioning in children: Views from developmental psychology. *Developmental Neuropsychology, 4,* 199–230.

Chapter **10**

Illiterates and Cognition: The Impact of Education

Alfredo Ardila
Florida International University

Mónica Rosselli
Florida Atlantic University

Illiterates represent a nonneglectable percentage of the world population (about one fifth of the world population; www.uis.unesco.org/en/stats/statistics/literacy2000.htm). Average educational level of contemporary man is about 3–4 years of school. Just a few centuries ago, reading and writing abilities were simply uncommon among the general population. Writing, as a matter of fact, has only existed during the past 5 to 6,000 of years of human history. It may be conjectured that the acquisition of these skills may have somehow changed the brain organization of cognitive activity in general.

It has been well established that educational attainment highly correlates with scores on standard tests of intelligence. This correlation ranges from about 0.57 to 0.75 (Matarazzo, 1979); thus, education accounts for nearly 50% of the intelligence test performance. Correlations with verbal intelligence subtests are usually higher (from about 0.66 to 0.75) than correlations with performance intelligence subtests (from about 0.57 to 0.61). Evidently, education represents the most crucial variable in cognitive test scores.

Several studies have demonstrated a similarly strong association between educational level and performance on various neuropsychological measures (e.g., Ardila, Ostrosky-Solis, Rosselli, & Gomez, 2000; Ardila, Rosselli, Ostrosky, & Puente, 1992; Ardila, Rosselli, & Puente, 1994;

Bornstein & Suga, 1988; Finlayson, Johnson, Reitan, 1977; Heaton, Grant, & Mathews, 1986; Ostrosky, Conseco, Quintanar, Navarro, & Ardila, 1985; Ostrosky et al., 1986; Ostrosky, Ardila, Rosselli, López-Arango, & Uriel-Mendoza, 1998; Ostrosky, Ardila, & Rosselli, 1999; Reis, Guerrero, & Petersson, 2003). Educational level accounts for a significant percentage of the variance in neuropsychological tests (Table 10.1). Ardila and Rosselli

TABLE 10.1
Percentage of the Variance Accounted by the Educational Variable in the Different NEUROPSI Subtests

Test	Correlation	Percentage of the variance
Verbal fluency: phonologic	0.62	38.5%
Language comprehension	0.59	35.3
Copy of a figure	0.57	32.9
Sequences	0.57	32.9
Digits backwards	0.54	29.5
Similarities	0.52	27.3
Verbal fluency: semantic	0.49	23.6
Calculation	0.48	22.6
Recall of a figure	0.46	21.1
Alternating movements	0.45	20.6
20 minus 3	0.44	19.0
Visual detection	0.41	17.1
Orientation: Time	0.35	12.0
Recall: Words	0.32	10.3
Coding: Verbal memory	0.31	9.7
Recall: Cuing	0.29	8.5
Language: Naming	0.28	7.9
Opposite reactions	0.27	7.2
Language: Repetition	0.26	7.0
Motor functions: Right-hand	0.26	6.9
Motor functions: Left-hand	0.24	5.7
Recall: Recognition	0.12	1.5
Orientation: Person	0.08	0.7
Orientation: Space	0.07	0.6

Note. From "Learning to Read Is Much More Than Learning to Read: A Neuropsychologically-Based Learning to Read Method," by A. Ardila, F. Ostrosky, and V. Mendoza, 2000, *Journal of the International Neuropsychological Society, 6,* 789–781. Adapted with permission of the authors.

(1989) reported that the educational variable was even more influential on neuropsychological performance than the age variable. As a matter of fact, Albert and Heaton (1988) argued that, when education is controlled, there is no longer evidence of an age-related decline in verbal intelligence. Clearly, formal education represents the most important variable accounting for score dispersion on cognitive test scores (Greenfield, 1997).

Some tests have been observed to be notoriously more sensitive to educational variables (e.g., language understanding) than others (e.g., orientation tests). Extremely low scores in current neuropsychological tests are observed in illiterate people (e.g., Ardila, Rosselli, & Rosas, 1989; Lecours et al., 1987a, 1987b; Ostrosky et al., 1985, 1998; Rosselli, Ardila, & Rosas, 1990). Reis et al. (2003) compared the performance of illiterates with literates with a similar socioeconomic status in a series of neuropsychological tests. The results indicated that naming and identification of real objects, verbal fluency using ecologically relevant semantic criteria, verbal memory, and orientation are not affected by literacy or level of formal education. In contrast, verbal working memory assessed with digit span, verbal abstraction, long-term semantic memory, and calculation (i.e., multiplication) are significantly affected by the level of literacy (Table 10.2).

Low scores on neuropsychological tests observed in illiterates can be partially due, not only to differences in learning opportunities of those abilities that the examiner considers relevant (although, evidently, they are not the really relevant abilities for illiterates), but to the fact that illiterates are not accustomed to being tested (i.e., they have not learned how to behave in a testing situation), and testing itself represents a nonsense (nonrelevant) situation.

Illiterates do not represent a homogenous group. Illiteracy has not the same causes in an industrialized and in a developing country. Quite often, in developing countries illiteracy is associated with poverty and lack of available schools. In industrialized countries, illiteracy is often associated with limited intellectual development. Illiteracy is also frequently increased in women due to some cultural attitudes found in some countries. By the same token, illiteracy has no the same causes in younger and older people. Today it is notoriously easier and more important to attend school than it was several decades ago. Illiteracy is also frequently associated with poverty and low socioeconomic status (SES). An association between nervous system disorders and low SES has been pointed out (e.g., Alvarez, 1983). Some research studies have shown that low SES subjects may receive quantitatively and qualitatively less stimulation at home in comparison with the high SES subjects. This differential stimulation contributes to the development of different behavioral styles (Cravioto & Arrieta, 1982). Some nervous system pathologies (for example, epilepsy) are significantly more frequent in developing countries and in low SES subjects than in industrialized countries

TABLE 10.2
Performance in the NEUROPSI Neuropsychological Test Battery Subtests in Different Educational Groups With Regard to the Group With the Highest Education

Test	\multicolumn{6}{c}{Years of school}					
	0	1–2	3–4	5–9	10–12	13–17	18–24
Orientation: Time	73	77	80	97	97	97	100%
Place	95	95	100	100	100	100	100%
Person	90	90	90	100	100	100	100%
Attention: Digits backwards	54	59	61	79	88	98	100%
Orientation: Time	73	77	80	97	97	97	100%
Place	95	95	100	100	100	100	100%
Person	90	90	90	100	100	100	100%
Attention: Digits backwards	54	59	61	79	88	98	100%
Visual detection	73	82	92	92	92	98	100%
20 minus 3	63	63	84	92	96	98	100%
Coding: Verbal memory	79	9	81	88	90	94	100%
Copy semi-complex figure	66	77	82	97	99	99	100%
Language: Naming	91	91	94	97	99	99	100%
Repetition	95	97	97	99	99	100	100%
Comprehension	62	73	77	93	97	97	100%
Verbal fluency: Semantic	63	68	72	86	93	98	100%
Phonol	23	47	51	57	92	100	100%
Conceptual functions: Similarities	37	61	68	87	91	96	100%
Calculation abilities	32	53	57	85	89	92	100%
Sequences	11	22	44	77	100	100	100%
Motor functions: left-hand	58	63	68	82	84	84	100%
right-hand	59	65	70	88	91	94	100%
Alternating movements	42	58	68	76	84	95	100%
Opposite reactions	94	94	100	100	100	100	100%
Recall: Words	57	63	77	88	88	96	100%
Cueing	77	81	89	90	92	92	100%
Recognition	96	98	100	100	100	100	100%
Semi-complex figure	59	66	79	87	92	96	100%

Note. Adapted from the information presented in the paper "Neuropsi: A brief neuropsychological test battery in Spanish with norms by age and educational level" by F. Ostrosky, A. Ardila, and M. Rosselli, 1999, *Journal of the International Neuropsychological Society*, 5, 413–433. Adapted with permission of the authors.

10. ILLITERATES AND COGNITION 185

and high SES individuals (e.g., Gomez, Arciniegas, & Torres, 1978; Gracia, Bayard, & Triana, 1988). It means that illiteracy is potentially associated with a diversity of variables.

Three different issues are approached in this chapter: (1) neuropsychological test performance of illiterates in different cognitive domains; (2) some characteristics of the neuropsychological syndromes observed in illiterate people; and (3) how neuropsychological testing could be approached in illiterate populations. In this last section, the issue of disadvantage of illiterates is analyzed, and some suggestions are presented.

NEUROPSYCHOLOGICAL TEST PERFORMANCE IN ILLITERATES

The significant schooling effect on neuropsychological test performance has been reported for different types of abilities. There is converging evidence that illiterate subjects obtain significantly low scores on most neuropsychological tests. Several research groups have approached the question of neuropsychological test performance of illiterates: Matute and Ostrosky in Mexico; Ardila and Rosselli in Colombia; Lecours, Mehler, and Parente in Brazil; Castro-Caldas and Reis in Portugal; Manly and Jacobs in the United States; Dellatolas, Caramelli, Braga, and colleagues in Brazil; Folia and Kosmidis in Greece.

Language

Language abilities are significantly correlated with socioeducational level. Robinson (1974) observed that low socioeconomic parents use more nonverbal strategies in their relations with children. Bernstein (1974) pointed out that the language used by low SES people is less fluent and has a simpler grammatical structure; it relies much more on emotional and contextual rather than logical strategies. Bruner, Oliver, and Greenfield (1966) suggested that rural unschooled children may lack symbolic representation skills because their linguistic ability is tied to immediate context of the referent. They proposed that formal education facilitates the development of language into a fully symbolic tool. Lantz (1979), however, showed that rural unschooled children performed better than Indian or American school children in coding and decoding culturally relevant objects, such as grain, seeds, and so forth. Thus, children without formal schooling are able to separate language symbols from the physical referent and to use those symbols for communicating accurately, but display of this ability depends on the stimuli used (Laboratory of Comparative Human Cognition, 1983). Luria (1976) pointed out that the significance of schooling lies not just in the acquisition of new knowledge, but in the creation of new motives and formal modes of discursive verbal and logical thinking divorced from the immediate practical experience.

Several studies have reported quite similar findings in language test performance of illiterates (da Silva, Petersson, Faisca, Ingvar, & Reis, 2004; Lecours et al., 1987a; Manly et al., 1999; Ostrosky et al., 1998; Reis & Castro-Caldas, 1997; Reis, Guerreiro, & Castro-Caldas, 1994). The single verbal test most sensitive to schooling effect is probably phonemic verbal fluency. Scores of illiterates are about 20% of the scores found in people with a university level of education (Ostrosky et al., 1998; Rosselli et al., 1990). Conversely, scores of illiterates in semantic verbal fluency are notoriously higher and closer to scores of educated people; they are about 60% of the scores found in highly educated people.

da Silva et al. (2004) compared literate and illiterate subjects in two verbal fluency tasks: "supermarket fluency task" (items that can be found in a supermarket), and animals. The quantitative analysis indicated that the two literacy groups performed equally well on the supermarket fluency task. In contrast, results differed significantly during the animal fluency task. They suggested that there is not a substantial difference between literate and illiterate subjects related to the fundamental workings of semantic memory.

Loureiro et al. (2004) analyzed the phonological and metaphonological skills in illiterate and semiliterate adults. Phonemic awareness was strongly dependent on the level of letter- and word-reading ability. Phonological memory was very low in illiterates and unrelated to letter knowledge. Rhyme identification was relatively preserved in illiterates and semiliterates, and unrelated to letter- and word-reading level. Phonetic discrimination (minimal pairs) was fairly good and marginally related to reading ability. Awareness is clearly and strongly dependent on the alphabetical acquisition.

Differences in naming ability between illiterate and educated people are also found, but the differences between both groups depend on two variables: (1) Word frequency differences are observed particularly in low and middle frequency words, not in high frequency words; and (2) stimuli presentation (naming line-drawn figures is harder for the illiterate than naming real objects; Reis et al., 1994). Illiterate subjects perform significantly worse on immediate naming of two-dimensional representations of common everyday objects as compared to literate subjects, both in terms of accuracy and reaction times. In contrast, there is no significant difference when the subjects named the corresponding real objects (Reis et al., 2001)

Language repetition can be normal for meaningful words, but abnormal for pseudowords or unfamiliar words (Reis & Castro-Caldas, 1997; Rosselli et al., 1990). Language understanding is also decreased in illiterates, particularly when relatively complex grammar is used (Lecours et al., 1987a;

Manly et al., 1999). A study by Ostrosky et al. (1998) that used a simplified Token Test version, revealed that language comprehension scores of illiterates were approximately 60% of the language-understanding scores observed in individuals with a university level of education.

Visuospatial and Visuoconstructive Abilities

Educational variables significant by impact visuospatial, visuoconstructive and visuoperceptual test performance (Rosselli & Ardila, 2003). Ardila et al. (1989) administered a basic neuropsychological test battery to two extreme educational groups: illiterate and professional individuals. Subjects were matched according to gender and age. All of the analyzed visuospatial tasks (copying a cube, a house, and Rey-Osterrieth Complex Figure; telling the time on a clock; recognizing superimposed figures; recognizing the national map; and drawing the plan of the room) showed highly significant differences between the two extreme educational groups. In all of these subtests, gender interacted with educational level. In the illiterate group, men outperformed women, but no gender differences were observed in the professional sample.

Ostrosky et al. (1998) reported defects in copying figures. The correlation between educational level and test performance was close to 0.60. Matute, Leal, Zaraboso, Robles, and Cedillo (1997) found significant differences in the ability to reproduce different stick constructions. The influence of literacy was most evident with regard to the fidelity of reproductions of the figures. Dellatolas et al. (2003) studied the effect of the degree of illiteracy (complete or incomplete) on visuospatial skills. Tasks tapping visual recognition of nonsense figures distinguished the best nonreaders and beginning readers.

Memory

Statistically significant differences between illiterates and professionals were reported in memory tests by Ardila et al. (1989). For instance, professionals memorized a 10-word list after an average of 3.22 presentations, whereas illiterates required 6.55 repetitions. Significant differences were also found in the 10-word delayed recall. There was a statistically significant interaction between age and educational level, with illiterates presenting a more notable variation across age groups. Immediate and delayed logical memory tests were also sensitive to educational level.

Differences in digits backward have been reported to be larger than differences in the digits forward test. Immediate and delayed recall of verbal and nonverbal information is significantly decreased in illiterates (Ardila et al., 1989). Nonetheless, differences are found under certain recall strategies (spontaneous recall and cueing recall), but not when using recognition techniques (Ostrosky et al., 1998).

Barltlett (1932) proposed that illiterates more frequently use procedures of rote learning, whereas literate people refer to more active information integration procedures (metamemory strategies). Cole and Scribner (1974) observed that, when memorizing information, literates and illiterates make use of their own groupings to structure their recall; for instance, high school subjects rely mainly on taxonomic categories, whereas illiterate farmers make little use of this principle.

Nitrini et al. (2004) compared the performance of illiterate and literate nondemented elderly individuals in two tests of long-term memory—the delayed recall of a word list from the CERAD and the delayed recall of common objects presented as simple drawings from the Brief Cognitive Screening Battery (BCSB). Fifty-one elderly subjects (23 illiterates) were evaluated, and the performance of the illiterates and literates differed in the CERAD memory test, but not in the BCSB memory test. In consequence, difficulties in memory test performance in illiterates depend on the specific memory test that is used. Illiterate people use different memory strategies, and our current evaluation instruments are not necessarily appropriate to test people with low levels of formal education.

Praxic and Motor Abilities

Education has shown to be an important variable on motor performance subtests (Ostrosky et al, 1985, 1986). Rosselli et al. (1990) observed differences according to educational level in the performance of buccofacial, ideomotor, and finger alternating movement tests. Illiterate subjects presented some errors in these tasks whereas subjects with a high educational level presented virtually no mistakes. Use of body part as instrument was the most common type of error found in illiterates. Interaction between education and age in performing buccofacial movements under verbal command was observed, and older illiterates presented the highest number of errors. In ideomotor praxis subtests, a significant interaction between education and gender was observed. Illiterate women presented roughly twice the number of mistakes of illiterate men. Illiterate subjects in the Rosselli et al. study poorly performed fine finger movements. The absence of training and practice in fine movements (particularly, writing) may account for the difference in fine movement test performance between the illiterates and highly educated subjects. Ostrosky et al. (1985, 1986) reported significant differences in performing programmed movements between subjects coming from different educational levels. Ostrosky et al. (1998) found that illiterates have very significant difficulties reproducing three positions with the hand (either) and alternating positions of the hands (right hand closed, left hand open, and switching). However, they perform normally on the "opposite reaction test" (If the examiner shows the finger, the subject must show the fist; if the examiner shows the fist, the subject must show the finger).

Executive Functions

Defects in performing executive function tests also have been documented in illiterate individuals. Finding similarities (Similarities test) has been the test most frequently administered in several studies (Manly et al., 1999; Ostrosky et al., 1998, 1999). According to Ostrosky et al. (1998), scores of illiterates are about one third of the scores found in people with a university level of education. Extremely low scores were found by Ostrosky et al. in the Sequences test (the subject is asked to continue a sequence of figures drawn on a paper; "what figure continues?"). Performance of illiterates was about one tenth of the performance found in people with high education. Of course, lack of practice in writing and drawing represents a significant confounding variable in this result. Phonemic verbal fluency can also be interpreted as an executive function test, and as mentioned before, it is a test extremely sensitive to the effect of educational variables.

To summarize, illiterate individuals present significant difficulties in neuropsychological tests directed to assess different domains. The magnitude of the educational effect, however, is variable.

BRAIN DAMAGE AND ILLITERACY

Two opposite points of view are found in neuropsychological literature regarding the influence of education on brain organization of language in particular and cognitive activity in general. Cameron, Currier, and Haerer (1971) reported that there is a lower frequency of aphasias associated with injuries of the left hemisphere among right-handed illiterate patients than among educated ones. The authors concluded that language is more bilaterally represented in the illiterate group. Damasio et al. (1976) claimed that there is no qualitative or quantitative difference between the aphasias of educated and illiterate patients. The aphasias of literates and illiterates did not differ in expectancy rate, distribution of clinical types, or semiological structure.

Matute's research studies (1988) provide some support to Damasio et al.'s conclusion. She compared three groups of right-handed Mexican subjects: brain-damaged illiterates, brain-damaged literates, and normal illiterates. An aphasia test was given to all three groups as part of a large neuropsychological assessment battery. All left-hemisphere damaged illiterate subjects presented aphasia, and no illiterates presented aphasia after right-hemisphere damage. The aphasia was, however, less severe in the illiterate group than in the literate one. The literate group presented a higher number of errors, with lower scores on the aphasia subtests than the illiterate brain-damaged individuals.

Lecours et al (1988) studied some relationships between brain damage and schooling with regard to aphasic impairments of language. The authors concluded from their results that: (1) There was a greater right-hemisphere language involvement in illiterates than in the well-educated subjects; and (2) school-educated left-stroke subjects seemed to be "sicker," as it were, than their illiterate counterparts. That is: (a) the classical symptoms of aphasia (suppression stereotype, jargonaphasia) are more apparent among left-stroke literates than among left-stroke illiterates; and (b) auditory comprehension was more frequently impaired among the literate left-stroke patients.

Lecours et al. (1987b) also studied the influence of education on unilateral neglect syndrome. They analyzed a large sample of right-handed unilingual brain-damaged subjects: illiterates (left stroke and right stroke) and literates (left stroke and right stroke). Evidence of unilateral neglect syndrome was found in both left and right brain-damaged literates and illiterates. Their results provided no indication that tropisms were globally stronger depending on the side of the lesion or on the educational level of the subjects. Rosselli, Rosselli, Vergara, and Ardila (1985), however, reported a higher frequency of right hemispatial neglect in low-educated subjects.

Interesting to note, it has been pointed out that brain functional organization can influenced by literacy. Castro-Caldas, Peterson, Reis, Stone-Elander, and Ingvar (1998), using PET, found that during the repetition of real words, literates and illiterates activated similar brain areas. In contrast, illiterates with more difficulty in repeating pseudowords did not activate the same neural structures as literates. Castro-Caldas et al. (1999) referred to some differences in the region of the corpus callosum where parietal fibers are thought to cross. This means that brain organization of cognition may be influenced by literacy.

Studies of brain-damaged illiterates when compared with brain-damaged literates indicate that: (1) Literacy does not change the dominance of the left hemisphere for language (illiterates as well as literates present aphasia most often after left-brain damage, and not after right-brain damage); and (2) it seems, however, that the right hemisphere has more participation in language in illiterate subjects. There is a general consensus that left-damaged literates present a higher number of errors on aphasia tests than do left-damaged illiterates (Lecours et al., 1988; Matute, 1988), and that right-damaged illiterates more frequently present lower performance on aphasia tests than do right brain-damage literates (Lecours et al., 1988).

ARE ILLITERATES NECESSARILY AT A DISADVANTAGE?

Cornelious and Caspi (1987) found that educational level has a substantial relationship with performance on verbal tests, but is not systematically related to everyday problem solving (i.e., functional criterion). This is an extremely important observation that is frequently overlooked. Illiterates are handicapped when using laboratory cognitive tests, but they can perform normally on functional intelligence tests.

The diagnosis of dementia or any other neuropsychological syndrome using psychometric procedures necessarily penalizes low-educated individuals. The use of psychometric instruments may inflate the severity of the cognitive defects, and hence, the prevalence of neuropsychological disturbances. The theoretical interpretation of this observation has been a matter of ongoing discussion during the last few years.

In 1988, Mortiner proposed that education provides protection against dementia. He assumed that psychosocial factors reduce the margin of "intellectual reserve" to a level where a minor level of brain pathology results in a dementia. He further supposed that "psychosocial risk factors" (i.e., no or low education) will present the strongest association in the late onset dementia of the Alzheimer type (DAT). During the last decade, several studies have in general, albeit not always, supported this hypothesis. A positive association between DAT and low education have been observed in research studies carried out across quite different countries: Brazil (Caramelli et al., 1997), China (Hill et al., 1993; Hsiu-Chih et al., 1994; Yu et al., 1989), Finland (Sulkava et al., 1985), France (Dartigues et al., 1991), Italy (Bonaiuto, Rocca, & Lippi, 1990; Rocca et al., 1990), Israel (Korczyn, Kahana, & Galper, 1991), Sweden (Fratiglioni et al., 1991), and the United States (Stern et al., 1994). Negative results, however, also have been reported (Christensen & Henderson, 1991; Knoefel et al., 1991; O'Connor, Pollitt, & Treasure, 1991).

Katzman (1993) has pointed out that, "when the very mild cognitive changes of normal aging are superimposed on lifelong cognitive impairment in some subjects with no or low education, an erroneous diagnosis of dementia could occur" (p. 15). Even though we certainly agree with his basic idea (mild cognitive changes in low-educated people may result in the erroneous diagnosis of dementia), we cannot share his departing point: Low educated people present a "lifelong cognitive impairment." This assumption supposes that what is normal is to be educated and that either no or low education is a kind of abnormality ("impairment"). It should be kept in mind that most of the world population is low educated, and even nowadays, about one fifth of the world people are illiterates. One hundred or 200 years ago, most of the world population was illiterate. One thousand to 2,000 years ago perhaps some 99% of the world population was illiterate. Low education or illiteracy obviously is not an abnormality, at least from the statistical point of view. The average educational level of contemporary man is about 3–4 years of school. We are afraid that Katzman is taking as "normal" what indeed is "abnormal" (or at least, "unusual"), and as "abnormal" what really is the norm. Further, we do not think that low-educated people are necessarily understimulated. Rather, we prefer to think that highly educated people are overstimulated from the point of view of some specific cognitive tasks. This preference, one may suppose, is just a matter of language nuance, but it may be crucial to perceiving and interpreting pathology. When dealing with low-educated individuals, functional scales, as Katzman pointed out (1993), obviously become crucial (Loewenstein et al., 1992). However, functional scales also need to be adapted to conditions of low-educated people.

Capitani, Barbarotto, and Laicana (1996) approached the question from a somewhat different perspective. They proposed that three different patterns of association could be expected between age-related decline and education: (a) parallelism (the age-related decline runs the same course in different educational groups, i.e., no interaction is observed); (b) protection (the age-related decline is attenuated in well-educated participants); and (c) confluence (the initial advantage of well-educated groups in middle age is reduced in later life). Ardila, Ostrosky, and Mendoza (2000) observed an even more complex pattern of interaction between education and cognitive decline associated with aging: parallelism, protection, confluence upward, confluence downward, and undefined. Regression curves were analyzed. Ardila and colleagues concluded that: (1) Lifelong changes in cognition are associated with education. Peak performance on neuropsychological tests by low-educated individuals is observed at an older age than in more highly educated subjects; and (2) there is no single relationship between age-related cognitive decline and education, but different patterns may be found, depending upon the specific cognitive domain.

The direct clinical observation of illiterates and low-educated populations does not seem to confirm the hypothesis that dementia is significantly higher in individuals with low education. For example, in neurological settings in developing countries, dementia seldom represents a reason for consultation in low-educated people. Of course, this can result from the interpretation that aging is associated with cognitive decline, and cognitive decline is not a disease but a normal process. Nonetheless, everyday observation indicates that most low-educated and illiterate individuals continue to be functionally active during their 60s, 70s, and even their 80s and 90s. As an illustration, in rural areas in developing countries, where most people have a very limited level of education, it is extremely unusual to find that somebody, regardless of his or her age, cannot participate to some extent in working and productive activities.

A significant misunderstanding may frequently exist with regard to the effects of education. School attendance does not mean that educated people simply possess certain abilities that low or noneducated individuals do not have. In other words, it does not mean that educated people have the same abilities that low-educated individuals have, plus something else. If comparing two children, one with 10 years of formal education, and the other one with zero schooling, it also means that the zero-education child was performing for 10 years certain activities (working or whatever) that the 10-year education child was not performing. The zero-education child was obviously obtaining certain knowledge that the 10-year education child was not obtaining. Nonetheless, formal cognitive testing is directed to evaluate those abilities that the 10-year education child was acquiring; thus it is not surprising that he or she will outperform the zero formal-education child. At this point, it has to be strongly emphasized that educational level is substantially related to performance on some cognitive tests, but is not systematically related to everyday problem solving (Cornelious & Caspi, 1987). Therefore, it is not totally accurate to assume that low-educated or noneducated people are somehow "deprived." It may be more accurate to assume that they have developed different types of abilities. If tests were based on knowledge associated with low or no education, highly educated people would be at a disadvantage. Regardless that the concept of "cognitive reserve" has become very popular in the dementia literature (e.g., (Sanchez, Rodriguez, & Carro, 2002; Scarmeas & Stern, 2003, 2004; Staff, Murray, Deary, & Whalley, 2004) it may be argued it simply represents a misunderstanding of what illiteracy means.

There is another important observation with regard to the diagnosis of dementia in low-educated people. In DAT, procedural memory (how to do things) is usually much better preserved than declarative memory (awareness of memories; Cummings & Benson, 1992). Quite often, low levels of education are associated with manual activities and procedural learning (e.g., farming, handcrafting, manual labor, etc.). Conversely, higher levels of education are strongly correlated with intellectual activities and declarative memory. Minor intellectual defects may be fatal for highly educated people. Nonetheless, low-educated people may continue working in a roughly normal way, despite minor or moderate cognitive defects. For example, in some rural areas in Colombia it has been observed that individuals with very significant cognitive defects ("dementia") can continue working as coffee collectors in a relatively normal way. The patient simply is taken to the coffee plantation (he cannot go by himself due to the spatial orientation defects), and once at the coffee plantation, he or she can perform the activity of collecting coffee in a roughly normal way. Obviously, this patient is significantly more impaired from the point of view of the neurologist/ neuropsychologist examiner than from the point of view of his own social group.

This observation raises an additional issue: When assessing DAT in manual laborers, procedural memory testing should be preferred. Or, at least, behavioral scales should emphasize the ability to perform lifelong procedural working activities.

Several authors (e.g., Folia & Kosmidis, 2003; Reis et al., 2003) have emphasized that low test performance in illiterates depends significantly on the types of instruments that are used. When the task is changed (e.g., instead of asking to tell animal names, to tell "items that can be found in the supermarket") differences in performance between literate and illiterate participants disappear. Of course, illiterates would perform higher than literate people if tested using the abilities best developed in illiterates (e.g., farming, handcrafting, certain spatial orientation abilities, etc.).

CONCLUSIONS

It is evident that literacy is strongly reflected in the performance of those tasks used not only in psychological, but also neuropsychological evaluation. Very important cognitive consequences of learning to read and write have been suggested: changes in visual perception, phonological awareness, logical reasoning, and remembering strategies (Ardila et al., 2000).

The analysis of performance of illiterate populations on neuropsychological measures suggests that cognitive abilities, as measured by standard neuropsychological tests, are significantly influenced by schooling. However, it is a mistake to assume that the inability to perform simple cognitive tasks, such as those incorporated in current neuropsychological test batteries, necessarily indicates abnormal brain function.

The influence of literacy seems to go farther: Literacy may somehow change the brain organization of cognition. We are far from correctly understanding the influence of external variables on brain organization of cognitive activity. However, it is a fact that educational and cultural variables may affect the degree of hemispheric dominance for language and most likely other cognitive abilities. Some studies about the consequences of brain damage in illiterate populations suggest a more bilateral representation not only for linguistic, but probably also for visuospatial abilities. Apparently, literacy does not change the direction of laterality in the brain organization of cognition, but the degree of this lateralization.

The use of psychometric testing instruments significantly penalizes illiterates. Low performance on neuropsychological tests may not only be due to the undertraining of those abilities included in most tests, but also to lack of familiarity, difficulties in understanding the testing situations, and other confounding variables. Functional scales and some specific tests with ecological significance can represent a more reliable and fairer procedure for assessing illiterate populations.

REFERENCES

Albert, M. S., & Heaton, R. K. (1988). Intelligence testing. In M. S. Albert & M. B. Moss (Eds.), *Geriatric neuropsychology* (pp. 10–32). New York: Guilford.

Alvarez, G. (1983). Effects of material deprivation on neurological functioning. *Social Science Medicine, 17,* 1097–1105.

Ardila, A., Ostrosky, F., & Mendoza, V. (2000). Learning to read is much more than learning to read: A neuropsychologically-based learning to read method. *Journal of the International Neuropsychological Society, 6,* 789–801.

Ardila, A., Ostrosky-Solis, F., Rosselli, M., & Gomez, C. (2000). Age related cognitive decline during normal aging: The complex effect of education. *Archives of Clinical Neuropsychology, 15,* 495–514.

Ardila, A., & Rosselli, M. (1989). Neuropsychological characteristics of normal aging. *Developmental Neuropsychology, 5,* 307–320.

Ardila, A., Rosselli, M., Ostrosky, F., & Puente, A. (1992). Sociocultural factors in neuropsychological assessment. In A. E. Puente & R. J. McCaffrey (Eds.), *Handbook of neuropsychological assessment: A biopsychosocial perspective* (pp. 181–192). New York: Plenum.

Ardila, A., Rosselli, M., & Puente, P. (1994). *Neuropsychological evaluation of the Spanish speaker.* New York: Plenum.

Ardila, A., Rosselli, M., & Rosas, P. (1989). Neuropsychological assessment in illiterates: Visuospatial and memory abilities. *Brain and Cognition, 11,* 147–166.

Barltlett, F. C. (1932). *Remembering.* London: Cambridge University Press.

Bernstein, B. (1974). Language and roles. In R. Huxley & E. Ingram (Eds.), *Language acquisition: Models and methods* (pp. 225–242). New York: Academic Press.

Bonaiuto, R., Rocca, E., & Lippi, A. (1990). Impact of education and occupation on the prevalence of Alzheimer's disease (AD) and multi infarct dementia in Appignano, Macerata Province, Italy [abstract]. *Neurology, 40* (Suppl. 1), 346.

Bornstein, R. A., & Suga, L. J. (1988). Educational level and neuropsychological performance in healthy elderly subjects. *Developmental Neuropsychology, 4,* 17–22.

Bruner, J., Oliver, R., & Greenfield, P. (1966). *Studies in cognitive growth.* New York: Wiley.

Cameron, R. F., Currier, R. D., & Haerer, A. F. (1971). Aphasia and literacy. *British Journal of Disorders of Communication, 6,* 161–163.

Capitani, E., Barbarotto, R., & Laicana, M. (1996). Does education influence age-related cognitive decline? A further inquiry. *Developmental Neuropsychology, 12,* 231–240.

Caramelli, P., Poissant, A., Gauthier, P., Bellavance, A., Gauvreau, D., Lecours, A. R., & Joanette, Y. (1997). Educational level and neuropsychological heterogeneity in dementia of the Alzheimer type. *Alzheimer Disease and Associated Disorders, 11,* 9–15.

Castro-Caldas, A., Miranda, P. C., Carmo, I., Reis, A., Leote, F., Ribeiro, C., & Ducla-Soares, E. (1999). Influence of learning to read and write on the morphology of the corpus callosum. *European Journal of Neurology, 6*(1), 23–28.

Castro-Caldas, A., Peterson, K. M., Reis, A., Stone-Elander, S., & Ingvar, M. (1998). The illiterate brain: Learning to read and write during childhood influences the functional organization of the adult brain. *Brain, 121,* 1053–1064.

Christensen, H., & Henderson, A. S. (1991). Is age kinder to the initially more able? A study of eminent scientists and academics. *Psychological Medicine, 21,* 935–946.
Cole, M., & Scribner, S. (1974). *Culture and thought.* New York: Wiley.
Cornelious, S. W., & Caspi, A. (1987). Everyday problem solving in adulthood and old age. *Psychology of Aging, 2,* 144–153.
Cravioto, J., & Arrieta, R. (1982). *Nutrición, desarrollo mental, conducta y aprendizaje* [Nutrition, mental development, behavior and learning]. Mexico, DF: UNICEF.
Cummings, J. L., & Benson, D. F. (1992). *Dementia: A clinical approach* (2nd ed.). Boston: Butterworth-Heinemann.
Damasio, A. R., Castro-Caldas, A., Grosso, J. T., & Ferro, J. M. (1976). Brain specialization for language does not depend on literacy. *Archives of Neurology, 33,* 300–301.
Dartigues, J. F., Gagnon, M., & Michel, P. (1991). Le programme de recherche PAQUID su l'epidemiologie de la demence methodes et resultats initiaux [Research program PAQUID on epistemology of dementia methods and initial results]. *Revue Neurologique, 145,* 225–230.
da Silva, C. G., Petersson, K. M., Faisca, L., Ingvar, M., & Reis, A. (2004). The effects of literacy and education on the quantitative and qualitative aspects of semantic verbal fluency. *Journal of Clinical and Experimental Neuropsychology, 26,* 266–277.
Dellatolas, G., Willadino Braga, L., Souza Ldo, N., Filho, G. N., Queiroz, E., & Deloche, G. (2003). Cognitive consequences of early phase of literacy. *Journal of the International Neuropsychological Society, 9,* 771–782.
Finlayson, N. A., Johnson, K. A., & Reitan, R. M. (1977). Relation of level of education to neuropsychological measures in brain damaged and non-brain damaged adults. *Journal of Consulting and Clinical Psychology, 45,* 536–542.
Folia, V., & Kosmidis, M. H. (2003). Assessment of memory skills in illiterates: strategy differences or test artifact? *The Clinical Neuropsychologist, 17,* 143–152.
Fratiglioni, L., Grut, M., Forsell, Y., Viitanen, M., Grafstrom, M., Holmen, K., et al. (1991). Prevalence of Alzheimer's disease and other dementias in an elderly urban population: Relationship with age, sex, and education. *Neurology, 41,* 1886–1892.
Gomez, J. G., Arciniegas, E., & Torres, J. (1978). Prevalence of epilepsy in Bogota, Colombia. *Neurology, 28,* 90–94.
Gracia, F., Bayard, V., & Triana, E. (1988). Prevalencia de enfermedades neurologicas en el corregimiento Belisario Potas [Prevalence of neurological diseases in Bolisario Potas town, Panama]. *Revista Médica de Panamá, 13,* 408–411.
Greenfield, P. M. (1997). You can't take it with you: Why ability assessments don't cross cultures. *American Psychologist, 52,* 1115–1124.
Heaton, R. K., Grant, I., & Mathews, C. (1986). Differences in neuropsychological test performance associated with age, education and sex. In I. Grant & K. M. Adams (Eds.), *Neuropsychological assessment in neuropsychiatric disorders* (pp. 108–120). New York: Oxford University Press.
Hill, L. R., Klauber, M. R., Salmon, D. P., Yu, E. S., Liu, W. T., Zhang, M., & Katzman, R. (1993). Functional status, education, and the diagnosis of dementia in the Shanghai survey. *Neurology, 43,* 138–145.
Hsiu-Chin, L., Teng, E. L., Lin, K. N., Hsu, T. C., Guo, N. W., Chou, P., et al. (1994). Performance on a dementia screening test in relation to demographic variables. Study of 5,297 community residents in Taiwan. *Archives of Neurology, 51,* 910–915.
Katzman, R. (1993). Education and the prevalence of dementia and Alzheimer's disease. *Neurology, 43,* 13–20.
Knoefel, J. E., Wolf, P. A., Linn, R. T., & Cobb, J. L. (1991). Education has not effect on incidence of dementia and Alzheimer's disease in the Framingham study. *Neurology, 41* (Suppl. 1), 322–323.

Korczyn, A. D., Kahana, E., & Galper, Y. (1991). Epidemiology of dementia in Ashkelom, Israel. *Neuroepidemiology, 10,* 100–120.
Laboratory of Comparative Human Cognition. (1983). Culture and cognitive development. In P. Mussen (Ed.), *Handbook of child psychology: Vol 1. History, theories and methods* (pp. 342–397). New York: Wiley.
Lantz, D. (1979). A cross-cultural comparison of communication abilities: Some effects of age, schooling and culture. *International Journal of Psychology, 14,* 171–183.
Loewenstein, D. A., Ardila, A., Rosselli, M., Hayden, S., Duara, R., Berkowitz, N., et al. (1992). A comparative analysis of functional status among Spanish- and English-speaking patients with dementia. *Journal of Gerontology, 47,* 389–394.
Lecours, A. R., Mehler, J., Parente, M. A., Caldeira, A., Cary, L., Castro, M. J., et al. (1987a). Illiteracy and brain damage 1: Aphasia testing in culturally contrasted populations (control subjects). *Neuropsychologia, 25,* 231–245.
Lecours, A. R., Mehler, J., Parente, M. A., Aguiar, L. R., da Silva, A. B., Caetano, M., et al. (1987b). Illiteracy and brain damage 2: Manifestations of unilateral neglect in testing "auditory comprehension" with iconographic material. *Brain and Cognition, 6,* 243–265.
Lecours, A.R., Mehler, J., Parente, M.A., Beltrami, M. C., Canossa de Tolipan, L., Castro, M. J., et al. (1988). Illiteracy and brain damage 3: A contribution to the study of speech and language disorders in illiterates with unilateral brain damage (initial testing). *Neuropsychologia, 26,* 575–589.
Loureiro, C. de S., Braga, L. W., Souza Ldo, N., Nunes Filho, G., Queiroz, E., & Dellatolas, G. (2004). Degree of illiteracy and phonological and metaphonological skills in unschooled adults. *Brain and Language, 89,* 499–502.
Luria, A.R. (1976). *Cognitive development.* Cambridge, MA: Harvard University Press.
Manly, J. J., Jacobs, D. M., Sano, M., Bell, K., Merchant, C. A., Small, S. A., & Stern, Y. (1999). Effect of literacy on neuropsychological test performance in nondemented, education-matched elders. *Journal of the International Neuropsychological Society, 5,* 191–202.
Matarazzo, J. D. (1979). *Wechsler's measurement and appraisal of adult intelligence* (5th ed.). New York: Oxford University Press.
Matute, E. (1988) El aprendizaje de la lectoescritura y la especialización hemisférica para el lenguaje [Learning to read and hemispheric specialization for language]. In A. Ardila & F. Ostrosky-Solis (Eds.), *Lenguaje oral y escrito* (pp. 310–338). Mexico: Trillas.
Matute, E., Lcal, F., Zaraboso, D., Robles, A., & Cedillo,. C. (1997). Influence of literacy level on stick construction in non-brain-damaged subjects [Abstract]. *Journal of the International Neuropsychological Society, 3,* 32.
Mortimer, J. A. (1988). Do psychosocial risk factors contribute to Alzheimer's disease? In A. S. Hendersen & J. H. Hendersen (Eds), *Etiology of dementia of Alzheimer's type* (pp. 39–52). Chichester, England: Wiley.
Nitrini, R., Caramelli, P., Herrera, E., Jr., Porto, C. S., Charchat-Fichman, H., Carthery, M. T., et al. (2004). Performance of illiterate and literate nondemented elderly subjects in two tests of long-term memory. *Journal of the International Neuropsychological Society, 10,* 634–638.
O'Connor, D. W., Pollitt, P. A., & Treasure, F. P. (1991). The influence of education and social class on the diagnosis of dementia in a community population. *Psychological Medicine, 21,* 219–234.
Ostrosky, F., Ardila, A., & Rosselli, M. (1999). NEUROPSI: A brief neuropsychological test battery in Spanish with norms by age and educational level. *Journal of the International Neuropsychological Society, 5,* 413–433.

Ostrosky, F., Ardila, A., Rosselli, M., López-Arango, G., & Uriel-Mendoza, V. (1998). Neuropsychological test performance in illiterates. *Archives of Clinical Neuropsychology, 13,* 645– 660.
Ostrosky, F., Canseco, E., Quintanar, L., Navarro, E., & Ardila, A. (1985). Sociocultural effects in neuropsychological assessment. *International Journal of Neuroscience, 27,* 53–66.
Ostrosky, F., Quintanar, L., Canseco, E., Meneses, S., Navarro, E., & Ardila, A. (1986). Habilidades cognoscitivas y nivel sociocultural [Cognitive abilities and sociocultural level]. *Revista de Investigación Clínica (México), 38,* 37–42.
Reis, A., & Castro-Caldas, A. (1997). Illiteracy: A cause for biased cognitive development. *Journal of the International Neuropsychological Society, 5,* 444–450.
Reis, A., Guerriero, M., & Castro-Caldas, A. (1994). Influence of educational level of non brain-damaged subjects on visual naming capacities. *Journal of Clinical and Experimental Neuropsychology, 16,* 939–942.
Reis, A., Guerreiro, M., & Petersson, K. M. (2003). A sociodemographic and neuropsychological characterization of an illiterate population. *Applied Neuropsychology, 10,* 191–204.
Robinson, W. P. (1974). Social factors and language development in primary school children. In R. Huxley & E. Ingram (Eds.), *Language acquisition: Models and methods* (pp. 000–000). New York: Academic Press.
Rocca, W. A., Bomaiuto, S., Lippi, A., Luciani, P., Turtu, F., Cavarzeran, F., & Amaducci, L. (1990). Prevalence of clinically diagnosed Alzheimer's disease and other dementing disorders: A door-to-door survey in Appignano, Macerata Province, Italy. *Neurology, 40,* 626–631.
Rosselli, M., & Ardila, A. (2003). The impact of culture and education on nonverbal neuropsychological measurements: A critical review. *Brain and Cognition, 52,* 226–233.
Rosselli, M., Ardila, A., & Rosas, P.(1990). Neuropsychological assessment in illiterates II: Language and praxic abilities. *Brain and Cognition, 12,* 281–296
Rosselli, M., Rosselli, A., Vergara, I., & Ardila, A. (1985). The topography of the hemi-inattention syndrome. *International Journal of Neuroscience, 20,* 153–160.
Sanchez, J. L., Rodriguez, M., & Carro, J. (2002). Influence of cognitive reserve on neuropsychologic functioning in Alzheimer's disease type sporadic in subjects of Spanish nationality. *Neuropsychiatry, Neuropsychology and Behavioral Neurology, 15,* 113–122.
Scarmeas, N., & Stern, Y. (2003). Cognitive reserve and lifestyle. *Journal of Clinical and Experimental Neuropsychology, 25,* 625–633
Scarmeas, N., & Stern, Y. (2004). Cognitive reserve: Implications for diagnosis and prevention of Alzheimer's disease. *Current Neurological Neurosciences Report, 4,* 374–380.
Staff, R. T., Murray, A. D., Deary, I. J., & Whalley, L. J. (2004). What provides cerebral reserve? *Brain, 127,* 1191–1119.
Sulkava, R., Wikstrom, J., Aromaa, A., et al. (1985). Prevalence of severe dementia in Finland. *Neurology, 35,* 1025–1029.
Stern, Y., Gurland, B., & Tatemichi, T. K.(1994). Influence of education and occupation on the incidence of Alzheimer's disease. *JAMA, 271,* 1004–1010.www.uis.unesco.org/en/stats/statistics/literacy2000.htm
Yu, E. S., Liu, W. T., Levy, P., Zhang, M. Y., Katzman, R., Lung, C. T., et al. (1989). Cognitive impairment among elderly adults in Shanghai, China. *Journal of Gerontology: Social Sciences, 44,* S97–106.

Chapter **11**

Relationship Between Functional Brain Organization and Education

Alexandre Castro-Caldas
Instituto de Ciencias da Saude
Universidade Catolica Portuguesa

Some 300 years ago, the British philosopher John Locke considered, in his "*Essay concerning Human Understanding*," that humans may attain all the knowledge they have without the help of any innate impressions. Since then, thousands of books and papers have been published but the question still remains open for research.

Nowadays we easily accept that the brain is an adaptative organ whose activity depends on its functional potential. This is the result of both genetic constraints and experiences obtained by means of sensory stimulation from the outside world. What we have to understand is how these processes interact and how they influence the outcome in the form of functional evidence.

Neural plasticity in response to changing circumstances, either physical or environmental, is now well documented in the literature (Buonomano & Merzenich, 1998; Kolb & Whishaw, 1998; Patterson & Lambon Ralph, 1999). This is particularly the case in brain regions involved in language processing that are plastic and adaptable to the characteristics of the information that is processed (Neville & Bavelier, 1998; Nobre & Plunket, 1997; Seidenberg 1997).

We have recently learned, after the work of Patterson and Lambon Ralph (1999; see also Bishop, 1999), that genetic effects on the profile of performance of certain cognitive functions were variable from childhood to adulthood. The authors studied children with Williams syndrome very early in their childhood. They showed that there was a dissociation between vocabulary and numerosity in favor of numerosity in their childhood. On the contrary, those children deal better with vocabulary later in life. This dissociation is the result of the interaction of the "natural" evolution of an abnormal brain, enframed by the stimulation of the sociocultural environment. Children developing normally tend to maintain the same pattern of skills along their lives. These findings also mean that an approach to cognitive functions based on fixed modularity, understood on the basis of adult behavior, is insufficient to understand how the brain acquires and processes information. In the case of Williams syndrome, or in the case of other genetic diseases affecting brain function, we can speculate that the biological abnormality becomes relevant only in a certain step of the maturative process of the brain, which is the moment when functional abnormalities become evident. After that, a cascade of events leads to a final abnormal arrangement in adult brain–behavior relationships. That means that the biologic substrate of behavior can have a certain shape until a certain moment and then it reorganizes itself due to the lack of structural support for more elaborate operations.

We have been considering exclusively the structural aspects related to neural tissues. However, we cannot forget that there are other important biological aspects that contribute to the normal or abnormal development of the brain. All the metabolic aspects related to the normal body function are important to support this development (for general review, see Sanes, Reh, & Harris, 2000).

Let us now consider another situation: the normal biologic development of the brain in the presence of serious deprivation. Recent studies (Bellin, Zatorre, Lafaille, & Pike, 2000) showed, by means of functional Magnetic Resonance, that in adult subjects the brain contains several regions that are sensitive to voices. These regions are arranged along the upper bank of the superior temporal sulcus in both hemispheres. They are selectively activated by vocal sounds whether speech or nonspeech. This fascinating finding together with the large corpus of information we have now about the adaptation to the sounds of language (Kuhl, 2000) and about the areas of the brain where different aspects of speech components are processed (Démonet et al., 1992; Price et al., 1996), certainly contribute to a better understanding of auditory comprehension. Most certainly the activation of these regions plays important roles in language processing and therefore in the cascade of acquisition of language-mediated information. Therefore, noneducated deaf subjects, unable to receive this type of information, also show in adult life a number of difficulties that are the cumulative effect of the auditory deficit. This means that the abnormal processing expands beyond the level of auditory comprehension (Neville & Bavelier, 2000).

Similar considerations could be made on what concerns visual deprivation (see, for instance, Mitchell, 1990). Therefore, the absence of a route to inform the brain may be compared to a genetic disease in a sense that an intervenient on the normal process of evolution is missing. Its absence prevents the brain from adapting harmoniously to the stimuli that constitute the environment and bring the information to the system.

Finally we have to consider the type of information vehiculated to the normal developing brain through the normal sensory processing systems. This seems to be an important intervenient in the way the brain adapts itself to the environment. Animal research showed that the quality of the environment matters for the organization of the brain. Animals whose environment was biased to certain forms of visual or auditory stimulation showed an adaptative behavior different from those that were raised in standard conditions. Neuropsychologic studies in these animals showed that the neuronal organization was different according to the type of sensory stimulation (see for general references Sanes et al., 2000).

In humans, we know, by means of the new techniques for brain imaging, how we adapt, for instance, to the exposure to a second language (Paulesu et al., 2000). Some evidence of this adaptation was also reported in aphasic patients (Paradis, 1998). Our main concern is the modification induced in behavior by formal education. The pattern of brain activation, as a result of learning to read and to write or of learning calculation rules can now be studied by means of the new image techniques.

THE ROLE OF FORMAL EDUCATION IN THE CONTEXT OF BRAIN-BEHAVIOR RELATIONSHIPS

In the classic literature, it was assumed that poorly educated subjects had low potential for tasks involving complex cognitive strategies, which is also a statement of common sense. We can find the reference to poor abstract thinking of low educated people in Luria's writings, for instance, and even Egas Moniz (1936) in his theoretical justification for the prefrontal leucotomy. Moniz considered that the frontal lobes were involved in the learning processes and that scholarization would change frontal function. These were simple opinions not based on empirical evidence. Therefore, it is important to understand the process of acculturation and select the best experimental paradigms. These paradigms must include a stimulus, an adaptative behavioral response to the stimulus, and a way to study the brain while responding to that stimulus. Furthermore, we need to know the structure of the stimulus well, that is, its components and the way they can be experimentally manipulated. We also need to know the expected behavior related to the stimulus and, finally, we should be able to analyze the biologic support of the operations. This can be done either through brain activation studies, or anatomic images, or by studying subjects with brain lesions.

For the past century, and particularly in the last 20 years, we have accumulated a great deal of information concerning language in its oral and written expression. We have the knowledge of the structure of the code, we understand the way humans acquire it, and we can now understand how the brain processes this type of information.

Oral language is "naturally" acquired by social exposure to speaking people. We know a lot about the way children start understanding and talking (Kuhl, 2000). On the contrary, written language requires a special teaching process and can only be acquired at the proper age, that is, when the system is ready to process this type of information.

If we are studying the implications of external stimulation on brain organization, we have to understand how the process started and grew in the history of humankind. The linkage of a writing activity to the very structure of language processing is a recent cultural acquisition. Writing is the result of the evolution of visually guided movement. We can consider that paintings on the walls of ancient caves are the first demonstration of that ability. Those paintings in a certain moment acquired meaning and became messages. Either a simple symbolic drawing had a specific signification, like some positions of the fingers painted on the walls, or a sequence of representative drawings were telling a story. The evolution of the first representation was toward pure symbols unrelated to known visual patterns, which gave birth to ideograms. These codes were later connected to a declarative representation of oral language. Orthography was then born. Isolated symbols represented sublexical components of oral language, either syllables or phonemes. The contextual meaning evolved to modern syntax (Morais, 1994). Brain regions related to this evolutive process are operators involved in the dorsal route that runs from the occipital to the parietal lobe of the left hemisphere. This route, which deals mainly with space and visually guided movement, became connected to the areas responsible for oral language. These latter areas are perisylvian regions of the left hemisphere. When children learn to read and to write, they start to activate these same pathways. Therefore, we may consider that if someone has never been exposed to this type of information, the evolutionary process of their brain will be different. We have thus a working hypothesis to explore and special regions of the brain at which to look.

The Target Populations for Studying

In certain regions of the world, as it was the case of Portugal in the past, illiteracy due to social reasons is a common finding. Our present figures indicate that around 10% of the population in Portugal (mainly those in their

60s and 70s) is unschooled because of social reasons. Indeed, until some 40 years ago, in rural areas it was common for the firstborn daughter of a couple to be kept at home instead of going to school at the age of 6. She was a caretaker for the younger siblings, who, on the contrary, at the age of 6 or 7 were sent to school. They spent all day at school and were fed there, which represented an economy for the meager budget of the family. In the communities that we have studied, mobility within the country is not common; literate and illiterate subjects live together in the same region influenced by the same sociocultural background. We cannot say that literate subjects included in most of the studies we review are sophisticated readers; on the contrary, they are generally poor and slow readers, but they learned how to do it at the proper age. This knowledge representing the main difference between the groups, makes them an interesting experimental population particularly for studies in which the "pure" effect of literacy is to be investigated. In certain studies, we may wish literacy to become the crucial effect and the general effect of schooling not to be so important. Then we raise several targeted questions enframed by a theoretical model. This theoretical model concerns the clarification of the biologic process of acquiring the skills of reading and writing. If the evidence becomes convergent to a certain result, we may assume that the results are related to literacy and not to other factors.

Some studies, mainly those coming from Mexico and South America, compared extreme groups, that is, unschooled subjects and subjects at the university level. In this case, the general effect of schooling becomes the kernel question and this may also be important mainly for developing neuropsychologic tests (Ardila, Rosselli, & Rosas, 1989; Rosselli, Ardila, & Rosas, 1990; Ostrosky-Solis, Ardila, Rosselli, Lopez-Arango, & Uriel-Mendoza, 1998).

Finally a word must be said about group comparisons. One of the most popular criticism to studies on literacy and schooling concerns the problem of IQ. There is a tendency to think that the illiterate or unschooled subjects are less intelligent than the schooled ones. We do not have tools to answer this question because in general, the performance in all tests is lower in noneducated subjects compared to educated ones. It is hard to find culture-free instruments. Therefore, if we compare subjects on the base of test results, we may be comparing the best illiterate with the worst literate, which does not reflect the reality. We have to rely on pragmatic questionnaires for daily living activities.

Hemispheric Competence for Language and Other Functions

The question of the influence of literacy on cerebral representation of functions goes back to the work of Cameron, Currier, and Haerer (1971) and to some anecdotal reports before that. These authors reported that lesions in the left hemisphere produced aphasia in 78% of literate subjects, 64% of semiliterate, and 36% of illiterate subjects. Although their illiterate subjects were not totally illiterate because they had attended school for a certain period of time, they claimed that schooling or learning to read and to write contributed to the left lateralization of verbal functions. Theoretically this is a difficult concept to accept. As we mentioned earlier, there is good evidence of functional lateralization of language processing independent from the written component. On the other hand, there is evidence that interhemispheric anatomical asymmetries are already present in the foetus brain (Tesnzer, Tzavaras, Gruner, & Hécaen, 1972; Gonçalves-Ferreira & Castro-Caldas, 1979) suggesting very early asymmetric biologic support for functions. Furthermore, we have to consider that most pioneers of the history of aphasia have been dealing mainly with illiterate subjects because literacy was reserved only for a few in the past. Nevertheless, Broca claimed that "we speak with left hemisphere" (Castro-Caldas, 1999). The work by Damásio, Castro-Caldas, Grosso, & Ferro (19786a) and Damásia, Hamsher, Castro-Caldas, Ferro, & Grosso (1976b) contradicted the assumption of cultural-induced changing of hemispheric competence, by showing that the percentage of cases with language disturbances following left and right cerebral lesions was similar both in illiterate and literate subjects. Finally, the presence of aphasia following right hemisphere lesions in dextral subjects (crossed aphasia) is absent in our experience of almost 200 cases of stroke aphasia in illiterate subjects (Castro-Caldas, Confraria, 1984 Castro-Caldas, Confraria, & Poppe, 1987).

The more recent work by Lecours et al. (1987, 1988) on literate and illiterate subjects with left and right hemisphere lesions suggested that the right hemisphere was more involved in the performance of some language tasks in illiterate subjects than in literate ones. What we can suggest is that problems can be solved by means of different types of strategies. The brain selects the most appropriate strategy in a certain moment according to the environmental constraints and to the previous experience of the subject. For unschooled subjects, a certain strategy may be based on a neural network involving mainly right hemisphere operators, whereas for schooled subjects, that same strategy may involve operators in both hemispheres or preferably those of the left side of the brain. This interpretation is also in accordance with some evidence from early-acquired cerebral lesions. Indeed, for instance, mathematical achievement is poorer in children with early right hemisphere lesions than in children with early left hemisphere lesions (Aram & Ekelman, 1988). This is different from what happens if the cerebral lesion occurs later in life after learning how to calculate. In this case, acalculia is related to lesions of the left cerebral hemisphere (Martins, Ferreira, & Borges, 1999; Martins, Parreira, Albuquerque, & Ferro, 1999).

This can be interpreted as the effect of formal learning. We can say that there are right hemisphere operators that are active for basic intuitive mathematical operations very early in life that support the necessary operations of problem solving in daily living. Learning new skills at school represents the activation of a new way of supporting the information that may have a different topographical distribution in the brain.

Consistent with this interpretation are the differences between schooled and unschooled subjects recently documented in an MRI study while subjects were performing contextual magnitude judgements (Braga, Castro-Caldas, Deloche, Dellatolas, & Campos da Paz, unpublished manuscript). In this study, unschooled subjects mainly activated structures of the right hemisphere whereas schooled subjects activated predominantly left hemisphere structures. In both groups the task was accurately accomplished.

On the other hand, taking in consideration the PET data that we discuss below and in which literate and illiterate subjects were scanned while repeating words and pseudowords, we selected Regions Of Interest (ROIs) with particular focus on the posterior parietal cortex. Left/right hemispheric differences were compared between groups averaging each subject's data over words, pseudowords, and word plus pseudowords, respectively. The three different analyses indicated the same pattern of between-group differences, all relating to the ROIs in the posterior parietal cortex (superior part of BA40 on the border of BA7, inferior part of BA39 extending into inferior part of BA40, and BA31 part of precuneus). The difference between groups indicated a dissociation between the superior and inferior parts of the angular–supramarginal regions, that is, the superior parts being more active on the left than on the right in illiterate compared to literate subjects, whereas the reverse was the case for the inferior parts and the precuneus. Therefore, it can be suggested that the knowledge of the visuospatial dimension of language (orthography) changes the pattern of interhemisphere distribution of operators involved in the task probably increasing the transfer of information between the two cerebral hemispheres Castro-Caldas, Petersson, Reis, Askelöf, & Ingvar, 1998a).

Language

In his seminal work, Morais, Cary, Alegria, and Bertelson (1979) called the attention to the fact that the capacity to conscenciously represent phonemes in isolation appears in the course of learning to read and write in the alphabetic system. Therefore subjects that never attended school and were never confronted with the need to match a segment of oral language to a written symbol, never developed the ability of consciously understanding that words can be segmented in small units of sound that belong to a comprehensive system. For these subjects, words are acquired on the basis of a semantic enframement like it happens with preschool children (Gathercole, 1999). Among the operations that adult illiterate subjects fail to achieve is the repetition of pseudowords (Reis & Castro-Caldas, 1997a). They tend to force a semantic analogy when they produce the word. This finding contributed to the argument of implementing a functional study with Positron Emission Tomography. A group of 12 women volunteered to travel from Portugal to Sweden, where the study was carried on. Six were illiterate and six were literate with an average of 4 years of schooling. Lists of real words with two and three syllables were prepared as well as lists of pseudowords. These were constructed by changing the consonants of the real words while maintaining the vocal components. Subjects were scanned while repeating lists of real words and while repeating lists of pseudowords. They were never informed about the content of the lists, they were only asked to repeat as close as possible what they were hearing. They were instructed that some words would be more difficult than others. They were also told that if they were unable to repeat the words, they should produce the word "passo," which means "pass" (Castro-Caldas, Petersson, Reis, Stone-Elander, & Ingvar, 1998b).

Results showed that the pattern of activation of both groups was very similar while they were repeating real words, activating brain areas of the sensory cortex of both hemispheres that can be related to the semantic processing. On the other hand, the pattern of activation while repeating pseudowords was rather different between the two groups. Illiterate subjects had a pattern of activation similar to the one that they activated for repeating words and literate subjects activated a complex network involving subcortical structures mainly on the left hemisphere, left insula, and cerebellum, a pattern that can be related to a procedural processing. We were able through this study to demonstrate that the failure to repeat pseudowords correctly was related to the absence of activation of the proper regions of the brain. These results were further analyzed by means of a network approach in which regions of interest were selected according to their theoretical relevance in the task of word and pseudowords repetition. Covariance analysis revealed that the pattern of interconnection of the different areas varied between groups and between tasks showing again that each group was using the brain in different ways (Petersson, Reis, Askelöf, Castro-Caldas, & Ingvar, 2000).

Having in mind these results, we went back to our files of illiterate aphasics (Castro-Caldas et al., 1997b). The first hypothesis we explored was related to the fact that illiterate subjects are unable to activate a phonological route to repeat and prefer a semantic one. In this case, when they have a comprehension defect due to aphasia, they will have a major defect in repetition. This was indeed the truth. There are very few illiterate aphasics who can repeat words without comprehending them. More recent results, still in preparation, showed that the improvement in repetition after 6 months of evolution of aphasia is worse in illiterate global aphasics than in literate ones. This also suggests that comprehension is crucial for recovering phonological skills.

The second hypothesis was related to the potentially different quality of the process of both groups in repeating words when a repetition defect is present. We compared literate and illiterate conduction aphasics and made an analysis of their performance in repeating words. Results showed that illiterate aphasics more frequently produced semantic paraphasias. The number and type of phonological paraphasias was similar in both groups. However, literate subjects made frequent corrections trying to produce the correct word whereas illiterate subjects rarely showed this behaviour. This is interpreted as the result of the absence of phonological awareness of illiterate subjects. The absence of a declarative representation of phonology prevents the trial and error behavior that is frequently observed in literate aphasics. Thus, these findings suggest a different strategy for processing repetition and cannot be explained on the basis of different lesion localizations because the brain lesions responsible for aphasias in all cases studied were vascular.[1]

Furthermore, in the same line of thought, we explored the hypothesis that the performance in digit span tasks by aphasics would give us more information. As a matter of fact, our previous results suggested that the semantic value of digits is of relevance for the performance in digit span tasks of illiterate subjects (Castro-Caldas, Reis, & Guerreiro, 1997a; Reis, Guerreiro, Garcia, & Castro-Caldas, 1995). Illiterate subjects have more difficulty in repeating series of digits composed of the digits 5 to 9 than repeating series composed of the digits 1 to 5. The group of aphasics we chose in this case was the one in which repetition is spared, that is, transcortical aphasics. In the case of transcortical motor aphasia, comprehension is spared whereas in transcortical sensory aphasia, comprehension is disturbed. In the literate group of aphasics, there was no difference in digit span performance between motor and sensory transcortical aphasia. This was not the case in the illiterate group in which the digit span was worse in sensory transcortical aphasics than in those with motor transcortical aphasia. These results also call attention to the importance of the semantic support for language processing by illiterate subjects. Different areas of the brain may be involved in language processing in subjects with different cultural backgrounds. Therefore, lesions in the same localizations produce different symptoms.

---

[1] In stroke aphasia, the different syndromes are related to the basic vascular anatomy. There is no reason to think that cultural aspects may interfere with the vascular anatomy.

The Corpus Callosum

Taking in consideration the previously reviewed findings, we can understand that schooling opens new opportunities for the brain to use new strategies. The acquisition of new strategies means an increase of the connectivity between neurons. The corpus callosum is the region of the brain that can be considered mainly an organ of connectivity. Therefore, the suggestion of an increase of the intra or interhemispheric communication made this region our target. Variations in the anatomy of the corpus callosum have been reported in several conditions, like gender and handedness. However, these differences were inconsistent across the studies (Duara et al., 1991; Hynd et al., 1995; Larsen, Hoien, & Odegaard, 1992). The study of monozygotic twins also suggested that the size and shape of the corpus callosum is influenced by both genetic and nongenetic factors (Oppenheim, Skerry, Tramo, & Gazzaniga, 1989). Another piece of important evidence comes from studies that showed a significant growing of the corpus callosum until late in life (Witelson, 1991; Cowell, Allen, Zalatimo, & Denenberg, 1992; Pujol, Vendrell, Junque, Marty-Vilalta, & Capdevilla, 1993), suggesting a prolonged interaction with environmental factors. Nothing is known about what really influences the morphological changes. One possibility is that they may be related to the acquisition of new skills, such as learning. We selected for our study 41 right-handed upper middle aged women, 18 being illiterate and 23 literate Castro-Caldas et al., 1999). The outline of each corpus callosum, as viewed in the midsagital section of MRI, was digitized by manually tracing over the film. The methodology used was a modification of what was proposed by Denenberg, Kertesz, and Cowell, (1991). In summary, the results of the comparison done between the two groups showed that there was a region of the corpus callosum that was smaller in illiterate subjects. This region corresponds to the area where interparietal fibers cross Pandya & Seltzer, 1986). These results are consistent with the behavioral studies that showed that some visuomotor tasks involving interhemispheric pathways are apparently more difficult for illiterate subjects (Reis & Castro-Caldas, 1997b). They are also consistent with the PET findings of an increased cross talk between the hemispheres at the parietal level when orthography is mastered, which were previously mentioned.

Dementia

Low education level has been shown to be associated with dementia in several studies (Katzman, 1993; Zhang et al., 1990). However, this was apparently not the result of schooling as suggested by a study conducted in India in which illiteracy was not found to be a risk factor (Chandra et al., 1998).

The several sources of information are still in conflict (Cobb, Wolf, Au, White, & D'Agostino, 1995; Stern, Albert, Tang, & Tsai, 1999; Stern, Alexander, Prokovnik, & Mayeux, 1992; Stein et al., 1994; Stein, Tang, Denaro, & Mayeux, 1995). The EURODEM incidence Research Group and Work Groups pooled European Studies to try to understand risk factors and found that the deleterious effect of lower education was more marked in women than in men (Launer et al., 1999). Ardila, Ostrosky-Solis, Rosselli, and Gómez (2000) studied a nondemented population of 883 subjects with ages raging from 16–85 years and schooling ranging from total illiteracy to over 10 years of schooling. They reported a protective effect of cultural level in some neuropsychological tests as in "Recall of the Words." This was not found, however, in most of the large number of tests that were used.

Several interpretations for these findings were proposed and were reviewed by Kukul and Ganguli (2000). Some are related to the possibility of higher educated subjects benefiting from a higher socioeconomic status and therefore better nutrition and health care. Intelligence was also called for explaining the cultural differences, which seems not to be a good explanation. Many of the explanations are included in the brain reserve model proposed by Katzman, (1993; Katzman et al., 1998). Finally, Kukul and Ganguli (2000) proposed a methodologic explanation. A better education may simply allow individuals to perform better on tests and thus may mask or delay the onset of dementia for a longer period of time. The use of MMSE (Folstein, Folstein, & McHugh, 1975) for Alzheimer's disease screening is, for example, a potential source of error. Our illiterate nondemented population scores below the cut-off score defined for the schooled population (Guerreiro, 1999). The absence of dementia in this group is well proven by follow-up studies in which the low score maintains and the subjects do not deteriorate.

The same line of thought that oriented our previous studies led us to consider the case of semantic memory in Alzheimer's Disease. Semantic memory becomes disturbed very early in the evolution of the disease, conversely, digit span is known to maintain longer. As we suggested earlier, illiterate subjects rely on semantics for their performance in digit span tasks. Therefore, the performance in digit span should be much worse in the early phase of illiterate demented subjects compared to literate ones. Indeed, our results showed that compared to normal controls, the performance on digit span tasks is much lower in illiterate that in literate demented subjects in the early stages of the evolution of the disease. We can thus consider that the biologic process affecting parietal regions is more devastating for subjects whose cognitive activity stems mostly from operations related with those areas of the brain (Guerreiro, Castro-Caldas, Reis, & Garcia, 1999; see also Castro-Caldas & Guerreiro, in press).

CONCLUSIONS

The development of the new image techniques to study the normal brain processing opened new opportunities to understand how the brain adapts itself to information. So far, we can say that a different pattern of activation of brain structures seems to be the base for a different performance when we compare groups of different educational level. We can still go back to brain lesioned cases and complete the information now in a different perspective. We can also study the normal anatomy of target regions by MRI and some histologic studies would be most welcome. There is still a long way to go before we fully understand these processes. However, we can foresee their interest for the understanding of the potential for learning in adult life and the way we have to adapt teaching techniques for adults. On the other hand, the description of diverse supports for information can be explored in rehabilitation of brain lesioned subjects.

REFERENCES

Aram, D. M., & Ekelman, B. L. (1988). Scholastic aptitude and achievement among children with unilateral brain lesions. *Neuropsychologia, 26,* 903–916.

Ardila, A., Rosselli, M., & Rosas, P. (1989). Neuropsychological assessment in illiterates: visuospatial and memory abilities. *Brain and Cognition, 11,* 147–166.

Ardila, A., Ostrosky-Solis, F., Rosselli, M., & Gómez, C. (2000). Age-related cognitive decline during normal aging: The complex effect of education. *Archives of Clinical Neuropsychology, 15,* 495–513.

Bellin, P., Zatorre, R. J., Lafaille, P., & Pike, B. (2000). Voice-selective areas in human auditory cortex. *Nature, 3,* 309–312.

Bishop, D. V. M. (1999). Cognition—An innate basis for language. *Science, 286,* 2283–2284.

Braga, L. W., Castro-Caldas, A., Deloche, G., Dellatolas, G., & Campos da Paz, A. A. *Culture and education generate alternative pathways in the functional anatomy of the brain.* Unpublished manuscript.

Buonomano, D. V., & Merzenich, M. M. (1998). Cortical plasticity: From synapses to maps. *Annual Review of Neuroscience, 21,* 49–186.

Cameron, R. F., Currier, R. D., & Haerer, A. F. (1971). Aphasia and literacy. *British Journal of Disorders of Communication, 6,* 161–163.

Castro-Caldas, A. (1999). Aphasia in atypical populations. (Book review). *Brain, 122,* 1200–1202.

Castro-Caldas, A., & Confraria, A. (1984). Age and type of crossed aphasia in dextrals due to stroke. *Brain and Language, 23,* 126–133.

Castro-Caldas, A., Confraria, A., & Poppe, P. (1987). Non-verbal disturbances in crossed aphasia. *Aphasiology, 5,* 403–413.

Castro-Caldas, A., & Guerreiro, M. (in press). Cultural background as a risk factor for dementia. In F. Boller & J. Grafman (Eds.), *Handbook of Neuropsychology* (2nd rev. ed.).

Castro-Caldas, A., Miranda, P., Carmo, I., Reis, A., Leote, F., Ribeiro, C., & Ducla-Soares, E. (1999). Influence of learning to read and write on the morphology of the corpus callosum. *European Journal of Neurology, 6,* 23–28.

Castro-Caldas, A., Petersson, K. M., Reis, A., Askelöf, S., & Ingvar, M. (1998a). Differences in inter-hemispheric interactions related to literacy, assessed by PET. *Neurology, 50,* A43.
Castro-Caldas, A., Petersson, K. M., Reis, A., Stone-Elander, S., & Ingvar, M. (1998b). The illiterate brain: Learning to read and write during childhood influences the functional organization of the adult brain. *Brain, 121,* 1053–1063.
Castro-Caldas, A., Reis, A., & Guerreiro, M. (1997a). Neuropsychological aspects of illiteracy. *Neuropsychological Rehabilitation, 7,* 327–338.
Castro-Caldas, A., Reis, A., Guerreiro, M., Leal, G., Farrajota, L., & Fonseca, J. (1997b). Illiteracy and aphasia revisited. *Journal of Neurology, 244*(3), S47.
Chandra, V., Ganguli, M., Pandav, R., Johnston, J., Belle, S., & Dekosky, S. T. (1998). Prevalence of Alzheimer's disease and other dementias in rural India: The Indo-US study. *Neurology, 51,* 1000–1008.
Cobb, J. L., Wolf, P. A., Au, R., White, R., & D'Agostino, R. B. (1995). The effect of education on the incidence of dementia and Alzheimer's disease in the Framingham Study. *Neurology, 45,* 1707–1712.
Cowell, P. E., Allen, L. S., Zalatimo, N. S., & Denenberg, V. H. (1992). A developmental study of sex and age interactions in the human corpus callosum. *Developmental Brain Research, 66,* 187–192.
Damásio, A. R., Castro-Caldas, A., Grosso, J. T., & Ferro, J. M. (1976a) Brain specialization for language does not depend on literacy. *Archives of Neurology, 33,* 300–331.
Damásio, A. R., Hamsher, K. DeS., Castro-Caldas, A., Ferro, J. M., & Grosso, J. T. (1976b). Brain specialization for language does not depend on literacy. *Archives of Neurology, 33,* 662.
Démonet, J.-F, Chollet, F., Ramsay, S., Cardebat, D., Nespoulous, J.-L., Wise, R., Rascol, A., & Frackowiack, R. (1992). The anatomy of phonological and semantic processing in normal subjects. *Brain, 115,* 1753–1768.
Denenberg, V. H., Kertez, A., & Cowell, E. (1991). A factor analysis of the human's corpus callosum. *Brain Research, 548,* 126–132.
Duara, R., Kushch, A., Gross-Glenn, K., Barker, W. W., Jallad, B., Pascal, S., et al. (1991). Neuroanatomic differences between dyslexic and normal readers on magnetic resonance imaging scans. *Archives of Neurology, 48,* 410–416.
Egas Moniz, A. (1936). *Tentatives opératoires dans le traitement de certaines psychoses* [Tentative treatment of certain psychoses]. Paris: Masson & Cie.
Folstein, M. F., Folstein, S. E., & McHugh, P. R. (1975). Mini-mental state: A practical method for grading the cognitive state of patients for the clinician. *Journal of Psychiatric Research, 12,* 189–198.
Gathercole, S. E. (1999). Cognitive approaches to the development of short-term memory. *Trends in Cognitive Sciences, 3,* 410–419.
Gonçalves-Ferreira, A. J., & Castro-Caldas, A. (1979). Assimetrias morfológicas inter-hemisféricas [Inter-hemispheric anatomic asymmetries]. *Análise Psicológica, IV,* 509–518.
Guerreiro, M. (1998). *Contributo da Neuropsicologia para o estudo das Demências.* Unpublished doctoral dissertation, University of Lisbon.
Guerreiro, M., Castro-Caldas, A., Reis, A., & Garcia, C. (1996). O Cérebro analfabeto: A questão da demência [The illiterate brain: The problem of dementia]. *Análise Psicológica, XIV,* 341–351.
Hynd, G. W., Hall, J., Novey, E. S., Eliopulos, D., Black, K., Gonzalez, J. J., et al. (1995). Dyslexia and corpus callosum morphology. *Archives of Neurology, 52,* 32–38.

Katzman, R. (1993). Education and the prevalence of dementia and Alzheimer's disease. *Neurology, 43,* 12–20.
Katzman, R., Terry, R., DeTeresa, R., Brown, T., Davies, P., Fuld, P., et al. (1998). Clinical, pathological, and neurochemical changes in dementia: A subgroup with preserved mental status and numerous neocortical plaques. *Annals of Neurology, 23,* 138–144.
Kolb, B., & Whishaw, I. Q. (1998). Brain plasticity and behavior. *Annual Review of Psychology, 49,* 43–64.
Kuhl, P. K. (2000). Language, mind and brain: Experience alters perception. In M. S. Gazzinaga (Ed.), *The new cognitive neurosciences* (pp. 99–115). Cambridge MA: MIT Press.
Kukull, W. A., & Ganguli, M. (2000). Epidemiology of dementia. *Neurologic Clinics, 18,* 923–949.
Larsen, J. P., Hoien, T., & Odegaard, H. (1992). Magnetic resonance imaging of the corpus callosum in developmental dyslexia. *Cognitive Neuropsychology, 9,* 123–134.
Launer, L. J., Andersen, K., Dewey, M. E., Lettenneur, L., Ott, A., Amaducci, L. A., et al. (1999). Rates and risk factors for dementia and Alzheimer's disease. Results from EURODEM pooled analyses. EURODEM Incidence Research Group and Work Groups. European Studies of Dementia. *Neurology, 52,* 78–84.
Lecours, A., Mehler, J., Parente, M. A., Aguiar, L. R., Silva, A. B., Caetano, M.., et al. (1987). Illiteracy and brain damage: 2. Manifestations of unilateral neglect in testing "auditory comprehension" with iconographic material. *Brain and Cognition, 6,* 243–265.
Lecours, A., Mehler, J., Parente, M. A., Beltrami, M. C., Tolipan, L. C., Cary, L., et al. (1988). Illiteracy and brain damage: 3. A contribution to the study of speech and language disorders in illiterates with unilateral brain damage (initial testing). *Neuropsychologia, 26,* 575–589.
Luria, A. R. (1970). The functional organization of the brain. *Scientific American, 222,* 66–78.
Martins, I. P., Ferreira, J., & Borges L. (1999). Acquired procedural dyscalculia associated to a left parietal lesion in a child. *Child Neuropsychology, 5,* 265–273.
Martins, I. P., Parreira, E., Albuquerque, L., & Ferro, J. M. (1999). Capacités de calcul chez des enfants scolarisés avec des lésions cérébrales acquises [Calculation capacities of educated children with acquired cerebral lesions]. *Approche Neuropsychologique des Apprentissages chez L'Enfant, 51,* 5–12.
Mitchell, D. E. (1990). Sensitive periods in visual development: Insights gained from studies of recovery of visual function in cats following early monocular deprivations or cortical lesions. In C. Blakemore (Ed.), *Vision coding and efficiency* (pp. 234–246). New York: Cambridge University Press.
Morais, J. (1994). *L'art de lire.* Paris: Éditions Odile Jacob.
Morais, J., Cary, L., Alegria, J., & Bertelson, P. (1979). Does awareness of speech as a sequence of phones arise spontaneously? *Cognition, 7,* 323–331.
Neville, H. J., & Bavelier, D. (1998). Neural organisation and plasticity of language. *Current Opinion in Neurobiology, 8,* 254–258.
Neville, H. J., & Bavelier, D. (2000). Specificity and plasticity in neurocognitive development in humans. In M. S. Gazzinaga (Ed.), *The new cognitive neuroscience* (pp. 219–234). Cambridge MA: MIT Press.
Nobre, A. C., & Plunket, K. (1997). The neural system of language: Structure and development, *Current Opinion in Neurobiology, 7,* 262–268.

Oppenheim, J. S., Skerry, J. E., Tramo, M. J., & Gazzaniga, M. S. (1989). Magnetic resonance imaging morphology of the corpus callosum in monozygotic twins. *Annals of Neurology, 26,* 100–104.

Ostrosky-Solis, F., Ardila, A., Rosselli, M., Lopez-Arango, G., & Uriel-Mendoza, V. (1998). Neuropsychological test performance in Illiterate subjects. *Archives of Clinical Neuropsychology, 13,* 645–660.

Pandya, D. N., & Seltzer, B. (1986). The topography of commissural fibers. In F. Lepore, M. Ptito, & H. Jaspar (Eds.), *Two hemispheres—one brain: Functions of the corpus callosum* (pp. 47–73). New York: Liss.

Paradis, M. (1998). Aphasia in bilinguals: How atypical is it? In P. Coppens, Y. Lebrun, & A. Basso (Eds.), *Aphasia in atypical populations* (pp. 35–66). Mahwah, NJ: Lawrence Erlbaum Associates.

Patterson, S. J., Brown, J. H., Gsödl, M. K., Johnson, M. H., & Karmiloff-Smith, A. (1999). Cognitive modularity and genetic disorders. *Science, 286,* 2355–2358.

Patterson, K., & Lambon Ralph, M. A. (1999). Selective disorders of reading. *Current Opinion in Neurobiology, 9,* 235–239.

Paulesu, E., McCrory, E., Fazio, F., Menocello, L., Brunswick, N., Cappa, S. F., et al. (2000). A cultural effect on brain function. *Nature Neuroscience, 3,* 91–96.

Petersson, K. M., Reis, A., Askelöf, S., Castro-Caldas, A., & Ingvar, M., (2000). Language processing modulated by literacy: A network analysis of verbal repetition in literate and illiterate subjects. *Journal of Cognitive Neurosciences, 6,* 475–782.

Price, C. J., Wise, R., Warburtan, E. A., Moore, C. J. Howard, D., Patterson, K., et al. (1996). Hearing and saying: The functional neuro-anatomy of auditory word-processing. *Brain, 119,* 919–931.

Pujol, J., Vendrell, P., Junque, C., Marty-Vilalta, J. L., & Capdevilla, A. (1993). When does human brain development end? Evidence of the corpus callosum growth up to adulthood. *Annals of Neurology, 34,* 71–75.

Reis, A., Guerreiro, M., Garcia, C., & Castro-Caldas, A. (1995). How does an illiterate subject process the lexical component of arithmetics? *Journal of the International Neuropsychologia Society, 1,* 206.

Reis, A., & Castro-Caldas, A. (1997a). Illiteracy: A cause for biased cognitive for development. *Journal of the International Neuropsychological Society, 3,* 444–450.

Reis, A., & Castro-Caldas, A. (1997b). Learning to read and write increases the efficacy of reaching a target in two dimensional space. *Journal of the International Neuropsychological Society, 3,* 222.

Rosselli, M., Ardila, A., & Rosas, P. (1990). Neuropsychological assessment in illiteraterater II: Language and praxic abilities. *Brain and Cognition, 12,* 281–296.

Sanes, D. H., Reh, T. A., & Harris, W. A. (2000). *Development of the nervous system.* San Diego, CA: Academic Press.

Seidenberg, M. S. (1997). Language acquisition and use: Learning and applying probabilistic constraints. *Science, 275,* 1599–1603.

Stern, Y., Albert, S., Tang, M.-X., & Tsai, W.-Y. (1999). Rate of memory decline in AD is related to education and occupation: Cognitive reserve. *Neurology, 53,* 1942–1947.

Stern, Y., Alexander, G. E., Prokovnik, I., & Mayeux, R. (1992). Inverse relationship between education and parietotemporal perfusion deficit in Alzheimer's disease. *Annals of Neurology, 32,* 371–375.

Stern, Y., Gurland, B., Tatemichi T. K, Tang, M. X., Wilder, D., & Mayeux, R. (1994). Influence of education and occupation on the incidence of Alzheimer's Disease. *JAMA, 271,* 1004–1010.

Stern, Y., Tang M.-X., Denaro, J., & Mayeux, R. (1995). Increased risk of mortality in Alzheimer's disease patients with more advanced educational and occupational attainment. *Annals of Neurology, 37,* 590–595.

Teszner, D., Tzavaras, A., Gruner, J., & Hécaen, H. (1992). L'asymétrie droite-gauche du planum temporale: À propos de l'étude anatomique de 100 cerveaux [Right-left asymmetry of the planum temporale: Anatomic study of 100 brains]. *Revue Neurologique, 126,* 444–449.

Witelson, S. F. (1991). Sex differences in neuroanatomical changes with aging. *The New England Journal of Medicine, 325,* 211–212.

Zhang, M., Katzman, R., Salmon, D., Jin, H., Cai, G., Wang, Z., et al. (1990). The prevalence of dementia and Alzheimer's disease in Shangai, China_: Impact of age, gender and education. *Annals of Neurology, 27,* 428–437.

Chapter **12**

Educational Effects on Cognitive Functions: Brain Reserve, Compensation, or Testing Bias?

F. Ostrosky-Solís
Universidad Nacional Autónoma de México

Several studies have postulated that education and literacy may protect not only against the effects of biological aging (Albert et al., 1995; Christensen & Henderson, 1991; Orell & Sahakian, 1995) but also against the clinical manifestation of cerebral neuropathology (Katzman, 1993; Stern, 2002; Stern et al., 1994; Zhang et al., 1990).

The relationship between education and dementia has been studied mainly in Alzheimer's disease (AD). It has been postulated that AD not only has a later onset but that it is less severe in highly educated people (Katzman, 1993; Stern et al.,1994). This association of high education with late age of onset of dementia has been considered as evidence of cognitive and/or brain reserve (Katzman, 1993; Mortimer 1988; Satz, 1993; Stern 2002). Several explanations for this effect have been postulated; for example, according to Mortimer (1988), lack of education reduces the margin of "intellectual reserve" to a level where a minor level of brain pathology results in a dementia and therefore people with higher education will have a late onset. Mortimer and Graves (1993) hypothesized three different mechanisms to explain the apparent association between educational attainment and dementia: (1) risk factor exposures related to low educational level and to socioeconomic status in adult life; (2) brain reserve capacity as determined by fetal or early-life exposure to factors associated with socioeconomic status of the family or origin; and (3) the effect of lifelong mental stimulation associated with education affects neuronal growth. Katzman (1993) suggested that "education increases brain reserve by increasing synaptic density in neocortical association cortex, leading to a delay of symptoms by 4 to 5 years in those with AD (and probably, other dementing disorders) hence halving the prevalence of dementia.

In a recent review, Stern (2002) discussed that the idea of reserve against brain damage stems from the repeated observation that there does not appear to be a direct relationship between the degree of brain pathology or brain damage and the clinical manifestation of that damage. He pointed out that one convenient subdivision of reserve models revolves around whether they envision reserve as a passive process, such as in brain reserve or threshold, or see the brain as actively attempting to cope with or compensate for pathology, as in cognitive reserve. However he further discussed that cognitive reserve may be based on more efficient utilization of brain networks or on enhanced ability to recruit alternate brain networks as needed.

COGNITIVE RESERVE AND OUTCOME MEASURES: EFFECTS OF TESTING BIAS

The relationship between education and dementia is controversial, although several epidemiological studies from different cultural settings have shown that the prevalence of dementia is higher in the poorly educated individuals (Obadia et al., 1997; Stern et al., 1994; Zhang et al., 1990). Other investigations have found no such evidence (Beard et al., 1992; Cobb et al., 1995; O'Connor et al., 1991). Therefore, it is important to take into account that when studying reserve, careful attention must be given to potential confounds. For example, typical correlates of reserve include IQ and education, both of which can directly affect test performance in the absence of reserve. Thus, several studies have suggested that differences associated with reserve could also be due to test bias because individuals with lower educational and occupational attainment perform worse on the clinical and neuropsychological tests used to diagnose dementia (Ardila, Rosselli, & Pinzón, 1989; Escobar et al., 1986; Ostrosky-Solís, López, & Ardila, 2000; Rosselli et al., 1990). One of the limitations of several of the epidemiological studies that had reported a higher prevalence of AD in individuals with lower education is that they used global mental status measures such as the Mini-Mental State Examination (MMSE) as a screening device.

The known correlation of mental status tests with education has led to concern as to whether the use of such tests in the screening phase of community investigation results in a spurious increase in dementia prevalence in those with no or low education (Katzman, 1993). The MMSE is one of the most frequently used rating instruments in the evaluation of the mental state in both clinical practice and research, therefore some authors have suggested adjusting the MMSE score as a way to take into account demographic variables, including age, education, and degree of dementia. Crum, Anthony, Bassett, and Folstein (1993), studied the distribution of MMSE scores by age and education in a population of 18,056 individuals in five states (New Haven, CT; Baltimore, MD; St. Louis, MO; Durham, NC; Los Angeles, CA). The MMSE scores were related to age and education level. They found an inverse relationship between MMSE scores and age, with a range of 29 for those aged 18 to 24, to 25 for individuals aged 80. The mean was 29 for individuals with fewer than 9 years of education, 26 for 5 to 8 years, and 22 for those with 0 to 4 years of education. They suggest adjusting the cutoff point according to these data.

The MMSE has been widely used as a screening instrument in both population and epidemiological studies for the detection of dementia, and although Spanish-speaking subjects are frequently included among the population sample (i.e., Crum et al., 1993; Stern, et al. 1994), there is a lack of normative data for the monolingual Spanish-speaking population as well as a lack of information about the sensitivity and specificity of the test for Spanish-speaking subjects. Therefore, Ostrosky, López, and Ardila (2000) applied the MMSE to 430 neurological intact monolingual Spanish-speaking subjects from 16 to 85 years of age. The sample was stratified by age into three groups: 16–50, 51–65, and 66–89 years, and four educational levels were considered within each age range: illiterates (none), low educational level (1–4), middle educational level (5–9), and high educational level (more than 10 years of education). They found that the educational level had a significant impact on the total score. Normal illiterate subjects obtained scores that classified them as within severe cognitive alterations ($\chi = 17.67$), whereas those with low education (1 to 4 years) classified within moderate cognitive alterations ($\chi = 20.61$). The sensitivity and specificity of the MMSE was established by using a sample of 40 patients with clinically diagnosed cognitive impairment. The subjects were matched with the control group according to age and education. Using the 23/24 cutoff point suggested by Folstein, Folstein, and McHugh (1975), low sensitivity and specificity levels were found for both the subjects with zero and 1 to 4 years of education, 50% and 72.73% respectively. The adjustment of the cutoff value according to the average performance of the neurologically intact group increased specificity (90%), but significantly reduced sensitivity (27.27%). In the subjects with more than 5 years of education, the specificity (86.3%) and sensitivity (86.6%) indices were higher.

These results confirm previous reports that the level of education plays a very important role in the MMSE performance. The performance of normal individuals with no education was as low as that of subjects with severe dementia, whereas the score for those with 1 to 4 years of education was similar to that of subjects with slight dementia.

With a cutoff point of 23/24, the sensitivity and specificity were acceptable (80% and 77.5% respectively), provided that the education factor was not included. However, when the sample was broken down into various education levels, a marked decline in the specificity among persons with no education or 1 to 4 years of education was noted (50%). On the other hand, although the adjustment of the cutoff point for the population with 0 to 4 years of education in terms of average performance (17 for the illiterate and 20 for those with 1 to 4 years of education) produced a significant increase in specificity (adequate discrimination of individuals without pathology), sensitivity declined significantly (detection of individuals with cognitive deterioration). Thus it can be concluded that varying the cutoff point is not sufficient to obtain adequate sensitivity and specificity indices, because one is favored to the detriment of the other. These results have significant implications for both research and clinical practice. Epidemiological studies that only include the MMSE as a rating instrument will classify normal subjects with low education as patients, which resultd in a higher rate of detection. It is possible that testing bias or lack of compensatory process, arising from greater strategies when confronted with difficulties, rather than brain or neuronal reserve, may overestimate the severity of cognitive decline and hence the estimates of the prevalence of dementia among the less educated individuals.

Diagnosis of dementia requires evidence of impaired social and/or occupational functioning, therefore, the assessment of functional capacity is regarded as an important part of a comprehensive diagnostic work-up for dementia; furthermore, evaluation of functional capacity has also become increasingly important to reduce the likelihood of spurious education and cultural effects. However, even functional capacities are prone to cultural biases. Loewenstein et al. (1992) compared Spanish- and English-speaking dementia patients and normal controls on a comprehensive functional assessment battery and found that, despite equivalent levels of cognitive impairment, Spanish-speaking dementia patients evidenced more difficulties on certain functional tasks relative to their English-speaking counterparts. They suggested that the extent of deterioration in specific functional subskills may be related to the degree to which they have been overlearned and practiced. Therefore, they pointed out, that not only for neuropsychological measures but also for functional scales, there is a need for normative data for older adults that belong to different ethnic and cultural groups.

EDUCATION AND AGE-RELATED COGNITIVE DECLINE DURING NORMAL AGING: PROTECTION, BRAIN RESERVE, OR COMPENSATORY STRATEGIES?

The association between education and cognitive change associated with normal aging has also been an important topic of research. Much debate has centered on whether the brain is more likely to degenerate as a result of overuse or underused. There is a popular belief that an active mental life may delay the cognitive deterioration associated with normal aging. Research with elderly rats exposed to an enriched environment showed that the brain had increased cortical thickness and weight and increased dendritic branching and that rats' general performance was better than that of control rats from a nonstimulating environment (Buell & Coleman, 1979).

In humans, a protective effect of education has also been reported during normal aging. Community longitudinal studies using a large number of subjects have reported an association between low educational attainment and decline in later life, noting that less educated people deteriorate to a greater extent than do better educated people over various follow-up periods (Christensen et al., 1997; Farmer, Kittner, Rae, Bartco, & Regier, 1995). It has also been reported that stimulating programs may be effective in reducing memory problems associated with normal aging (Yesavage, 1985).

As with the studies of dementia, it has been suggested that the protective effect arises from slower biological aging in the highly educated (Albert et al., 1995; Evans et al., 1993; Orell & Sahakian, 1995). An alternative explanation is that higher scores among the highly educated is the result of compensation due to the fact that education and stimulating mental activity may help improve coping skills and strategies for solving problems (Christensen et al., 1997). Based on the last explanation, another way to approach the question of the protective effect of education has been to study in what areas of cognitive function the protective effect is manifested and what is the effect of other biological variables that can influence cognitive functioning.

In a recent meta-analysis, Anstey and Christensen (2000) reviewed 14 longitudinal studies conducted since 1985 that examined the relationship between years of education and cognitive change and analyzed published findings on genetic, health, and lifestyle predictors of cognitive change in late adulthood. Studies reporting data on education, activity, health, blood pressure, and Apoliprotein E alles (APOE) as predictors of cognitive change were reviewed. Results showed that education, hypertension, objective indices of health and cardiovascular disease, and APOE were associated with cognitive change, and that the results regarding the effect of physical activity were inconclusive. They pointed out that education was the most important nonbiological correlate of cognitive performance in many of the studies reviewed. The authors categorized the results into those reporting one of four outcomes: (1) studies reporting the rate of decline being less rapid for the highly educated, (2) studies failing to find an effect of education on cognitive change, (3) studies where the effect was restricted to a subgroup or subgroups (women or age subgroups), and (4) studies that were restricted to types of outcomes such as measures of verbal intelligence. They pointed out that the outcomes of these studies could be due to the type of cognitive test included in the study; therefore studies that used brief cognitive measures such as the MMSE or measures related to memory and crystallized abilities such as vocabulary, similarities, information, and reading found a protective effect of education, but studies that used fluid measures and processing speed, choice reaction time, and symbol digit substitution did not find protective effects.

Because educational attainment is an important variable that must be considered when interpreting scores on cognitive measures, another important factor that could affect the results reviewed by Anstey and Christensen (2000) is the range of years of education of the population studied. In the studies reviewed, the range of the educational variable was very small. For example, some studies included subjects with an average of 6 years in the low education group and an average of 12 years or more in the high education groups or they simply divided them as less than 10 years, and more than 11 years. As Ardila, Ostrosky-Solis, Rosselli, and Gómez (2000) pointed out, the educational effect in not linear, but rather is a negatively accelerated curve, tending to a plateau. Differences between 0 and 3 years of education are highly significant; differences between 3 and 6 years of education are lower, between 6 and 9 are even lower, and virtually no differences are expected to be found between, for example 12 and 15 years of education. There is also evidence that literacy level affects cerebral organization. Reis and Castro-Caldas (1997) reported that illiterate women from Southern Portugal performed worse than literate women on repetition of pseudowords, on recall of phonologically related word associates, and on fluency tasks involving generation of words beginning with specific phonemes. Using neuroimaging studies, the authors reported different areas of activation between the two groups (Castro-Caldas & Reis, 2003; Reis & Castro-Caldas, 1997).

Results of the neuropsychological and neuroimaging studies with illiterates and subjects with low levels of education, point out that there is a different brain organization in normal illiterate subjects; therefore, it is not only important to explore if the rate of decline in cognition varies as a function of age but also how the educational level affects or interacts with the rate of decline. Ardila, Ostrosky-Solis, Rosselli, and Gómez (2000) analyzed the effects of education on cognitive decline in normal aging. They studied 806 neurologically intact subjects age 16 to 85 years. Subjects were grouped into four educational levels—completely illiterate (no education), 1–4, 5–9 and 10 or more years of education. Subjects were studied with a Brief Neuropsychological Test in Spanish, NEUROPSI (Ostrosky-Solís, Ardila, & Rosselli, 1996, 1999), which is a brief neuropsychological battery evaluating a wide spectrum of cognitive functions including crystallized and fluid type of measures. It includes the evaluation of orientation, attention, memory, language, visual and space functions, and executive and motor functions. The battery contains items that are sensible and relevant for Hispanic population and that can be used in illiterate people. They reported that there are different patterns of association between age-related decline and education. In some cognitive functions, such as copy of a complex figure, the age-related decline was the same in the different educational groups. In other cognitive functions, such as verbal memory, the age-related decline was attenuated in well-educated participants; and furthermore, in other cognitive domains, such as semantic verbal fluency, the initial advantage of well-educated groups was reduced in later life. The authors concluded that the protective effect of education is not always observed but depends on the specific cognitive ability that is measured and that the diagnosis of dementia using psychometric procedures penalized low-educated individuals. A minor cognitive decline in illiterates may be extremely deleterious whereas a similar raw decline in high education may be virtually unnoticed. Testing bias may overestimate the severity of cognitive decline and hence the estimates of prevalence of dementia among the less-educated individuals.

From the literature review, we can conclude that the protective effect of education is not always observed but depends on the specific cognitive ability measure. It seems that education affects crystallized abilities, memory, and global cognitive function, but not other measures related to fluid or frontal lobe type abilities. As postulated by Horn and Cattell (1976), crystallized abilities include those aspects of intelligence influenced by educational and cultural opportunities, whereas fluid intelligence is composed of abilities acquired as a result of genetic factors. As Christensen et al., 1997 pointed out, protection or age-related decline attenuation in well-educated participants appears to extend primarily to verbal abilities and/or crystallized abilities. However, in other measures related to fluid intellectual ability and/or frontal lobe functions (i.e. cue recall, alternating movements, opposite reactions, processing speed, symbol-digit substitution), parallelism or similar levels of decline in high- and low-educated groups are observed. Because mainly verbal abilities, and not frontal lobe type tasks, which are the ones affected by biological aging, show a protective effect, education may provide the individual with greater compensatory resources rather than protection.

A limitation of the brain or neuronal reserve hypothesis is that most measures of reserve are influenced by cultural and educational factors. This includes measures of socioeconomic status, such as income or occupational attainment, literacy, and IQ. All these variables can affect test performance and/or our ability to accurately detect the symptoms in the absence of a concept of "brain reserve." Furthermore, lower education and low socioeconomic level are associated with increased risk for toxic or environmental exposures, nutritional deficiencies, or perinatal insult. Recent studies have reported an association between education and vascular and alcohol related dementia but not AD. Del Ser, Hachinski, Merskey, and Munoz (1999) studied 87 patients with pathologically confirmed degenerative dementia. They found that less-educated patients became demented later and died later, but cognitive function declined at the same rate in all educational groups and there was no difference in the burden of neurodegenerative lesions between them, but less-educated patients had more vascular lesions. They concluded that higher education does not modify the course of AD, but lower education relates to the occurrence of cerebral infarcts. They suggested that individuals with greater educational attainment and associated higher socioeconomic status are exposed to fewer toxins, enjoy a healthier lifestyle, and have greater quality care, all of which would tend to spare their brains from lesions contributing to dementing illness. Small vascular lesions in less-educated individuals may explain their increased risk of dementia described by epidemiological studies better than the brain reserve hypothesis.

CONCLUSIONS

As Stern (2002) pointed out, cognitive reserve is a rich concept that has great heuristic value for research, however the concept of brain reserve might not be related to the actual number of neurons or brain size, but may be based on more efficient utilization of brain networks or of enhanced ability to recruit alternate brain networks as needed but only for certain abilities. Rather than a physical or a protective process that slows biological aging in normal aging or that delays the start of decline, education and verbal advantage could serve as a means of compensatory strategies, such as using verbal cues to aid recall or encoding visuospatial tasks with language. These are the strategies provided by formal education. The use of these strategies could mask otherwise similar rates of biological aging among different educational groups and this advantage coupled with the effects of several important variables such as good health, appropriate occupation, and active engagement with surrounding environment could explain why cognitive stimulation can provide some moderating influence on the complex changes in cognitive performance associated with aging. As Ardila, Ostrosky-Solis, Rosselli, and Gómez (2000) pointed out, it is also important to consider that in humans, lack of education is not equivalent to deprivation or total lack of stimulation, because although not attending school, illiterate and low-education subjects are doing different type of activities and have to develop different types of learning. If tests were based on the knowledge and skills of those with low levels of formal education, highly educated people might be at a disadvantage.

In clinical neuropsychology, it is important to consider that there is a strong association between educational level and performance on several neuropsychological measures including memory and executive functions, and these are the measures that are currently used in the diagnosis of dementia. Testing bias has implications for the diagnosis of dementia and for the notion that low level of education and occupational attainment is associated with increased risk of developing dementia. Studies with Spanish-speaking subjects of different educational levels indicate that in many of the studies that had included in their sample subjects with less than 4 years of education, the higher rates of dementia detected could be due to testing bias. Furthermore, dementia involves a decline in cognitive skills from a premorbid level. However, assessment of premorbid ability is seldom available among the low socioeconomic individuals, and without knowledge of premorbid ability, there is a danger that in some individuals, low education or illiteracy is related to a history of learning disabilities or limited intellectual ability and therefore they are mistakenly diagnosed as demented. Although several authors have suggested adjusting for education when screening for dementia, our study with the MMSE showed that the level of education plays a very important role in the total score. The performance of normal individuals with no education was as low as that of subjects with severe dementia, whereas the score for those with 1 to 4 years of education was similar to that of subjects with slight dementia. Although the adjustment of the cutoff point for the population with 0 to 4 years of education in terms of average performance produced a significant increase in specificity, the sensitivity declined significantly. The assessment of functional capacity is an important part of a comprehensive diagnostic work-up for dementia, however, there is data that supports the notion that functional abilities are also affected by culture and education. Therefore, there is the need for normative data of functional abilities of older adults that belong to different and ethic and cultural groups.

Further studies that take into account the interaction of culture, education, and brain pathology could help to understand how active stimulation as well as pathological conditions affect brain structure and functions.

ACKNOWLEDGMENT

This work was supported in part by a grant from Consejo Nacional de Ciencia y Tecnología (CONACYT) and Programa de Apoyo a Proyectos de Investigación e Innovación Tecnológica Universidad Nacional Autónoma de México (PAPITT).

REFERENCES

Albert, M. S., Jones, K., Savage, C. R., Berkman, L., Seeman, T., Blazer, D., & Rowe, J. W. (1995). Predictors of cognitive change dementia in older persons: MacArthur studies of successful aging. *Psychology and Aging, 10*, 578–589.

Anstey, K., & Christensen, H. (2000). Education, activity, blood pressure and apolipoprotein E as predictors of cognitive change in old age: A review. *Gerontology, 46*, 163–177.

Ardila, A., Ostrosky-Solis, F., Rosselli, M. & Gómez, C. (2000). Age related cognitive decline during normal aging: The complex effect of education. *Archives of Clinical Neuropsychology, 15*, 495–514.

Ardila, A., Rosselli, M., & Pinzón, O. (1989). Alexia and agraphia in Spanish speakers: CAT correlations and interlinguistic analysis. In A. Ardila & F. Ostrosky (Eds.). *Brain organization of language and cognitive processes* (pp. 147–175). New York: Plenum.

Beard, C. M., Kokmen, E., Offord, K., & Kurland, L. T. (1992). Lack of association between Alzheimer's disease and education, occupation, marital status or living arrangement. *Neurology, 42*, 2063–2068.

Buell, S. J., & Coleman, P. D.(1979). Dendritic growth in the aged human brain and failure of growth in aedile dementia. *Science, 206*, 864–866.

Castro-Caldas. A., & Reis, A. (2000). Neurobiological substrates of illiteracy. *Neuroscientist, 6*, 475–482.

Christensen, H., & Henderson, A. S. (1991). Is age kinder to the initially more able? A study of eminent scientists and academics. *Psychological Medicine, 21*, 935–946.

Christensen, H., Korten, A. E., Jorm, A. F., Henderson, A. S., Jacomb, P. A., & Rodgers, B. (1997). Education and decline in cognitive performance: Compensatory but not protective. *International Journal of Geriatric Psychiatry, 12*, 323–330.

Cobb, J. L., Wolf, P. A., Au, R., White, R., & D'Agostino, R. B. (1995). The effect of education on the incidence of dementia and Alzheimer's disease in the Framingham Study. *Neurology, 45*, 1707–1712.

Crum, R. M., Anthony, J. C., Bassett, S. S., & Folstein, M. F. (1993). Population-based norms for the Mini-Mental State Examination by age and educational level. *JAMA, 269*, 2386–2390.

Del Ser, T., Hachinski, V., Merskey, H., & Munoz, D. G. (1999). An autopsy-verified study of the effect of education on degenerative dementia. *Brain, 122*, 2309–2320.

Escobar, J. I., Burnam, A., Karno, M., Forsythe. A., Landsverk. J., & Golding, J. M. (1986). Use of the Mini-Mental State Examination (MMSE) in a community population of mixed ethnicity. *Journal of Nervous and Mental Disorders, 174*, 607–614.

Evans, D. A., Beckett, L. A., Albert, M. S., Herbert, L. E., Scherr, P. A., Funkenstein, H. H. & Taylor, J. O. (1993). Level of education and change in cognitive function in a community population of older persons. *Annals of Epidemiology, 3*, 71–77.

Farmer, M. E., Kittner, S. J., Rae, D. S., Bartco, J. J., & Regier, D. A. (1995). Education and change in cognitive function: The epidemiologic catchment area study. *Annals of Epidemiology, 5*, 1–7.

Folstein, M. F., Folstein, S. E., & McHugh, P. R. (1975). "Mini Mental State": A practical method for grading the cognitive state of patients for clinician. *Journal of Psychiatric Research, 12*, 189–198.

Horn, I. L., & Cattell, R. B. (1976). Age differences in fluid and crystallized intelligence. *Acta Psychologica, 26*, 107–129.

Katzman, R. (1993). Education and the prevalence of dementia and Alzheimer's disease. *Neurology, 43*, 13–20.

Lowenstein, D., Ardila, A., Rosselli, M., Hayden, S., Duara, R., Berkowitz, N., Fuentes, P., Mintzer, J., Norville, M., & Eisdorfer, C. (1992). A comparative analysis of functional status among Spanish- and English-speaking patients with dementia. *Journal of Gerontology, 47*(6), 389–394.

Mortimer, J. A. (1988). Do psychosocial risk factors contribute to Alzheimer's disease? In A. S. Hendersen & J. H. Hendersen (Eds). *Etiology of dementia of Alzheimer's type* (pp. 39–52). Chichester, England: Wiley.

Mortimer, J. A., & Graves, A. B. (1993). Education and other socioeconomic determinants of dementia and Alzheimer's disease. *Neurology, 43*(4), 39–44.

Obadia, Y., Rotily, M., Degrand-Guillaud, A., Guelain, J., Ceccaldi, M., & Severo, C. (1997). The PREMAP Study: Prevalence and risk factor of dementia and clinically diagnosed Alzheimer's disease in Provence, France. *European Journal of Epidemiology, 13*, 247–253.

O'Connor, D. W., Pollitt, P. A., & Treasure, F. P. (1991). The influence of education and social class on diagnosis of dementia in a community population. *Psychological Medicine, 21*, 219–224.

Orell, M., & Sahakian, B. (1995). Education and Dementia. Research evidence supports the concept "use it or lose it." *British Medical Journal, 310*, 951–952.

Ostrosky-Solis, F., Lopez, G., & Ardila, A. (2000). Sensitivity and specificity of the Mini-Mental State Examination in a Spanish-speaking population. *Applied Neuropsychology, 7*(1), 25–31.

Ostrosky-Solís, F., Ardila, A., & Rosselli, M. (1999). NEUROPSI: A brief neuropsychological test battery in Spanish with norms by age and educational level. *International Journal of Neuropsychology, 5*, 413-433.

Ostrosky-Solís, F., Ardila, A., & Rosselli, M. (1996). Examen Neuropsicológico Básico en Español: NEUROPSI [Neuropsychological evaluation in Spanish]. San Antonia, TX: Psychological corporation.

Reis, A,. & Castro-Caldas, A. (1997). Illiteracy: A cause for biased cognitive development. *Journal of the International Neuropsychological Society, 5*, 444–450.

Rosselli, M., Ardila, A., & Rosas, P. (1990). Neuropsychological assessment in illiterates II: Language and praxic abilities. *Brain and Cognition, 12*, 281–296.

Satz, P. (1993). Brain reserve capacity on symptom onset after brain injury: A formulation and review of evidence for threshold theory. *Neuropsychology, 7*, 273–295.

Stern, Y. (2002). What is cognitive reserve? Theory and research application of the reserve concept. *Journal of the International Neuropsychological Society, 8*, 448–460.

Stern, Y., Gurland, B., Tatemichi, T. K., Tang, M. X., Wilder, D., & Mayeux, R. (1994). Influence of education and occupation in the incidence of Alzheimer's disease. *Journal of the American Medical Association, 271*, 1004–1010.

Yesavage, J. A. (1985). Non-pharmacological treatment for memory loss with normal aging. *American Journal of Psychiatry, 142*, 600–605.

Zhang, M., Katzman, R., Salmon, D., Jin, H., Cai, G., Wang, Z., et al. (1990). The prevalence of dementia in Alzheimer's disease in Shanghai, China: Impact of age, gender and education. *Annals of Neurology, 27*, 428–437.

Chapter **13**

Visuospatial Assessment in Cross-Cultural and Nonwestern Settings

Roy Sugarman
University of New South Wales, Australia

At its most negative, testing in nonwestern settings may fall short of the discrepant views held by the person who takes the test, and the person who made the test. Tests in general have only face validity (Walsh, 1992), and there are strong indicators in cross-cultural settings that the test-taker and test-maker may look for, and respond to, different test content (Nell, 1999a), failing for reasons different from the one in the tester-maker's mind.

To illustrate: A 14-year-old boy with a nonwestern language background and education is given a complex figure to copy. He does so, abysmally, with a less than 10th percentile performance. His father returns with him the next week to continue the testing and shows the tester a beautifully constructed model of a Harley-Davidson motorcycle. The model is a three-dimensional wire construction with triangles, circles, and squares, all linked in a single manipulation of light-gauge wire. The elements on the complex figure that baffled this child in two dimensions pose no problem for him in three dimensions. He also has no problem with the object assembly subtest of one of the western-normed IQ tests, finding the jigsaws easy in contrast.

Furthermore, later on in the assessment, despite having done well generally, the child manages equal times for the ungrouped and grouped dots on Rey's 1941 test, strongly suggesting poor motivation (Lezak, 1995).

When the test is redone with the psychometrist and tester present, the child does just as poorly. On questioning, it is clear he knows that, for instance, the 4 × 2 dots make up 8, but he counts each dot individually, as he did on the 7-dot card before. On investigation, it appears that the translating psychometrist told him in the vernacular to "count the dots," instead of using the phrase "tell me how many dots there are, as quickly as possible," to which he then responded instantly and correctly. He explained that he was simply "doing what the boss told me to do," apparently in awe of the psychometrist in the suit, who had to be obeyed explicitly and who clearly had status in the western paradigm test situation, which the testee did not.

In this way, many test situations in the western paradigm fall foul of the distant and silent tester using prescribed language, as a failure of the more sociable and tactile approach of many other testers in nonwestern test paradigms. Stated thus, many test situations serve as a form of gatekeeping, favoring the advantaged and test-wise western subject, in the service of the tester and not the subject (Taylor, 1999). What then is being measured is unclear.

One issue is that the measurement of such complex functions occurs on many levels at once, falling foul of what Bateson called "epistemological error," confusing an entire class of abilities with abilities that are members of that class (Sugarman, 2002). The mere act of observing and testing culturally determined abilities may have a profound effect on the way the ability and its overarching cortex interact, thus producing an action that allows the test to measure its own effect on itself in a recursive feedback loop, but not the supposed capacity of the subject. To illustrate: An aboriginal woman with multiple admissions for suicidal and aggressive behavior was assessed with conventional western tools and found to be retarded, deranged, and dangerous, with several multiaxial psychiatric diagnoses. A simple approach to the interactions between the community care team and the patient resulted in her never returning to the hospital ward and making a full recovery to her previous position in society (Sugarman, 2001). She was found to be most hostile to formal assessment, because she had had assessments frequently since she was a child, had been institutionalized as a result, and had her two children removed from her care as a result of these assessments.

Conventional western tests deliberately minimize the interactions between tester and testee and focus on correct answers rather than processes, such as those important to learning (Taylor, 1999). In this way, western test procedures focus on overlearned information, not on the potential to learn, thus working to the advantage of those who have actualized their potential, and against those who have potential that has yet to be realized. In the words of Fanon (1968), western social interaction, as epitomized by the neuropsychological assessment, empties the native brain of all form and content that it finds to have no conventional value. Global IQ scores and the component scores of various batteries ignore domains of mental functioning that are capable of further development in the future, especially (in response to what Taylor, 1999, proposes, namely, the well-designed teaching programs that a more dynamic testing approach could create), programs that fulfill Vygotsky's (1978) desire to foster the functions that have not yet matured, but are still embryonic.

Uncritical universalism thus dominates assessment of visuospatial abilities in western test settings, and most critics are now arguing for a more humane relativism, with the expectation that wide variations in normative performances will occur (Nell, 1999b). Therefore, test instruments can be constructed that do not show statistical evidence of bias (Taylor, 1999) or assume species-wide comparisons (Lezak, 1995), a criticized approach (Nell, 1999a).

As seen in the previous vignette, there is no clear link between stimulus material and the dimension or process being measured, and heavy demands are thus placed on the interpreter and tester (Taylor, 1994, 1999) to extract diagnostically meaningful information, the goal of neuropsychological assessment (Matarazzo, 1990). This is not unique to visuospatial assessments in nonwestern settings, and the inferences drawn by clinical neuropsychologists on such tests define the speciality itself. Walsh (1992) warns against such face validity pronouncements on performance evaluations; Franzen (1989) found that many tests in the visuospatial batteries share little in the domain of main effects variance anyway, and the inferential skill of the tester is still a factor, western setting or not.

THE VISUOSPATIAL ARENA

Many significant authors imply in their approaches that the more neurological-specific a test is, the less the chance that it will run foul of the cross-cultural trap. This would imply that born-with skills are the best to assess, as done in the neurological assessment of motor performance, and that tasks that demand the later genotype–phenotype transformation within the environment would be more prone to western–nonwestern inference conundrums. Vygotsky (1978) indeed took intelligence to represent primarily a social phenomenon: This approach has more recently been applied by Barkley (1998) in his definitions of frontal-based functioning as having emerged from the interaction of environment with genetically determined structures in the process of evolution (Sugarman, 2002). Like Nell (1999a, 1999b), Barkley (1998) has examined social Darwinism for its "buds and fruits," as well as for its thorns. In Barkley's formulation, the brain's executive systems have developed in tandem with evolutionary physiological changes; the organism is in competition with its peers and environment, with ultimate success depending in "wresting" control from the environment by the application of visuospatial and verbal internalized simulators that predict outcome.

In this way, Barkley (1998) describes the first aspect of the brain that emerges in the infant as the visuospatial—or at least the nonverbal—working memory, enabling the infant to embark on the process of internal mediation so that the social intellectual property of the culture is taken over by the individual and turned into personal intelligence or social competency. Thus, any damaged brain will respond either with social aggression or with social withdrawal (Sugarman, 1999).

Feuerstein (1979), Budoff (1987), Campione and Brown (1987), Carlson and Wiedl (1979, 1992), and others have attempted to apply and develop Vygotsky's original formulations of the zone of proximal development (see Nell, 1999a, 1999b), but with mixed and much criticized success (Taylor, 1994, 1999).

The difficulty is that many dynamic instruments, using verbal or nonverbal modalities, are not well-grounded in theory, with tasks not designed to extract meaningful diagnostic information about the dimension (Taylor, 1994) or process (Nell, 1999a) being measured. This is as crucial for the assessment of visuospatial abilities as it is for executive functioning, given that tests so often have only face validity, and that many testees fail in the same way for multiple reasons (Walsh, 1992). The problem is one of validation, even in normal populations (Matarazzo, 1990).

If diagnostically meaningful information is to emerge from the testing situation, then nonverbal procedures must have novelty (Nell, 1999b), but must still fulfill the dynamic test procedures' goal in bringing a nontestwise subject to the point of familiarity, the starting point of the testwise subject.

Conventional visuospatial testing imposes almost no learning demands on the individual, and learning for the testwise subject is usually limited to the instructional phase. The assumption of the western approach is that there is no need for instruction, because these skills are cultural universals (see Nell, this volume). In contrast, the hallmark of a learning potential instrument is that the testee learns a new skill or competency in the process of taking the test. In many ways, this dichotomy defines the difference between tests that are nonwestern testee unfriendly and those that are, by virtue of design.

The failure of so many to apply this criterion thus far, despite following on Vygotsky and Feuerstein's formulations, emerges from failures to apply theory correctly in translating western tests into nonwestern settings, with poor grading of difficulty, reliance on linguistic processing, limited tester–testee interaction, and so on (Taylor, 1999).

There are, nevertheless, test batteries in existence that are grounded in theory; are graded in difficulty from illiterate to business executive; use the

13. VISUOSPATIAL ASSESSMENT

visuospatial skills common to all genotypes, namely symbol transformations; and are learning potential measures where the differences between individuals are minimized so that all testees have the same level of familiarity with the test material before testing commences. This is leveling the playing field (Nell, 1999b), the goal of cross-cultural assessment in order to create valid tests with valid criteria.

The successes of such unbiased instruments, many operating in the visuospatial arena, are worthy of study, if novel instruments are to be developed that are not mere linguistic translations of existing western paradigm tests and that operate in the visuospatial arena.

THE TRAM-1, TRAM-2, AND APIL-B BATTERIES: USING THE VISUOSPATIAL GENOTYPE WITHOUT STATISTICAL BIAS, AND WITH PREDICTIVE VALIDITY

Using the theoretical formulations of Taylor (1994), three tests have been developed over the past two decades. The first, the TRAM-1 Battery (1999), is designed for the assessment of learning potential in illiterates and semiliterates. The second, the TRAM-2 (1998), is a slightly higher level battery for literates, and the third, the APIL- B (1997), is a high-level learning potential assessment instrument. The titles are loose acronyms for TRansfer, Automatization, Memory-learning, and Ability, Processing of Information, and Learning Battery, respectively. All three use the same modality, namely visuospatial puzzles. More importantly, the tests are created uniquely from the ground up, without reference to established procedures and within the context of the multicultural population where they will be applied. These are novel tests, not language-altered clones.

The tests are most complex in construction, and in order to evaluate them further, they will be examined briefly here to introduce them as paradigms for how novel, culture-fair tests should be created *de novo*, and to test them for statistical shortcomings.

The TRAM-1

The battery, revised in its current manual format in 1999, is a learning potential test. It is designed in such a way as to minimize the effect of the administrator's interventions in applying help to the illiterate or semiliterate testee, in the 0–9 years of education range. In contrast to many developed countries, where such education may confer literacy, in many developing countries this may not reflect on any useful application of anything beyond the vernacular, with little graphic skill at all attained across the school years. Instructor assistance will thus never boost the performance of the poor learners to the point where they outstrip the more gifted individual who does not require help, and thus both typologies will begin the test with the playing field leveled (Nell, 1999b).

In the visual format, these tasks are novel to everyone taking the test, and help is available to all in the postinstruction phase, a new approach to testing, making it fulfill dynamic criteria. The actual task involves the testee translating symbols into other symbols using a specially supplied dictionary. The symbols are quasi-geometric, displaying only highly familiar objects, such as items of clothing, natural phenomena, and common household items (see Fig. 13.1). The symbol-to-symbol transformations are not arbitrary, and embody some underlying rule, such as being opposite or used together, or analogues in the man-made realms, and so on. Given significant correlations statistically, younger respondents and those with more years of formal education will do somewhat better.

The battery scores on five dimensions, namely Automization, Transfer, Memory and Understanding, Speed, and Accuracy. Most of these dimensions are found across the three batteries just named.

Automization is defined as the effect of repeated exposure to a task, monitoring the progress from initial slow and inefficient processing to speed and efficiency. Utilizing the principles of Sternberg (1984), one of the two major processes of learning is this, the other being transfer. This test focuses on measuring the speed of acquisition of a new skill *once it has been taught*, a measure of the learning curve.

Transfer, the other of the major processes, thus occurs when the individual masters a new challenge using a skill newly acquired by automization, reflecting on capacity to adapt to new environments using previously mas-

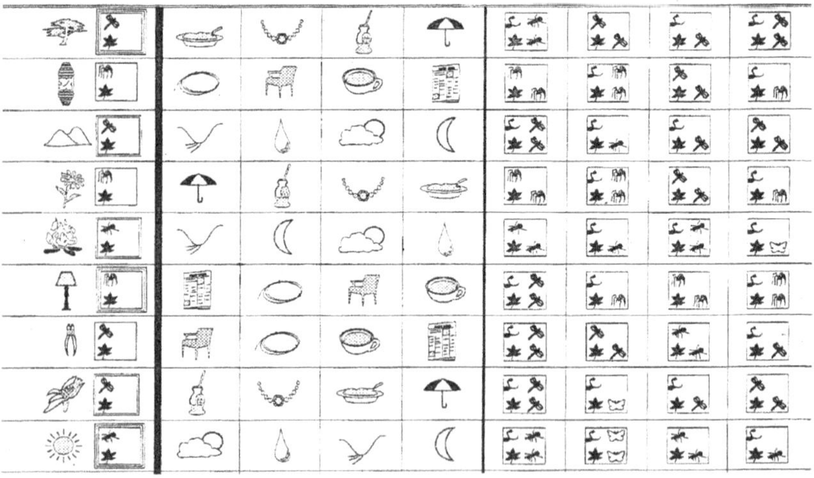

FIG. 13.1. The TRAM-1 format: The problem stimuli are to the left of the bolder line. Reproduced with permission of the author, copyright AProLab cc.

13. VISUOSPATIAL ASSESSMENT

tered skills, perhaps the core of intelligence (Biesheuvel, 1972) and a good place to begin assessment.

Memory and Understanding is not a test of rote learning, because this skill as tested here relies on implicit, not declarative use of knowledge, and thus is not part of the learning potential paradigm. Rather, this is a measure of the extent to which the testee can form underlying algorithms from appreciating the symbol-to-symbol relationships in the dictionaries provided. Later items in the Memory and Understanding test are not drawn from the dictionaries, but are analogous, and thus require the testee to use newly formulated declarative rules of understanding to solve them. The validity statistics support this latter contention.

The composite score that thus emerges incorporates scores on all of the previously named dimensions, but the memory and understanding part is given double weight.

The Material. Each page of the test booklets has nine rows and each row is delineated into nine sections by vertical lines (see Fig. 13.1). Two of the vertical lines are thicker to demarcate the position of the problem stimuli, and the zones in the row where the two response crosses must be made. A pair of problem stimuli appears side by side on the left of the row, with the first practice items having only one problem stimulus in each row in contrast: Again the need for leveling the field is paramount.

The problem stimuli are separated from the other stimuli by the first and thicker of the two lines. Four stimuli then appear between this and the next thick line. Then, another four stimuli appear to the right of this line, making up the rest of the row.

In Phase A, for example, the first row in Fig. 13.1, the tree and a small box (three-line outline) with a leaf and an insect are the stimuli to be considered. The tree, in this case, is to be paired with the umbrella, and a cross is made over the umbrella, the stimulus being man-made objects that arise from the concept of the *function of natural objects*.

The three lines of the box will indicate (from the dictionary) a different transformation to a box with a two-line outline, different again from a single-line outline box. The rules of transformation involve the single-line box directing that the insect in the upper left corner will be replicated in the lower right corner of the box. In a stimulus with a two-lined box, the insect in the upper left corner becomes a snake, but in the lower right corner. In the three-line box, the insect in the upper left corner also transforms into a snake, but the original creature is replicated in both upper right and lower left corners. The subject is thus trained to appreciate the rules of transformation.

Like the categories type of test in neuropsychology, Phase B of this test will be easier if the testee transfers the logic learned in Phase A, and then goes on to the memory and understanding part, given last.

A full manual is provided with the rules in the language to be used and can be translated into any vernacular without difficulty, in theory. Even so, in its Dutch translation for the Netherlands, the word/picture *buck* would have implied an American $, and not a small antelope. Even in such a test, regional language variations and concepts override the test universalism.

The results are processed via computer software running in PC/Windows format. The computer generated report supplies graphs of testee versus norm performances, with transfer and automatisation graphs based on correct transformations.

The TRAM-2

This test is designed for use with those who have 10 to 12 years of education, at the level, say, of reading a local western language newspaper. It was revised to its present format in February 1998. Unlike trainability tests, the TRAM-2 is a generic instrument designed to predict success on a number of work-related activities that impose appreciable conceptual demands on the individual, and it requires a mastery of new learning challenges. Motor coordination and manual dexterity are not measured in any meaningful way. The test thus gives a prospective view of how the person is likely to do in any setting requiring these skills. In many ways, this test fulfils David Wechsler's formulation of intelligence as the global measure of an individual's ability to act purposefully, think rationally, and deal effectively with the environment (Walsh, 1992), as do the TRAM-1 and APIL-B.

The Material. The test booklet has three main sections, namely the Concept Formation Test (standard level); the SymTran test; and the Memory and Understanding Test, which is based on the SymTran material. SymTran itself is divided into Parts A and B, with Part A divided into two parts separated again by a lesson. Again, two dictionaries are provided, and they list symbol–word equivalences. The pairs of symbols that confront the testee have to be translated into two simple words (see Fig. 13.2). Initially the testees will have to look up all the answers in the dictionary, but as they learn the symbol–word transformations, they will ultimately discard that aid, resulting in an increase in work output.

The TRAM-2 produces scores on six dimensions: Conceptual Reasoning, Automization, Transfer, Memory and Understanding, Speed, and Accuracy. The first, different from the TRAM-1, refers to the capacity to think abstractly and detect underlying commonalties while ignoring superficial differences. Stimulus material is again nonverbal or quasi-geometric, or diagrammatic. This test material conforms to Cattell's (1971)

13. VISUOSPATIAL ASSESSMENT

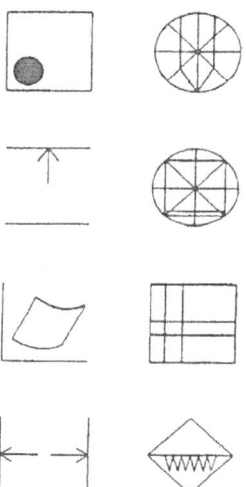

FIG. 13.2. The TRAM-2 format: The top two symbols will translate as "4 ties." Reproduced with permission of the author, copyright AProLab cc.

concept of fluid intelligence. The other dimensions are those measured in the TRAM-1.

The Concept Formation Test. As in Fig. 13.3, and identical in fact to the APIL-B, there is a row of drawings, in this case six, labeled A through F. Five of the six share some conceptual similarity, while the sixth is different. The testee's task is to find the anomalous diagram. Once it has been isolated, the testee crosses out one of the six letters A through F on the answer sheet. In Fig. 13.3, B is anomalous because the three similar shapes are in the top left, top right, and bottom right quadrants of the circle. In all the others, the three similar shapes are in the top left, top right, and bottom left quadrants. There are 36 items, with the more difficult problems occurring later in the test.

The SymTran Test. Pairs of drawings in Part A stand for highly familiar objects and concepts, designed for easy acquisition (see Fig. 13.2). The dictionaries describe the words that each symbol stands for, and the top two symbols in Fig. 13.2 can then be translated into "four ties" so that the testee will rapidly learn that a square with a black dot in the bottom left corner will always stand for the number "four," and then two vertical lines with horizontal arrows pushing them outward will represent "wide" (fourth pair), and so on. The testee may have to search several pages of the dictionary, then mark which of the words apply on the answer sheet, without having to write anything. Part B is very similar structurally, but the drawings are different and the testee must recall contextual boundaries without confabulation from one set to the next.

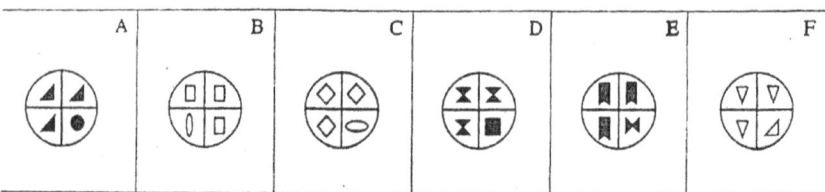

FIG. 13.3. The TRAM-2 format: Design 3 is anomalous because the others have only the bottom right quadrant odd compared to other designs. Reproduced with permission of the author, copyright AProLab cc.

The Memory and Understanding Test. Here, the question and answer format is reversed, and the testee is asked to formulate what the pairs of symbols might mean, as in Fig. 13.4. Thirty problems are given in this way, often involving whole sentences in which the words are replaced by symbol sequences. Finally, 14 scores are produced and fed into a computer program running in PC/Windows format to produce TRAM-2 reports. Secondary raw scores are computer generated on the six dimensions already mentioned, and these scores are referred to norm tables built into the software; the resulting stanines are reflected in the report.

The APIL-B

This is an edition last revised in December 1997. It is designed to assess an individual's core or fundamental cognitive capacities and potentialities, but it does not measure specific skills and is likely to identify those individuals who are able to master new, cognitively demanding material in a formal educational or training context, with industrial and educational applications.

The battery provides a profile of eight scores as well as a learning curve. It is suitable for those with 12 years of education or even with tertiary education, including also those currently in their 11th or 12th year of secondary school, with aspirations of going further.

The Material. There are five types of stimulus material contained in a main test booklet, and two ancillary booklets. The eight domains are Abstract Thinking, Speed of Information Processing, Accuracy of Information Processing, Cognitive Flexibility, Performance Gain in a learning task, Overall Work Output on this task, Processing Depth (concept memorization and mastery), and Transfer of Learning.

The concept formation test (see Fig. 13.5) again uses alphabetically labeled line drawings with the same approach as the TRAM-2, with a need to determine essential from inessential detail, as one does with absurdities or picture completion tasks.

The speed of information processing is determined by four short tests, named FAST (see Fig. 13.6). This is an acronym for flexibility, accuracy, and speed. These four tests yield three secondary scores when reworked. Almost no testee can reach the final item, given the level of speed required, although the content is not that difficult to solve. All four tests share the same geometrical stimulus material, as per Fig. 13.6, producing a universe of these 16 figures, which are manipulated for the test items.

The next set of material is a learning test in which the same task occurs on four occasions, and also allows for three study periods. The first and second exposures are equally difficult, but the third and fourth are equal to each

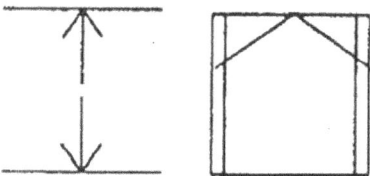

FIG. 13.4. The TRAM-2 format: This pair would be translated to mean "tall houses." Reproduced with permission of the author, copyright AProLab cc.

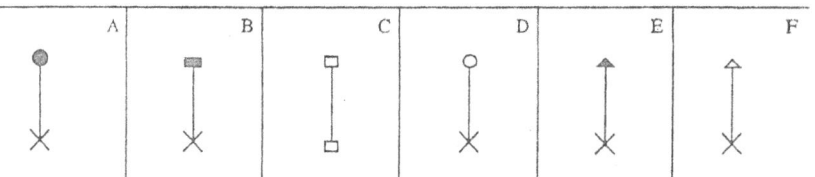

FIG. 13.5. The APIL-B format: This sample item indicates, as with Fig. 13.3, that Item C is anomalous. Reproduced with permission of the author, copyright AProLab cc.

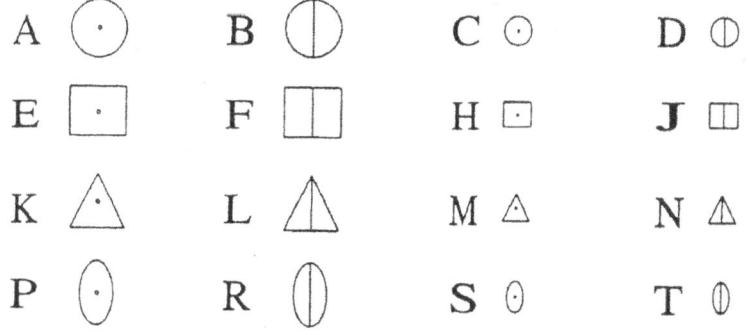

FIG. 13.6. The APIL-B FAST subtest has the above 16 designs as its universe, and all four subsubtests of the FAST share the above designs. Reproduced with permission of the author, copyright AProLab cc.

other and harder than the first two. The scores yield a learning curve. Various measures apply to the repeated exposure with difference in output between first and fourth sessions, and the total amount of work in all four sessions. As in Fig. 13.7, double transformations of pairs of geometrical designs have to be solved, with the left-hand figure always a color or number, and the right-hand figure an item of clothing or a means of transport. In Fig. 13.7, the two exercises translate as "brown canoes" and "three ties," respectively, using the eight-page dictionary supplied. The sequel to this learning test measures the trainees retention of the material learned previously, and relies on encouraged learning of the dictionary symbol–symbol and symbol–word transformations used previously, hence drawing on extensive memory and learning skills in both modalities. Rote learning is, however, not easy, and conceptual mastery of executive memory tasks is required for success here, with prospective memory encouraged.

Another learning exercise and mastery task follows, with knowledge transfer activities supported. The previous task was analogous to Sternberg's (1984) concept of *automatisation*, that is, the ability to become efficient on a cognitive task with practice, but here the concept is one of transfer of this acquired skill to another task, different but related (Nell, 1999a; Taylor, 1994). According to these authors, these tasks are an essential part of the test-teach-test approach in cross-cultural settings.

The APIL-B does not have to be administered in its entirety, but is more reliable when done so.

Constructs Measured. In keeping with its goal of measuring the individual's ability to think abstractly and conceptually, the APIL-B Construct Formation subtest also demands the ability to form abstract concepts, reason hypothetically (i.e., as Barkley, 1998, formulates it, to utilize mental tracking to simulate outcomes), theorize, build scenarios (again Barkley's

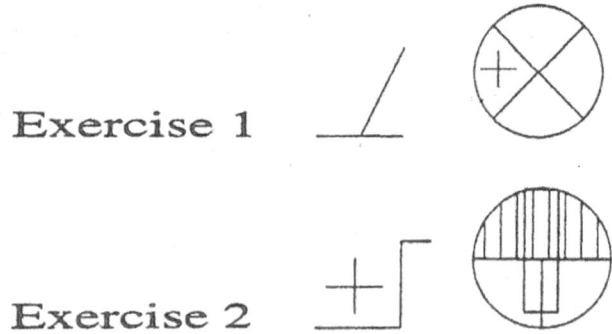

FIG. 13.7. The APIL-B learning components: the two exercises here translate as "brown canoes" and "three ties," respectively. Reproduced with permission of the author, copyright AProLab cc.

simulator is echoed), and trace causes. This all involves more than mere routine and rule-following such as one finds in IQ tests, and requires rather the executive functions of simulation, self-regulation, self-monitoring, error utilization, and inhibition. Creativity is also demanded in the form of generating algorithms, or the unpacking and repacking of chains of behavior, a form of fluid intelligence thought to be the engine behind the development of new skills and abilities (Barkley, 1998; Snow, Kyllonen, & Marshalek, 1984). The emphasis is therefore not on crystallized intelligence or overlearned material, but rather on novel situations, a core demand of neuropsychological assessment tools (Matarazzo, 1990).

The next subtest measures speed (or rather quickness), as well as accuracy of information processing and cognitive flexibility, again, rather than overlearned skills. Given as stens, the cutting point between 5 and 6 is used to distinguish *slow* from *quick*, *inaccurate* from *accurate*, and *low flexibility* from *accomplished*. Scores from 1–3 and 8–10 are further graded by the use of uppercase letters, to demonstrate where they lie in the distribution of these skills. In this way, 16% of the scores of a norm sample fall in the extreme ranges, and about 34% in each of the medium range abilities. In this way too, the individual can be placed in one of 64 categories in the FAST subtest (see earlier), an astonishing versatility of classification that makes this test unique. What this also assumes, in essence, is a normal distribution, even in such disparate populations.

Hence, processing speed can be determined for moderately difficult material, namely series, mirror images, and transformations, in strings of geometric shapes with one member missing in each string.

Processing accuracy, subjected to logarithmic transformation in order to make the distribution more symmetrical, is a measure here of failure to control quality of response, as well as lapses in mental tracking (hence the utilization of error feedback). The ratio of correct work output in the fourth subtest in relation to the correct output in the first three subtests, weighted with the output in the fourth test, gives the index of cognitive flexibility.

The curve of learning construct emerges again from the refusal of this nonwestern paradigm to measure abilities that are assumed to have attained a stable level in the individual, as with most conventional tests available to the neuropsychologist in most settings, even when inappropriate.

In nonwestern societies, this assumption is highly questionable, since great discrepancies in opportunities have existed, and continue to exist, not only in Africa (Nell, 1999a, 1999b) but in North America as well (Hohl, Grundman, Salmon, Thomas, & Thal, 1999; Llorente, Ponton, Taussig, & Satz, 1999; Perez-Arce, 1999; Ponton & Ardila, 1999). From a practical and ethical point of view, it becomes important to assess dynamic aspects of the individual's cognitive endowment. This will then include the capacity to acquire and utilize new competencies and ultimately to automate them into the individual's portfolio. Automization is thus an indicator of culture-fair intelligence assessment (Neubauer, 1990).

An additional element measured here is the individual gain score, which indicates the extent to which the individual's later performances represent a gain on the initial scores at baseline. A slow starter is rewarded, as is one who works fast throughout. At the upper end of scoring is the fast learner who also improves rapidly. Again, the benefits for neuropsychological inference are clear.

The memory and understanding tests that follow immediately after, and as already noted, have scoring that rewards those who have internalized the material, rather than those who still look up the answers in the dictionary, much as coding/digit symbol transformation speed is enhanced by learning which symbol goes with which digit on Wechsler-type IQ battery subtest items.

Part of error monitoring and error utilization involves the adaptation and application of newly obtained skills and the transfer of this knowledge to analogous, and even not so analogous, situations. This skill of adaptation is essential to cognitive development and is disrupted in so-called adaptive behavior syndromes (Snow, Kyllonen, & Marshalek, 1984; Walsh, 1991). This is all accomplished in the last part of the test (Fig. 13.8) where features must be matched to designs in a complex, now learned set of responses.

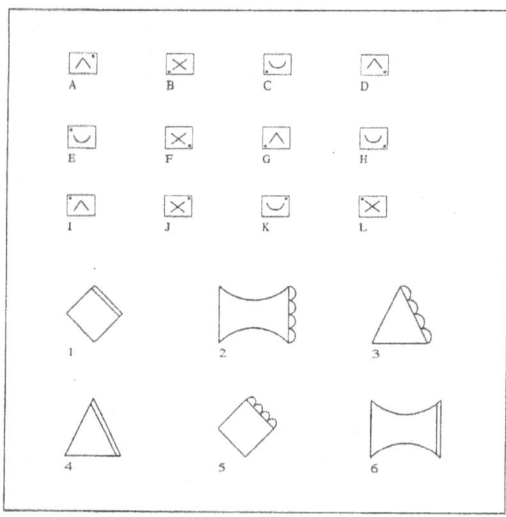

FIG. 13.8. The APIL-B concludes with a complex test requiring the classification of the designs (1–6) under the rules guiding the properties of the symbols (A–L: e.g., a dot in the upper-right-hand corner indicates scalloping). Reproduced with permission of the author, copyright AProLab cc.

13. VISUOSPATIAL ASSESSMENT

STATISTICAL PROPERTIES

The TRAM-1

Many tests lack statistical validity. Content validity, ecological validity, and reliability are often absent as well (Franzen, 1989; Nell, 1999a). This rules out most tests evaluated in the nonwestern settings.

The TRAM-1 was first administered to 176 illiterate and semiliterate subjects, with an average age of 38.3 years ($SD = 7.3$) and average education (in a poor system) of 4.5 ($SD = 3.0$) years. It was also administered to government employees ($n = 135$; average age 43.4, $SD = 7.9$, with education 8.7 yrs, $SD = 1.8$). Means, standard deviations, and intercorrelations for each dimension of automization, transfer, memory, speed, and accuracy scores are given. More recently, 490 service and support workers in a large parastatal company were administered the test, mean age 38.9 ($SD = 6.2$) and mean education 8.9 ($SD = 1.8$) years. Memory and speed correlated negatively with age, but .38 and .47 with education. One hundred and one graduates of a course presented by an in-house training company, mean age 35.1 ($SD = 5.1$) and education 7.1 ($SD = 1.4$) years, raised the means on the TRAM-1 substantially, confirming that its dynamic nature and the correlations of speed and memory were low, at .13 and .09, respectively.

In terms of reliability, each dimension is evaluated with a unique measure, because the tests are novel and unusual. For automization, the score is a regression line deviation, and there is no standard method of calculating the reliability of such a score. A correlation with the improvement score was made, and found to be .78 in the first group and .94 in the second. The reliability of the transfer score was estimated in the same way, and found to be .86 and .93, respectively, in the two groups. Split-half reliability on a special trial with 84 mineworkers yielded a reliability estimate of .87 for the first part and .67 for the second.

The reliability of the transfer scores was estimated the same way with split-half methodology, leading to a reliability estimate of .91 for the first half; the second half yielded a reliability estimate of .74 on the same 84 mineworkers.

For memory and understanding, statistically un-unique in format, a KR20 formula, an index of internal consistency was found to yield .94 (mining sample) and .91 in another sample. A KR21 reliability estimate (an underestimate of KR20) was found to be .92 in one group (parastatal above) and .88 (previous in-house training group), a very reliable set of tests of memory and understanding.

For speed, the work done in each of the two parts was correlated, and found to be .81 in both first groups (see earlier). This is noted to be an underestimate because of the idiosyncrasies of the test scoring. Halving the test length because of this and recalculating, the correlated reliability estimate improves to .90 for both sample groups. On the mining group, reliability estimates for various intercorrelation combinations of the test yielded .87, .95, and .95, respectively, without adjusting for test shortening.

Accuracy correlated in the same way as .83 and .66 for the two groups, and correcting this for speed, the reliability improves to .91 and .79 for the sample groups. Redoing the estimates as intercorrelation combinations yielded .68, .62, and .73, respectively, again without corrections for test shortening.

Validity ratings on a group of 52 subjects in a training college show that testing TRAM-1 results against training course scores predicts mathematics exam scores very well, with lowest scores on automization. The correlations are otherwise very satisfactory, with most scores above .25 at the .05 level of significance. The more elite the group, the better the validity rating, as preselection predicts the results.

On 54 miners, the ratings were similar, with TRAM-1 results correlating at 0.59 with the overall outcome of their training scores, again with high correlations on mathematics, less so on English, with math scores correlated at .62. Math improvement scores correlated with the global TRAM-1 score at .38 and with the memory score at .39, remarkable since the ranges of the improvement scores are limited, giving credence to the idea that the TRAM-1 is a learning potential instrument.

On semiliterate miners who had been pre-selected ($n = 101$), the TRAM-1 composite score correlates with the total variable at .54. The simple difference is that automization and transfer scores outperform the regression deviation alternatives, and when these latter are used, the correlation of the TRAM-1 composite score with the total drops from .54 to .46, hence the use of simple difference scores.

Overall, the TRAM-1 statistics prove that in illiterate or semiliterate individuals, the assessment modality is valid and reliable, predicts outcome academically and vocationally, and as a dynamic tool fulfills the requirements of the literature on cross-cultural assessment. From the neuropsychological perspective, the dimensions and constructs of the test are familiar, and easily translate into the dimensions of neuropsychological inference.

The TRAM-2

A sample of 208 employed subjects was assessed. These subjects had an education level ranging from 9–12 years, with a mean of 10.9 years. Means and standard deviations are given for the six dimensions, and intercorrelation tables are also given. Age correlated negatively for all of the dimensions, and poorly with acquisition, automation, and transfer, but highly with concept formation, memory, and speed.

Scale reliabilities for the concept formation and memory/understanding, given that these are power tests, were computed with the KR20 formula, with .86 and .91, respectively.

Speed and accuracy, using split-half methodology, and corrected for test shortening, yielded .98 and .94 for the two, respectively.

The reliability of the automation and transfer dimensions was based on regression line deviations, again a little unfair to the test, as in the TRAM-1. This yields .72 and .78, respectively, but analysis of the means and standard deviations of the various parts of these two dimensions clearly indicates that SymTran is a learning test.

Validity data were obtained on 151 applicants at a local municipality. Most had 12 years of education, and none less than 9, with an average 9.3 years of education and 22.74 years old. Another sample group of 102 military recruits of average age 20.5, all with 12 years of education, was also considered.

Reliabilities of the scales were found to be .98, .86, .98, .88, .90, and .90 for the dimensions of concept formation, memory, speed, accuracy, automation and transfer, respectively. The trainers divided the groups into a high trainability and low trainability selection, and the groups' scores were then found to be different at the .001 level of significance. An examination of all theoretical aspects of their training was then given, and the TRAM-2 scores correlated with very good concurrent validity regarding the group and examination variables. Speed was the best predictor, at .61, and the composite TRAM-2 score at .61 was compared to examination results.

Based on surname, 65% of the sample group were assumed to be Black South Africans, but the difference in their mean TRAM-2 scores from other surnames was less than 1 SD. The mean difference in the composite scores was .55, which is better than most similar test results in that country, where 1 SD differences are usually found. This is a satisfactory sign. Most importantly, where tests are verbal, differences of more than 2 SDs are frequently found. Again, it is encouraging to see that the lowest differences were with dynamic learning scores.

With regard to predictive bias, the slopes and intercepts did not differ significantly, but the samples are small after all.

On other groups, of police trainees ($n = 202$), training facilities students ($n = 50$), and technical job applicants ($n = > 500$), similar impressive results were obtained.

On the latter group, Scheuneman methodology was used to check for *ethnic bias*. This reveals that not a single item in the concept formation and memory/understanding dimensions emerged as biased. This again is a remarkable finding when other test batteries are considered.

The APIL-B

Six sample populations, intercorrelation tables, and the means and standard deviations are given, for a total of $n = 1,245$ across the six populations. As before, KR 20 statistics for the concept formation and memory dimensions are high, ranging across the six sample groups from .78 to .87 for concept formation, and .70 to .82 for memory. Similar results for the other dimensions are also obtained using various statistical methods. There is unfortunately no way that the reliability of the flexibility scores can be estimated. There is, however, large variance, which is a prerequisite for good reliability.

Validity. Supervisors of 30 individuals filled in a questionnaire and compared these results with APIL-B data; all were significant at the 5% level. Substantial correlations with skills such as learning ability, technical knowledge, communications skills, judgment and the like indicate that individuals with measured high potential tend to acquire superior job-relevant skills. More astoundingly, zero correlations were found with psychological variables such as motivation: Potential thus does not always equal actualization, and such individuals would require specialized intervention.

On 33 first-year students, correlations with success were at .44 ($p = .012$) on 110 employees in a beverage factory. Correlations with performance ratings and certain of the subtest dimensions of the APIL-B were at > .90. With 43 candidates for a mini-MBA course, evaluated in-house and at a local university, the correlations for the two institutions' appraisals were .67 and .79 at a highly significant level.

On 2,400 first-time university students, against a local test somewhat like the American scholar's aptitude tool, the correlations were .67 and .68 for verbal and nonverbal scores on the aptitude test. The composite scores of the APIL-B and aptitude test were correlated at .71, with about 50% of the variance thus in common. In June, exam scores of those who succeeded in obtaining admission were at .29, creditable when it is realized that Physics and Social Work, for instance, are poorly correlated in skill dimensions. However, correlated by subject, it was clear that the strongest correlations were with lower subject scores, suggesting that the more the individual struggled with the subject, the greater the reflection on cognitive endowment; but with subjects such as Mathematics, Physics, and Statistics, the preselection was much more strict with regard to ability. Hence, memory dimensions are poorly correlated with Physics and Zulu, but with higher correlations in Psychology, Education, and Social Work.

A predictive racial bias study was done on the psychology students' June exam mark, because there were a substantial number of students there with home languages less likely to be of western origin; 66 students with obviously African names were identified. Of the remainder of the 400 students, a few with Asian names were also identified. The slope and intersect values for the Black subsample were .349 and 34.868, respectively, and the White subsample were at .354 and 41.131, respectively. These values are relatively similar. A t value of .033 was obtained with 462 DF, which is nonsignificant for the slope values. Although the intercept values appear discrepant, the t = 1.443 with 462 DF is not significant either.

In another sample of 263 applicants for B Comm degree bursaries, some still at secondary school, correlations with the APIL scores of .533 were obtained, some three times greater than with other local, conventional test instruments. The longer administration time of the APIL yields three times the predictive power, another reason to adapt these tests to neuropsychological batteries.

DISCUSSION

It is clear that "the development of valid and reliable test measures for the assessment" of individuals from nonwestern ethnic groups must be "based on empirical investigations" (Rey, Feldman, Rivas-Vaquez, Levin, & Benton, 1999, p. 593).

This call is mirrored in Nell (1999a, 1999b) and Taylor (1994). Neuropsychological instruments that are designed to measure, or utilize visuospatial modalities, must not only fulfill the criterion of being fair to nonwestern groups, but also not discriminate between western and nonwestern groups, as already noted. Culture fair does not mean the translation of western test into nonwestern language, because what is culturally acceptable in one instance, such as that speed indicates intelligence, may not be acceptable in another, where speed is equated with sloppiness, and slowness with being meticulous.

The call has been to create novel tests that do not emanate, say, from U.S. Army testing in the pre-World War I years (Lezak, 1995) nor present African Americans, Caucasian and Asian subjects with highly discrepant results that imply some inherent bias in the test battery, as in The Bell Curve (Herrnstein & Murray, 1994). The latter authors did, after all, try to eliminate test entities that were overtly biased, but nevertheless some groups in society must be left with the sense that on the attribute supposedly measured, they are somewhat on the wrong side of the bell curve. In both developed and developing societies, this must lead to the inevitable sidelining of growing but impotent populations. Such populations cannot always draw on overlearned skills, as do the psychometrics of IQ tests.

Despite the idea that visuospatial skills are present in some form from birth (Barkley, 1998), especially with regard to mental tracking skills, a vital prerequisite of executive functioning, the application of that genotype in the early moments of life to the environment leads to a developing phenotype that can bedevil test administrators in the cross-cultural setting.

In the previous discussion and investigation of the geometric-figure based tests, the empirical designs have held up well in terms of bias. Clearly, the minds of the test-takers can be dynamically linked to the test-makers, and the results show up as statistically hopeful in the extreme. The generally poor validity and reliability measures that plague neuropsychological instruments in general (Franzen, 1989) are not present when the test-maker swaps to a largely visuospatial format, despite the fact that most tests in neuropsychology load largely on one underlying general ability factor, namely Spearman's "g" (Matarazzo, 1990), even if under the rubric of memory, or coding, or some other title.

In cross-cultural assessment of visuospatial ability, it probably does not matter that very little overt verbal reasoning takes place, and that the already mentioned assessment tools purport to utilize only one modality at face value. The reliability loadings clearly indicate that the general ability factor is being measured, but utilizing a domain that allows for:

1. Culture fair appraisal.
2. Low racial bias.
3. Predictive and criterion validity.
4. Application across a wide spectrum of racial groups and languages.
5. Application across widely discrepant contexts.
6. Dynamic assessment with good empirical and statistical support.
7. Internal consistency and ecological validity.
8. The application of the visuospatial modality from zero to superior levels of education.
9. Low verbal loading and hence low susceptibility to language bias, while it:
10. Avoids the literal translation of English instruments.
11. Avoids the necessity for translators as interlocutors.
12. Avoids blind reliance on adapted measures without scientific validation.
13. Allows for negation of the test-wiseness bias.
14. Allows for the possibility of multiple inference with regard to neuropsychological substrates being measured, especially the vexing executive functions.

The concern of many authors in South Africa such as Taylor (1994, 1999) and Nell (1999a, 1999b), North and Central America, for example, Rey et al. (1999) and others in Brazil and China (discussed later) is thus addressed.

13. VISUOSPATIAL ASSESSMENT

This does not imply that the TRAM and APIL test are neuropsychological batteries *per se*, but it does imply that the historical failure of most attempts to create unbiased or low-bias instruments is remediable, with good attributes emerging. This fulfills further the criterion that any test should be scientifically validated as reliable for the intended purpose, can be applied to anyone regardless of culture, and is not biased against anyone from any designated group (Nell, 1999b). What is clear is that functional and cultural equivalence (Perez-Arce, 1999) is demonstrated by adopting a dynamic assessment approach that will allow for neuropsychological inference as well (Walsh, 1992).

APPLICATIONS TO VISUOSPATIAL ASSESSMENT TOOLS

It must therefore be accepted that many tools in neuropsychological assessment, applied to the search for quantification of visuospatial abilities, must foul of the western-bias paradigm, even though the genetic basis for such skills might be one of what Lezak (1995) calls "species-wide." Even though visuospatial activity should be strongly neurologically based, it is not free from cultural bias, with the west outperforming the rest, for example, in South America (Brito, Alfradique, Pereira, Porto, & Santos, 1998).

It is clear from Walsh (1991) that even complex figures have a strong verbal loading, as seen in the beginning of this chapter. Block design subtests thus may also seem innocuous, but yet many African children may never see a set of blocks in their lives, until confronted in the test situation. Nell (1999a, 1999b) and others have called for modifications in the approaches to testing, such as advising repeated learning trials until the subject is as test-wise as possible with regard to the instrument. There are many alternative versions of each test design and training is possible.

Far from presenting simply a visuospatial array, machinery such as the Austin Maze may represent just a piece of unfamiliar machinery and load novelty in such a way as to preclude any criterion validity assumptions. The idea that the Milner pathway is unchanging does not automatically occur to many nonwestern patients, nor do they become convinced even when told so. Their failures may suggest to them that the tester is unethical, taking advantage of them, and trying to remove them from, or exclude them from, the fruits of the western world—in a word, gatekeeping. In one instance, a patient in my practice could not manage the pathway in 40 trials. A photostat of the Austin Maze was managed in 12 trials, because the patient felt I could not manipulate the paper image.

Another patient refused to use the blocks unless the underside, blue-yellow option was used. Another could not do block test items with embedded designs; when trained on another set of items, and then returned to the original, he had no problems. He was too embarrassed to assume that the changes from one card example to the next were part of the test and not a mistake.

Three-dimensional items may also produce surprising findings. Using the Tinker Toy Test (Lezak, 1995), a young township (*barrio*) child produced a scattering of items with some long sticks with roundels tastefully distributed after nearly a half hour of fiddling. Yet on questioning, she had utilized every piece to create a masterpiece of visuospatial fantasy, with streetlights, an overturned truck, scattered goods of all kinds, houses, animals, and multiple vignettes, all meticulously generated. The construction of this representation of her internal mental offering would have done any sculptor proud, and clearing the items away left a sadness that was poignant: A gallery owner would have understood. On the Lezak scoring, she did surprisingly well.

The allure that visuospatial assessment, in its pure form, calls in no large measure on verbal reasoning is also spurious, as noted earlier. A patient, shot by the police at point-blank range with a high velocity rifle, lost nearly his entire right, dominant hemisphere, but scored at the 90th percentile on a complex figure copy and recall tasks. His psychometrist, a blind student, had never seen the figure, but she could draw it faultlessly on command.

The reasons that all these scenarios can occur are neurological. At the level of the primary visual cortex, the brain is able to register that something has been seen, and this is then recognized by the association cortex that surrounds that area. It is in these posterior areas that the brain reassembles perception as reality, and the further the impulse moves from the primary area, the greater the parallel input from neighboring modalities, namely the heteromodal association cortex, from temporal to parietal to frontal area, namely multiple sensory modalities (Koopowitz, 1999). Psychiatry too is undergoing a revolution, as this last cited article asserts.

In essence, in cross-cultural concerns, what the brain processes is heteromodal, rather than specifically visual-spatial-unimodal, and neuropsychology remains a science of inference of brain output. It can be safely assured that the nonwestern subject is of the same species neurologically, but the processing of information at the level of temporo-parietal-limbic pathways, under the influence of the frontal-executive areas clearly influences what the patient sees as fact, as this has been culturally mediated (Bukowski & Sippola, 1998; Sugarman, 2002). This cultural mediation is always a dynamic process, as trial and error species are not successful (Barkley, 1998; Sugarman, 2002).

Consequently, what the rest of the western world has found to be appropriate is not necessarily universal, and visuospatial assessment tools fall foul of the same translation problems as the verbal, in China, as in everywhere else (Chang, Chau, & Holroyd, 1999).

What the TRAM and APIL test instruments tell us, however, is that totally novel visuospatial assessment tools must be created that meet the now well-established criteria for cultural equivalence.

Nucci (1997) noted that the case could be made for the individual construction of a personal domain of choice and privacy that generalizes across cultures, maintaining a differentiated personality identity and a sense of personal agency. The personal is thus expressed with considerable social class and cultural variation, and therefore the sense of brain, and its visuospatial domain (Koopowitz, 1999) is constructed out of social interactions as well.

Testing of this domain is thus likely to require social interaction between the test-maker and test-taker at a much greater level than previously, and more practice, and the aspects of this that emerge in analyzing the WAIS-III and WMS-III are encouraging (Nell, 1999b).

Most encouraging, however, is the nature of the recursive feedback allowed for in such testing and indeed inherent in it, which confronts the problem of the linearity of other less sensitive testing, and work on the many levels of second order cybernetic abstraction that confront the tester in the transcultural interface.

ACKNOWLEDGMENTS

The author is indebted to Terry Taylor, PhD, of AProLab CC, P.O. Box 91866, Auckland Park, South Africa 2006, to whom all queries regarding the TRAM and APIL instruments should be addressed. E-mail: Aprolab@icon.co.za

REFERENCES

APIL-B. (1997). *Assessment instrument for those with 12 years of education or more* [Manual]. Johannesburg, South Africa: Aprolab.

Barkley, R. A. (1998). *Attention-deficit hyperactivity disorder: A handbook for diagnosis and treatment* (2nd Ed.). New York: Guilford.

Biesheuvel, S. (1972). Adaptability: Its measurement and determinants. In L. J. Cronbach & P. D. Denth (Eds.), *Mental tests and cultural adaptation*. The Hague: Mouton.

Brito, G. N., Alfradique, G. M., Pereira, C. C., Porto, C. M., & Santos, T. R. (1998). Developmental norms for eight instruments used in the neuropsychological assessment of children: Studies in Brazil. *Brazilian Journal of Medicine and Biological Research, 31*(3), 399–412.

Budoff, M. (1987). Measures for assessing learning potential. In C. S. Lidz (Ed.), *Dynamic testing* (pp. 52–81). New York: Guilford.

Bukowski, W. M., & Sippola, L. K (1998). Diversity and the social mind: Goals, constructs, culture and development. *Developmental Psychology 34*(4), 742–746.

Campione, J. C., & Brown, A. L. (1987). Linking dynamic testing with school achievement. In C. S. Lidz (Ed.), *Dynamic testing* (pp. 82–115). New York: Guilford.

Carlson, J. S., & Wiedl, K. H. (1979). Toward a differential testing approach: Testing the limits employing the raven matrices. *Intelligence, 3,* 323–344.

Carlson, J. S., & Wiedl, K. H. (1992). The dynamic testing of intelligence. In H. C. Haywood & Dd Tsuriel (Eds.), *Interactive assessment* (pp. 114–143). New York: Springer-Verlag.

Cattell, R. B. (1971). *Abilities: Their structure, growth, and action.* Boston: Houghton Mifflin.

Chang, A. M., Chau, J. P., & Holroyd, E. (1999). Translation of questionnaires and issues of equivalence. *Journal of Advanced Nursing, 29(2),* 316–322.

Fanon, F. (1968). *Wretched of the earth.* London: Penguin.

Feuerstein, R. (1979). *The dynamic assessment of retarded performers: The learning potential assessment device. Theory, instruments and techniques.* Baltimore: University Park Press.

Franzen, M. D. (1989). *Reliability and validity in neuropsychological assessment.* New York: Plenum.

Herrnstein, R. J., & Murray, C. (1994). *The bell curve: Intelligence and class structure in American life.* New York: The Free Press.

Hohl, U., Grundman, M., Salmon, R. G., Thomas, & Thal, L. J. (1999). Minimental state examination and Mattis Dementia Rating Scale Performance differs in Hispanic and non-Hispanic Alzheimer's disease patients. *Journal of the International Neuropsychological Society 5(4),* 301–307.

Koopowitz, L. F. (1999). The role of the brain in psychiatry: Implications for the specialist practice of psychiatry. *Australasian Psychiatry, 7,* 253–265.

Lezak, M. D. (1995). *Neuropsychological assessment* (3rd ed.). Oxford, England: Oxford University Press.

Llorente, A. M., Ponton, M. O., Taussig, I. M., & Satz, P. (1999). Patterns of American immigration and their influence on the acquisition of neuropsychological norms for Hispanics. *Archives of clinical Neuropsychology, 14(7),* 603–614.

Matarazzo, J. D. (1990). Psychological assessment versus psychological testing: Validation from Binet to the school, clinic and courtroom. *American Psychologist, 45(9),* 999–1017.

Nell V. (1999a). *Cross-cultural neuropsychological assessment: Theory and practice.* Mahwah, NJ: Lawrence Erlbaum Associates.

Nell, V. (1999b). Standardising the WAIS-III and the WMS-III for South Africa: Legislative, psychometric, and policy issues. *South African Journal of Psychology 29(3),* 128–137.

Neubauer, A. C. (1990). Coping with novelty and automatisation of information processing: An empirical test of Sternberg's two-facet subtheory of intelligence. *Personality and Individual Differences 11,* 1045–1052.

Nucci, L. (1997). Culture, universals, and the personal. *New Directions in Child Development 76,* 5–22.

Perez-Arce, P. (1999). The influence of culture on cognition. *Archives of Clinical Neuropsychology, 14(7),* 581–592.

Ponton, M. O., & Ardila, A. (1999). The future of neuropsychology with Hispanic populations in the United States. *Archives of Clinical Neuropsychology, 14(7),* 265–580.

Rey, G. J., Feldman, E., Rivas-Vasquez, R., Levin, B. E., & Benton, A. L. (1999). *Archives of Clinical Neuropsychology, 14(7),* 593–602.

Snow, R. E., Kyllonen, P. C., & Marshalek, B. (1984). The typography of ability and learning correlations. In R. J. Sternberg (Ed.), *Advances in the psychology of human intelligence* (Vol. 2). Hillsdale, NJ: Lawrence Erlbaum Associates.

Sternberg, R. J. (1984). Towards a triarchic theory of human intelligence. *Behavioural and Brain Sciences, 7,* 269–287.

Sugarman, R. (1999). The phenomenology of social withdrawal after traumatic brain injury. *Spanish Journal of Neuropsychology [Revista Espanola de Neuropsicologia], 1*(4), 83–112.

Sugarman, R. (2001). A neurobehavioural-informed approach to the use of clinical competencies in supporting the community based care of individuals with multi-axial diagnoses. *Australian Health Review 24*(4), 197–201.

Sugarman, R. (2002). Evolution and executive function: Why our toolboxes are empty. *Spanish Journal of Neuropsychology [Revista Espanola de Neuropsicologia] 4*(4), 351–377.

Taylor, T. R. (1994). A review of three approaches to cognitive assessment, and a proposed integrated approach based on a unifying theoretical framework. *South African Journal of Psychology, 24,* 184–193.

Taylor, T. R. (1999). *Proposed approach for the development of a dynamic assessment instrument for 6 to 9 year old children.* Unpublished manuscript.

TRAM-1. (1999). *Instrument to assess learning potential in illiterates and semiliterates* [Manual]. Johannesburg, South Africa: Aprolab.

TRAM-2. (1998). *Assessment of learning potential of literate testees* [Manual]. Johannesburg, South Africa: Aprolab.

Vygotsky, L. S. (1978). *Mind in society: The development of higher psychological processes* (M. Cole, V. John-Steiner, S. Scribner, & E. Souberman, Eds. & Trans.). Cambridge MA: Harvard University Press.

Walsh, K. W. (1991). *Understanding brain damage: A primer of neuropsychological evaluation* (2nd ed.). London: Churchill Livingstone.

Walsh, K. W. (1992). Some gnomes worth knowing. *The Clinical Neuropsychologist, 6,* 119–133.

Chapter **14**

Neural Circuit of Reading and Writing in the Japanese Language

Makoto Iwata
Neurological Institute, Tokyo Women's Medical University

Kanji and Kana are two distinct and parallel systems of letters that have been used in the Japanese language for more than 1,200 years (Iwata, Sugishita, & Toyokura, 1982; Iwata 1984). Kanji letters were imported from China around the 6th century. Because Kanji letters correspond to morphemes of the spoken Japanese language, each individual Kanji letter has several phonetic as well as semantic values. However, when more than two Kanji letters are combined to represent a single word, the phonetic value of each Kanji letter becomes strictly fixed and the entire string of letters should be read in a particular way. As Kanji letters have both semantic and phonetic values when they are used to represent words, they are different from true ideograms that have only meaning without definite phonetic value. Consequently, Kanji letters should be considered as morphograms. Nowadays, most of the nouns, roots of the verbs, adjectives, and adverbs are usually written in Kanji.

Kana letters are phonograms invented in 9th century by the Japanese ancestors abbreviating or simplifying the original Chinese characters. Because each Kana letter almost precisely corresponds to mora, or the syllable of the spoken Japanese language, Kana should be called syllabogram, but is usually called Japanese phonogram. Although any Japanese word or phrase can be written entirely in Kana letters, Kana is usually used to write grammatical words and inflections, foreign words, and onomatopoeia. The system of Kana letters is further divided into Hiragana and Katakana.

These two sorts of Kana are entirely parallel systems of phonogram, Hiraganas are currently used to write grammatical elements. The use of Katakana is restricted to represent foreign words and onomatopoeia.

IRRELEVANCY OF THE ANGULAR GYRUS HYPOTHESIS

In 1891 and 1892, Dejerine reported successively two different types of alexia. Based on the clinicopathological studies on these two types of alexia, he proposed that the left angular gyrus (AG) serves as the center of reading and writing. The currently accepted hypothesis, further refined by Geschwind (1965), of cerebral mechanism of reading and writing in the western languages is that the left AG is the center of the cross-modal association of visual, auditory, and somatosensory engrams. According to this theory, reading is the visual–auditory engram association and writing the auditory–somesthetic or -kinesthetic engram association, both of which are realized by the left AG.

The universal validity of this angular gyrus hypothesis has been repeatedly criticized in Japan. At first, the left AG lesion corresponding to the classical clinical picture of alexia with agraphia has been known to spare Kanji word reading, whereas alexia of Kana is very severe (Iwata, 1984; Yamadori, 1975). Another argument has arisen from the clinical observations of pure alexia caused by left medial occipital lesion in the Japanese patients. In contradiction to the name of the syndrome, pure alexia in the Japanese is almost constantly accompanied by agraphia of Kanji (Iwata, 1984; Iwata et al, 1982).

The last challenge to the angular gyrus hypothesis also came from the studies of Japanese alexics (Iwata, 1986; Sakurai, Sakai, Sakuta, & Iwara, 1994). The present author reported a nonaphasic patient with severe alexia and agraphia only for Kanji (Iwata, 1984, 1985, 1986; Iwata & Toyokura, 1982). CT scan of the patient showed a hemorrhagic lesion affecting the left posterior inferior temporal (PIT) area; the detailed analysis of alexia and agraphia in the patient is presented later in this chapter.

In summary, localized lesions on the various left hemispheric areas produce three distinct types of alexia and agraphia without aphasia in the Japanese (Table 14.1; Iwata, 1984). A left AG lesion causes alexia and agraphia

TABLE 14.1
Varieties of Alexia and Agraphia Caused by Localized Left Hemispheric Lesions in the Japanese Language

Site of lesion	Kana Reading	Kanji Reading	Kana Writing	Kanji Writing
angular gyrus (AG)	affected	preserved	affected	affected
medial occipital lobe	affected	affected	preserved	affected
posterior inferior temporal area (PIT)	preserved	affected	preserved	affected

of Kana, but only agraphia for Kanji. A left medial occipital lesion that causes alexia without agraphia in the westerners produces pure alexia of Kana and alexia with agraphia of Kanji in the Japanese. The third variety of reading and writing disturbances caused by left PIT lesion produces alexia and agraphia specific to Kanji letters (Iwata, 1984, 1985, 1986).

ALEXIA AND AGRAPHIA OF KANJI

The first patient reported by the present author (Iwata, 1984, 1985, 1986; Iwata & Toyokura, 1982) as a case of alexia and agraphia specific for Kanji caused by focal lesion affecting left PIT did not show any difficulty in reading and writing Kana, but Kanji reading was very severely affected. There are several types of errors in Kanji reading (Iwata, 1985, 1986) as shown in Fig. 14.1. The patient often failed to recognize the whole character and read only a part of it. Figural confusion, and semantic paralexia were also noted. One of the most characteristic type of errors was the error in selecting appropriate phonetic value. As mentioned earlier, each Kanji letter has usually more than two phonetic values among which the appropriate one should be chosen according to the meaning of the word. The patient with left PIT lesion showed great difficulty in this ability (Iwata, 1985, 1986).

The patient also showed severe agraphia in Kanji (Iwata, 1985, 1986). When he was asked to dictate phrases using Kanji letters, he wrote using only Kana letters and said that he could not write Kanji letters. When he was asked, however, to copy the phrase using Kanji, he could copy it without any difficulty (Fig 14.2). The Kanji characters that he produced in the copying task were not the slavish copies of the model, but the writings of the patient showed his own calligraphy. In order to analyze the mechanism of agraphia in this patient with PIT lesion. a Kanji letter construction test was designed,

Reading errors in PIT patient

(1) Incomplete recognition of whole letter form

森→木   青→月

(2) Confusion with graphically similar letter

鍵→銀   毛→手

(3) Confusion with semantically similar letter

象 (elephant)→ 猪 (wild boar)

(4) Incorrect selection of phonetic values

言葉 [kotoba] → [gen.....]

FIG. 14.1. Different reading errors in a patient with left PIT lesion.

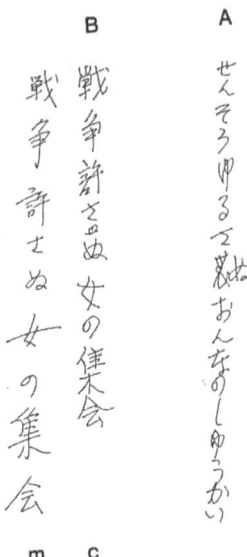

FIG. 14.2. Agraphia specific for Kanji in a patient with left PIT lesion. Column A is dictation; column B is copy writing of the model (m) by the patient (c).

in which the patient was presented several cards on which an element of a complete Kanji letter was written. He was asked to combine two cards to form the complete Kanji character that he could not write under dictation. The patient tried to combine two cards rather randomly to construct the target letter until he attained a correct combination. Figure 14.3 shows an example of such a trial. He was asked to write under dictation the Kanji letter "場" which he could not write in Kanji and wrote in Kana as "じょう" Then he was asked to construct the Kanji letter "場" using two of the six cards shown in the second row. He tried to construct the target letter 12 times but he could not come across the correct combination. At the 13th trial, he happened to make the correct combination and recognized that he could finally attain to the target. The test revealed that he could recognize the target letter he could not write down under dictation when he happened to make a correct combination of cards. Consequently, the visual engrams of Kanji letters were apparently preserved in his brain but they could no longer be evoked by auditory presentation of Kanji letters. However, the phonological processing of Kanji letters did not seem to be totally lost because the patient could correctly recognize the letter he had constructed as the target. The results of the analysis of agraphia in the patient imply that Kanji letter writing requires the selection of the visual engram of Kanji according to the semantic processing of the target morphemes and the left PIT plays an important role in this process of morpheme–grapheme transfer.

14. NEURAL CIRCUIT OF READING AND WRITING 257

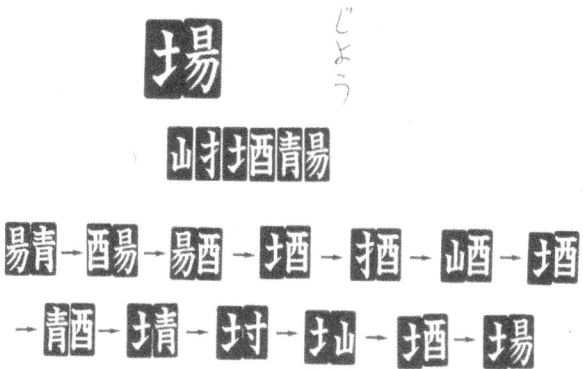

FIG. 14.3. Kanji letter construction test in a patient with left PIT lesion.

Figure 14.4 shows an infarct affecting PIT in another patient who developed a right superior quadrantanopsia and alexia with agraphia only for Kanji. Reading and writing of Kana were remarkably well preserved. She had no aphasia and the infarcted area in this patient was located on the left fusiform gyrus involving its cortex as well as the underlying white matter. Part of the inferior temporal gyrus seemed to be involved, too. Table 14.2 shows the results of reading aloud and dictation tests of the patient, using 416 Kanji letters that must be learned in Japan by the end of the second year of primary school education and the corresponding words written in Kana. There is a striking dissociation between Kana and Kanji, both in reading and writing tasks.

From these neuropsychological analyses, the present author proposed a dual pathway model of cerebral mechanism of reading and writing (Fig. 14.5; Iwata, 1984, 1986). From the visual area that receives visual inputs of letter strings, two parallel association pathways convey the information to the speech area; the dorsal pathway via the left AG and the ventral one going through the left PIT. The former is assumed to be the phonological reading pathway and the latter the semantic pathway. As to the process of writing, Kana letter writing is realized by auditory-to-somatosensory engram association by way of the left AG. In order to write Kanji letters, however, visual engram of letters must be evoked from the auditory engram, and the process mediated by the left PIT. Then visual-to-somatosensory engram association by way of the AG takes place to complete Kanji writing. As a consequence, a localized lesion of left AG produces alexia and agraphia of Kana with agraphia of Kanji, whereas that of left PIT causes alexia and graphia of Kanji, sparing the ability to read and write Kana letters.

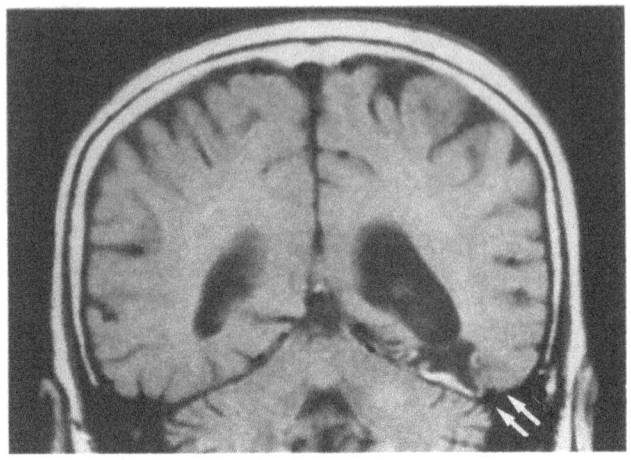

FIG 14.4. MRI (T1-weighted image) of a patient with left PIT lesion (arrows).

TABLE 14.2

Reading Aloud and Dictation in a Patient With Left PIT Lesion: Correct Responses in Reading Aloud and Dictation of 416 Kanji Letters That Must Be Learned in Japanese Primary School Before Age 8 and the Corresponding Kana Letters

	Kanji Reading	Kana Reading	Kanji Writing	Kana Writing
Correct Responses	216 / 416 (51%)	408 / 416 (98%)	265 / 416 (61%)	413 / 416 (99%)

PET SCAN STUDIES ON READING PROCESS

In order to confirm the previously mentioned dual pathway hypothesis, Sakurai, Momose and I did $H_2{}^{15}O$ PET scan studies. The detailed descriptions of the method were reported elsewhere (Momose, Sasaki, Sakurai, & Iwata, 1992; Sakurai et al., 1992, 1993). For the activation study, we used ^{15}O as a tracer in the form of intravenous bolus injection of $H_2{}^{15}O$ saline. Subjects were normal right-handed Japanese adult volunteers, undergraduate university students.

In our experiments, two different tasks, a fixation task and an activation task were applied to the subjects (Sakurai et al, 1992, 1993). in the fixation task, the subjects were asked to fixate their gaze on a central white spot projected on the dark screen 2 m forward. The activation task was to read aloud one of the following materials; two-letter Kanji words, three-letter Kana

14. NEURAL CIRCUIT OF READING AND WRITING

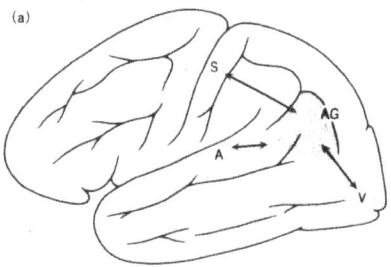

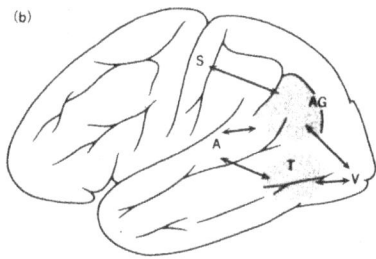

FIG. 14.5. Angular gyrus model (a) and dual pathway model (b) of reading and writing. S = somatosensory engram of writing action; V = visual engram of letters; A = auditory engram of words; AG = left angular gyrus; and T = left posterior inferior temporal area.

words, or three-letter nonsense strings of Kana letters. The reading materials were tachistoscopically presented in vertical fashion on the dark screen for 300 msec duration every 2 sec. These two tasks were alternately applied to each subject. The rCBF was measured by 90 sec scan six times in each subject, three times during fixation task and three times during reading-aloud task. The obtained rCBF values were normalized so that the mean whole CBF was constant (40 ml/100 g/min), and the mean rCBF during each task was calculated by intrasubject averaging of 3 measurements. Subtraction images were obtained in each subject by subtracting the mean rCBF during the fixation task from that during the activation task.

For the anatomical identification of the activated areas, subtraction PET images were superimposed on MR images of each subject. In order to precisely analyze the activated areas, 40 circular ROIs (16 mm in diameter), from which rCBF changes were to be sampled, were determined according to the superimposed PET-MR images of each cerebral area. The rCBF increase of more than 5% of the whole CBF (2 ml/100 g/min) was regarded as significant activation.

Figure 14.6 shows the cortical areas that showed significant rCBF increase by activation tasks (Sakurai, 1994). One of the most striking findings

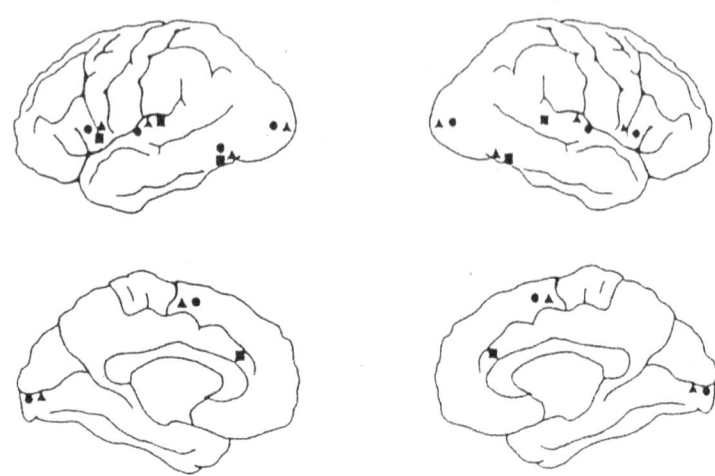

FIG. 14.6. Cortical areas showing significant rCBF increase in reading Kana nonword (circle), Kana word (triangle), and Kanji word (square).

is the activation of the left PIT in all three activation tasks. The PIT of the right hemisphere was also activated by reading tasks of both Kanji and Kana words. But the activation of the right PIT was always far less significant than that of the left PIT in every task. On the other hand, the activation rate of the left PIT was far more significant in reading either Kana or Kanji words as compared with meaningless nonsense Kana letter strings (Fig. 14.7; Sakurai et al., 1993). As a consequence, the left PIT is thought to play a certain role in semantic reading process.

On the contrary, both left and right AGs showed significant decrease in rCBF during activation tasks (Sakurai, 1994). This may be due either to the real deactivation of AG by the reading aloud task as compared with the fixating task, or due to the artifactual apparent rCBF reduction by the normalization of the whole CBF in the activation state. Anyhow, the role of the left AG in phonological reading was not confirmed by PET studies.

Recently, Sakurai et al (2000) applied statistical parametric analysis (SPM) to the previously mentioned data. They demonstrated using cognitive conjunction analysis that the main area activated by Kanji reading was the lateral fusiform gyrus (Area 37) whereas the Kana reading showed the greatest activation in the middle and inferior occipital gyri (Areas 18 and 19). They also found that the deep perisylvian temporoparietal area (Area 40/22 and 22/21) was definately activated by Kana reading.

Of interest is the significant increase of rCBF on bilateral lateral occipital areas, especially on the left side, in reading either Kana words and Kana

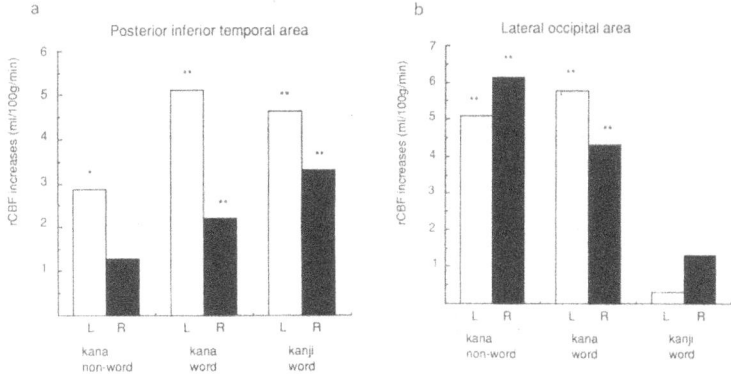

FIG. 14.7. Mean rCBF increases in PIT (a) and lateral occipital area (b) in reading Kana nonword, Kana word, and Kanji word tasks. $*p < 0.05$, $** p < 0.01$.

nonsense letter strings, whereas no significant activation was noted during Kanji-word reading. It implies that the lateral occipital area, especially on the left side, which is located just behind the AG, might play a certain role in phonological process of reading. Kleist pointed out, in his famous monograph on the higher cortical dysfunction caused by war injuries, that the cortical center for reading process is located in the left lateral occipital area, whereas he gave no particular role in reading to the left AG (Kleist, 1934). According to Kleist, the classical clinical pictures of alexia with agraphia in left AG lesion is actually caused not by the damage of the AG cortex itself but by the damage of the underlying white matter that connects left lateral occipital cortices with Wernicke's area. Our results obtained from PET scan studies seem to support the hypothesis of Kleist.

CONCLUSION AND SUMMARY

Japanese patients with alexia without aphasia caused by focal left hemispheric lesion show the dissociation between Kanji and Kana functions. Recently discovered in Japan was a clinical syndrome of left PIT lesion that produces alexia and agraphia selective for Kanji. We carried out activation studies using $H_2^{15}O$ PET scan and confirmed the role of the left PIT, especially Area 37 on the lateral fusiform gyrus in semantic reading process. Although the role of left AG has been regarded as crucial in reading process from the classical clinicoanatomical studies, our PET scan studies did not show any significant activation of that area in reading-aloud of both Kanji and Kana. On the other hand, the adjacent left lateral occipital areas (Areas 18 and 19) were found to be significantly activated by Kana reading no matter whether the presented letter strings have meaning or not. Consequently, it might be postulated that the left lateral occipital area plays an important role in phonological reading process, as Kleist (1934) had suggested in his monumental book on the studies of focal brain damage. According to these findings, the author proposed a newly modified diagram of reading process in the Japanese language as shown in Fig. 14.8. The neural circuit or circuits responsible for writing Kanji and Kana letters are still to be analyzed in more detail based on both clinicopathological correlation studies on the patients with focal brain damage and on activation studies on normal subjects.

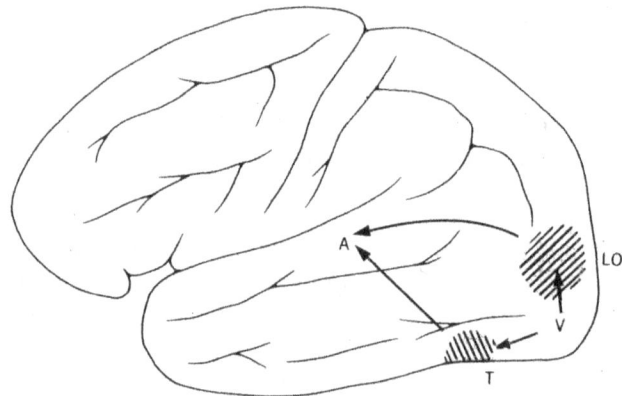

FIG. 14.8. New model of neural circuit of reading process in the Japanese language. V = visual engram of letters; A = auditory engram of words; LO = left lateral occipital area; and T = left posterior inferior temporal area.

REFERENCES

Dejerine, J. (1891). Sur un cas de cécité verbale avec agraphie [About a case of alexia with agraphia]. *Comptes Rendus de la Société de Biologie, 3,* 197–200.
Dejerine, J. (1892). Contribution à l'étude anatomo-pathologique et clinique des différentes variétés de cécité verbale [Contribution to the anatomopathological and clinical study of different varieties of alexia]. *Comptes Rendus de la Société de Biologie, 4,* 61–90.
Geschwind, N. (1965). Disconnexion syndrome in animals and man. *Brain, 88,* 237–294, 585–644.
Iwata, M. (1984). Kanji versus Kana: Neuropsychological correlates of the Japanese writing system. *Trends in Neurosciences, 7,* 290–293.
Iwata, M. (1985). Neural mechanism of reading and writing; Neurogrammatological approach. In Y. Tsukada (Ed.), *Perspectives on neurosciences: From molecule to mind* (pp. 299–312). Tokyo: University of Tokyo Press.
Iwata, M. (1986). Neural mechanism of reading and writing in the Japanese language. *Functional Neurology, 1,* 43–52.
Iwata, M., Sugishita, M., & Toyokura, Y. (1982). The Japanese writing system and functional hemispheric specialization. In S. Katsuki, T.Tsubaki, Y.Toyokura Y

(Eds.), *Neurology. Proceedings of 12th World Congress of Neurology* (pp. 53–62). Amsterdam: Excerpta Medica.

Iwata, M., & Toyokura, Y. (1982). Neural mechanism of alexia due to left cerebral hemispheric lesion [Abstract]. *Japanese Journal of Medicine, 21,* 308.

Kleist, K. (1934). Kriegsverletzungen des Gehirns in ihrer Bedeutung für die Hirnlokalization und Hirnpathologie. In K. Bonhoeffer (Ed.), *Handbuch der Ärztlichen Erfahrungen im Weltkriege 1914/1918* (pp. 553–558). Leipzig: Barth.

Momose, T., Sasaki, Y., Sakurai, Y., & Iwata, M. (1992). Functional studies with $H_2^{15}O$ PET. *Biomedical Research, 13*(1), 77–82.

Sakurai, Y. (1994). Mechanism of reading analysed by PET scan. (in Japanese) *Brain Medical, 6,* 63–69.

Sakurai, Y., Momose, T., Iwata, M., Sudo, Y., Ohtomo, K., & Kanazawa, I. (2000). Different cortical activity in reading of Kanji words, Kana words and Kana nonwords. *Cognitive Brain Research ,9,* 111–115.

Sakurai, Y., Momose, T., Iwata, M., Watanabe, T., Ishikawa, T., & Kanazawa, I. (1993). Semantic process in Kana word reading: Activation studies with positron emission tomography. *Neuroreport, 4,* 327–330.

Sakurai, Y., Momose, T., Iwata, M., Watanabe, T., Ishikawa, T., Takeda, K., Kanazawa, I., & Sasaki, Y. (1992). Kanji word reading process analysed by positron emission tomography. *Neuroreport, 3,* 445–448.

Sakurai, Y., Sakai, K., Sakuta, M., & Iwata, M. (1994). Naming difficulties in alexia with agraphia for *kenji* after a left posterior inferior temporal lesion. *Journal of Neurology, Neurosurgery, and Psychiatry, 57,* 609–613.

Yamadori, A. (1975). Ideogram reading in alexia. *Brain, 98,* 231–238.

Chapter **15**

Cross-Cultural Issues in Neuropsychology: Assessment of the Hispanic Patient

Marcel Pontón
Harbor-UCLA Medical Center

Marta Elena Corona-LoMonaco
Private Practice

The question of what term is appropriate to define this population has been discussed at length elsewhere (Pontón, 2001a; Pontón & Ardila, 1999; Pontón et al., 1996; Taussig & Pontón, 1996). For the purposes of this chapter, the terms Hispanic/Latino are used interchangeably.

Demographics speak clearly of a dramatic change in the U.S. population in terms of the number of working people from non-English speaking households. Major urban settings throughout the United States have experienced a significant growth of non-English speaking peoples in their population. This is also true of counties and suburban areas that have grown above the national average in the past decade. Although different ethnic groups have experienced dramatic growth, none has grown as fast as the Hispanic population. Of note, the Hispanic population accounted for half of all the growth in the U.S. population from April 2000 to April 2002, according to the U.S. Census Bureau (2003a). By 2005, the Hispanic population reached 41.8 million people, becoming the largest minority in the U.S. (14% of the total population) (U.S. Census Bureau, 2006). Among people residing in the United States, 47,000,000, ages 5 and older, speak a language other than English. That is about 1 in 5 Americans. Over 28 million of those people speak Spanish at home, according to the U.S. Census Bureau (2003b). Therefore, it is reasonable to expect that neuropsychologists will find themselves providing services to this population. How should the neuropsychologist conduct his or her evaluation of an individual whose language he or she does not speak and whose culture he or she does not know?

The clinician needs several tools to conduct an appropriate evaluation of the Hispanic patient. The reader may be eager to acquire norms and to obtain tests to assess this population. But these are only one set of tools. The critical tools the clinician needs are more personal and demand critical attention. For instance, language and culture, both multifaceted constructs, require careful consideration in neuropsychological assessment of the Hispanic patient.

LANGUAGE

Language is a very diverse construct that needs to be assessed and understood at several levels (e.g., cultural "subjective" and linguistic "objective" levels). The cultural "subjective" assessment of language is typically addressed in culture measures such as the Short Acculturation Scale for Hispanics (Marin, Sabogal, Marin, Otero-Sabogal, & Perez-Stable, 1987) and the Cultural Identity Scales (Felix-Ortiz, Newcomb, & Myers, 1994). The linguistic "objective" assessment of language is emphasized in bilingual research and theory (e.g., metalinguistic abilities: Bialystok, 1986 & 1988; threshold theory: Ricciardelli, 1992; First Language interference theory: Pialorsi, 1981; interdependence hypothesis: Cummins, 1989) and is assessed with normed tests of language proficiency (e.g., Woodcock Language Proficiency Battery–Revised, 1991).

A review of the literature shows that research efforts have focused on comparing linguistic ability to cognitive functioning. Specifically, attempts to understand the linguistic diversity of Hispanics and other racial groups has revealed discrepancies between monolingual and bilingual test results (Bialystok, 1986; Cervantes & Acosta, 1992; Garcia, 1986). Other cross-cultural research findings have shown that bilingualism, as compared to English monolingual speakers, increased a child's ability to solve problems involving high levels of control (fluid ability); (Bialystok, 1986, 1988). Similarly, an analysis of cognitive complexity and attentional control of cognitive development in a child sample suggests that bilingual children exhibit stronger executive functioning skills over monolingual children (Bialystok, 1999). In the context of these important findings, the neuropsychologist must consider how bilingual language functioning is defined. Differing levels of bilingualism have been studied and suggest differences between

15. ASSESSMENT OF THE HISPANIC PATIENT

groups (Bialystok, 1988; Corona-LoMonaco, 2000; Diaz, 1985). Language proficiency is a complex subject for the bilingual population, for example some subjects may be Spanish-dominant bilinguals whereas others may be English-dominant bilinguals. The concept of a balanced bilingual (someone who has equal mastery of both languages) can be quite elusive.

Although the need to be sensitive to language and culture differences throughout the assessment process are mentioned in the American Psychological Association ethical guidelines (APA, 2003), and despite continued attention to bilingualism and language representation in the literature (Genesee, Nicoladis, & Paradis, 1995; Paradis, 1996, 2000, 2001; Roberts, 1998), studies examining the impact of bilingualism on neuropsychological test performance seem less available. In fact, the issue of language proficiency (subjective and objective) has not been directly addressed in recent efforts to provide normative data for the neuropsychological assessment of Hispanics (e.g., Artiola i Fortuni & Mullaney 1998; Pontón & Ardila, 1999; Pontón et al., 1996; Taussig, Henderson, & Mack, 1992). Yet, the impact of language proficiency on test performance has been noted as important (Harris, Cullum, & Puente, 1995). One study looked at the impact of language and culture on a neuropsychological screening battery for Hispanics (Corona-LoMonaco, 2000) and found that neurocognitive assessment of Hispanic patients should always consider language proficiency, including language dominance, as part of the testing and interpretation process. Corona-LoMonaco operationalized five objective language categories, including balanced bilingualism. All bilingual groups (Spanish-dominant bilinguals; English-dominant bilinguals; balanced bilinguals) demonstrated at least average level functioning on assessment of Spanish and English language proficiency. Controlling for gender, age, and education, significant differences were noted between bilingual groups on the following neuropsychological domains: reasoning, language, memory, executive functions/attention-concentration. English dominant bilingual subjects generally produced significantly lower scores. Moreover, compared to Spanish monolingual subjects, bilingual skills presented as a cognitive benefit on the executive functions/attention-concentration domain.

Neuroimaging research supports the notion that when faced with language activation tasks, bilinguals recruited additional "brain regions." Thus, there is a beneficial dimension to bilingualism in cognitive performance, however, this depends on the proficiency of subjects in each language (De Bleser et al., 2003). Marrero, Golden, and Espe-Pfeifer (2002) have suggested that bilingualism may be a factor that aids in cognitive rehabilitation following head injury, whereas Gollan, Montoya, and Werner (2002) suggested that voluntary language switching in cognitive tasks incurs a processing cost for bilingual subjects (where bilinguals tend to process information worse than monolinguals). This is an area that requires much research because the relationship between language proficiency of Hispanic individuals and its influence on neurocognitive functioning remains poorly understood. However, research and theory to date suggest that a critical assessment of language proficiency of the bilingual speaker is essential to the interpretation of neuropsychological functioning.

CULTURE

Although language functioning has obvious relevance to the process of cognitive assessment, the cultural dimension of cognition is also important to the neuropsychological interpretation process (Artiola i Fortuny & Mullaney, 1997; Rosselli & Ardila, 2003; Teng, 2002; van de Vijver, 2002). From the time of Vygotsky's cross-cultural work on perception (Vygotsky, 1978), culture has been considered an important element affecting perception and cognitive development. Culture determines what cognitive activities are valued by a society (Ardila, 1995). Moreover, cultural experiences are known to impact performance on measures of language, intelligence, visuospatial functioning, memory, executive functioning, and creativity (Arnold, Cuellar, & Guzman, 1998; Grigsby et al., 2002; Manly et al., 1998; Selby, Jeffrey, & Laver, 2001; Touradji, Manly, Jacobs, & Stern, 2001; Westwood & Low, 2003). Research by Corona-LoMonaco (2000) assessed the impact of culture on neuropsychological test performance of a Hispanic sample and found that although bicultural assessment of language and behavior (English/American & Spanish/Latino) showed a significant relationship with neurocognitive functioning, these confounds were considerably reduced when other demographic variables were taken into account (e.g., gender, age, education). However, specific neuropsychological domains remained significantly correlated with culture following demographic controls (nonverbal reasoning, language, executive-functions/attention-concentration). More research is needed to advance our understanding of culture as a moderator variable on neuropsychological test performance of monolingual and bilingual Spanish-speaking Latinos. However, available research suggests that culture measurement requires consideration of multiple domains (Felix-Ortiz et al., 1994); therefore, the need to look beyond language as a single variable is essential.

It is suggested that neuropsychologists consider the impact of cultural identity (e.g., language, behavior, and values; Felix-Ortiz et al., 1994) and acculturation when interpreting neuropsychological test performance (Manly et al., 1998; Pontón, 2001b; Pontón & Ardila, 1999).

THE ASSESSMENT PROCESS

Having identified the critical elements in the assessment of this population, we turn to the issue at hand; how to conduct a neuropsychological evaluation of a Hispanic patient with the available tools. The following guidelines are offered.

Determine the Patient's Preferred Language

How should the clinician proceed when the patient's English language skills are questionable? Clinicians ought to begin their assessment with a clear sense of the most basic fact: Can *this* patient be tested in English? The following steps can assist the clinician in arriving at their decision:

1. Ascertain the patient's actual level of language functioning. The clinician needs to determine whether the patient is monolingual (English or Spanish) or bilingual.

    a. For the monolingual patients, this will not be complicated. It will be evident to the clinician whether patients can only speak English or Spanish.
    b. The problem lies with the bilingual patient, as degrees of bilingualism vary considerably (Corona-LoMonaco, 2000; Pontón & Ardila, 1999; Pontón, 2001b). This issue is addressed in detail later (see #5).

2. If the Hispanic patient is monolingual English speaking, then testing can proceed in English. However, an assessment of acculturation should be included. Such assessment would screen for the individual's history of exposure to English and Spanish languages (e.g., home, school, work, social) as well as Latino and American culture (e.g., history, music, media). Examples of acculturation measures are offered later. Acculturation data are important to the interpretation section of the neuropsychological evaluation, particularly when determining whether cognitive discrepancies could be explained by cultural factors.
3. If the patient is monolingual Spanish speaking, then the patient should be tested in Spanish by a bilingual, bicultural clinician. The ethical thing to do is to refer the patient to a Spanish-speaking clinician (APA, 2002).
4. If the patient cannot be referred and the only option is to test him or her via an interpreter, use the following approach:

    a. Make an attempt to acquaint yourself with the interpreter.
    b. To use an interpreter:

        i. Contact him or her ahead of time.
        ii. Make an effort to ascertain the qualifications of the interpreter (certified interpreters are the standard). Utilizing "interpret-

ers" who have little to no formal training invalidates the neuropsychological evaluation because they introduce significant random error in the assessment process. It is critical that the credentials of the interpreter be clarified before the evaluation.

    iii. When possible, the clinician asks for an interpreter familiar with psychological/ psychiatric evaluations (Melendez, 2001).

    iv. The clinician meets with the interpreter ahead of time and familiarizes the interpreter with the materials of the evaluation.

    v. The clinician allows the interpreter the opportunity to become familiar with the instructions of the tests and to write down such instructions in Spanish so as to maintain the standardization elements of the test.

    vi. The clinician warns the interpreter against making value judgments and filtering information either in favor or against the patient.

    vii. Prior to the actual testing, the interpreter is allowed to clarify any details about the testing instructions and how to handle ambiguities that may arise during the evaluation.

    viii. The clinician instructs the interpreter to avoid "becoming the psychologist" at any time during the evaluation (i.e., providing suggestions to the patient or making assumptions or inferences about the information relayed by the patient or his/her behavior).

  c. The use of family members, office staff, nurses, janitorial staff, or any other staff that are not certified interpreters will bring a significant amount of error into the evaluation, invalidating the results. The use of such people in the evaluation process is also unethical as the confidentiality of the patient's clinical history may be compromised. Therefore, it is suggested that whenever using an interpreter, the clinician review confidentiality with both the certified interpreter and the patient at the start of the evaluation.

  d. As discussed earlier (see number 2 above), assessment of acculturation should be completed with the Spanish monolingual speaker.

5. When assessing a bilingual patient, follow these basic guidelines: [Figure 15.1 provides a decision tree to assist the clinician (Pontón, 2001b)]:

  a. Assess English language functioning qualitatively (during conversation and the interview), and quantitatively using appropriate tests (see table of neuropsychological tests for suggestions).

b. If poor for testing (i.e., below the 25th percentile on the WLPB-R), refer patient to bilingual clinician.
c. If adequate for testing (i.e., equal to or greater than the 25th percentile on the WLPB-R), then determine level of acculturation using the Marin and Marin (1991) scale.
   i. If acculturation is high and the patient was educated in the United States, proceed with testing in English.
   ii. If acculturation is low and the patient had a foreign education, then the patient should be evaluated in Spanish.
   iii. If acculturation is moderate to low and the patient has been educated in the United States and/or a foreign country, proceed with bilingual assessment and compare performance (i.e., allow the patient to answer test items in either language and administer select tests in English and/or Spanish).
   iv. Suggested scales of acculturation include:

   1. Short Acculturation Scale for Hispanics (Marin et al., 1987).
   2. Cultural Identity Scales (Felix-Ortiz et al., 1994).

d. As a general rule, if educated in the United States and a foreign country, proceed with bilingual assessment and compare performance.

Psychologists should assess patients in the language of their choice (APA, 1992, 2003). However, it is conceivable that a patient may choose a language (English or Spanish) as the language of choice for testing when in fact they are better in their native language. It is up to the clinician to assess this issue carefully and to allow for bilingual assessment when appropriate. In other words, the patient's best performance can be obtained and the evaluation will reflect his or her actual level of functioning when credit is given for answers in either language.

The Use of Measures

Multiple tests either have been developed or are currently under development. Some of these measures are batteries of tests with appropriate norms, independent tests, or screening batteries. Table 15.1 provides a cursory list of some of these tests. The reader is referred to Pontón and Leon-Carrion (2001a) for an extended discussion of some of these tests. This is an area of great fluidity as test publishers have decided that "there is a market" with this population and new measures seem to be appearing constantly. Therefore, no list can be considered exhaustive or even up to date. By the time this chapter is published, many more measures heretofore unknown may already be available.

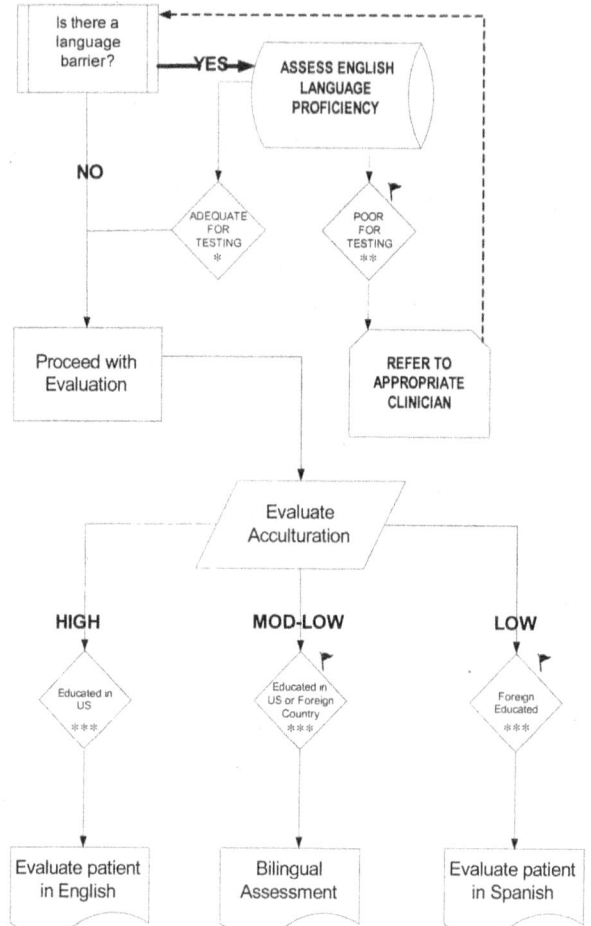

FIG. 15.1. Adapted from "Research and Assessment Issues With Hispanic Populations," by M. O. Pontón, 2001, in *Neuropsychology and the Hispanic Patient: A Clinical Handbook*, p. 47. Copyright by Lawrence Erlbaum Associates.
*(i.e., equal to or greater than the 25th percentile on the WLPB-R)
**(i.e., below the 25th percentile on the WLPB-R)
***If educated in the United States and a foreign country, proceed with bilingual assessment and compare performance.

Among the measures listed in Table 15.1, we are intimately familiar with the Neuropsychological Screening Battery for Hispanics (NeSBHis; Pontón et al., 1996). This measure has been used with several patient groups in clinical and research activities (dementia, epilepsy, HIV, brain injury) and can be easily adapted to the needs of the patient. Upcoming revisions of the battery include expanded normative datasets as well as new tests. The normative set provided later (Table 15.2) is based on 300 subjects and provides data stratified by age and education.

Pediatric Assessment. Are there any special considerations that should be taken into account when evaluating the Hispanic child or adolescent? This section provides guidelines for the process of assessment with this population. Unfortunately, it is not intuitive among many clinicians to recognize that a thorough assessment of language usage is critical. Hence, at the risk of sounding redundant, we must emphasize the importance of obtaining a history of exposure to English and Spanish languages (e.g., home/family/siblings, daycare, school, travel, friends/play, media—radio, television, movies, prayer/church) in addition to performing an objective assessment of their language proficiency. Of note, the level of acculturation of the primary care giver(s) should be assessed. This may be accomplished by completing the acculturation measures described in the adult section. If

TABLE 15.1
List of Tests Available in Spanish

Test	Age Groups	References
Bateria III Woodcock Muñoz	2–90	Woodcock & Muñoz-Sandoval, (2005)
Neuropsychological Screening Battery for Hispanics (NeSBHIS)	17–75	Pontón et al. (1996), Pontón, Gonzalez, Hernández, & Igareda (2000)
Cognistat, Spanish Version	18+	Kiernan, Mueller, & Langston (1998)
Batería Neuropsicológica en Español	Adults	Artiola i Fortuny (2000)
Computerized Seville Neuropsychological Test Battery	Adults	Leon-Carrion, (1997)
Neurologically Related Changes in Personality Inventory	Adults	Leon-Carrion (1998a)
NEUROPSI	16–85	Ostrosky-Solís, Ardila, Rosselli (1997)
Woodcock Language Proficiency Battery—Revised, Spanish Form	2–90	Woodcock & Muñoz-Sandoval, 1993

Note. Although the Spanish version of the Wechsler Adult Intelligence Scale-III is available in Spanish with Mexican norms (Manual Moderno), this test can only be found in Mexico. This table obviates the multiple tests with norms for Spanish-speaking subjects, and focuses on batteries instead. Because this is a fluid process, many more efforts are forthcoming and will be available in the future.

TABLE 15.2
Normative Data Stratified by Age and Education for the
Neuropsychological Screening Battery for Hispanics

NeSBHis Subtest	Age 16–29		Age 30–49		Age 50–75	
Years of Education	≤ 12	≥ 13	≤ 12	≥ 13	≤ 12	≥ 13
	n = 32	n = 45	n = 73	n = 78	n = 46	n = 23
	M (SD)	M (SD)	M (SD)	M (SD)	M (SD)	M (SD)
FAS Total	25.8 (8.5)	28.8 (9.5)	26.0 (9.3)	35.4 (10.2)	23.3 (12.7)	33.1 (9.2)
Pontón-Satz BNT	20.9 (2.7)	22.4 (3.9)	22.5 (2.9)	25.9 (2.9)	22.5 (3.6)	24.8 (3.0)
AVLT—List 5	13.2 (1.6)	13.3 (2.0)	12.8 (1.7)	13.6 (1.5)	12.0 (1.9)	13.0 (1.4)
AVLT—Total	52.1 (7.3)	55.4 (9.1)	50.9 (7.1)	56.3 (6.8)	47.0 (6.8)	52.1 (7.3)
(AVLT—Recall	12.0 (1.7)	12.2 (2.6)	11.5 (2.3)	12.1 (2.1)	10.5 (2.4)	10.7 (2.3)
AVLT—Delay	12.5 (2.0)	12.7 (2.4)	11.8 (2.2)	12.8 (1.9)	10.7 (2.2)	12.4 (1.9)
Rey-O Memory	20.8 (6.6)	19.9 (5.4)	16.8 (6.7)	20.6 (6.3)	12.5 (5.4)	17.9 (5.7)
Pin Test Dom-Tot	95.3 (16.1)	100.8 (14.4)	94.9 (19.9)	105.2 (16.1)	78.5 (19.5)	92.4 (15.0)
Pin Test Ndom-Tot	75.5 (17.1)	77.8 (13.7)	77.2 (18.2)	81.1 (15.1)	62.3 (17.1)	74.9 (13.9)
Digit Span—F	4.9 (.8)	5.2 (1.1)	4.8 (.8)	5.3 (1.2)	4.7 (.9)	5.1 (.7)
Digit Span—B	3.8 (1.0)	4.0 (1.0)	3.6 (1.0)	4.3 (1.2)	3.5 (.9)	4.0 (.9)
Digit Span—Total	8.8 (1.3)	9.1 (1.8)	8.4 (1.5)	9.7 (2.1)	8.3 (1.5)	9.1 (1.1)
Digit Symbol	49.1 (11.6)	64.2 (11.6)	44.5 (14.1)	62.4 (11.6)	34.3 (14.2)	53.8 (15.3)
Color Trails 1	44.2 (16.2)	34.4 (11.6)	50.8 (14.5)	35.8 (10.5)	34.4 (11.6)	46.4 (17.6)
Color Trails 2	103.2	82.8	119.5	84.3	82.8	103.0

	(26.1)	(27.1)	(43.1)	(24.8)	(27.1)	(30.9)
Block Design	32.0	37.3	29.4	37.5	25.9	32.5
	(7.4)	(5.9)	(9.2)	(5.1)	(8.0)	(7.8)
Rey-O Copy	31.1	31.9	29.0	31.7	25.0	30.2
	(4.3)	(2.6)	(5.1)	(4.2)	(6.9)	(5.0)
Ravens SPM Total	39.0	42.4	34.8	43.9	27.5	44.2
	(11.5)	(11.3)	(12.3)	(9.3)	(9.1)	(8.0)

Note. FAS = Controlled Oral Word Association Test; Pontón-Satz BNT = Modified version of the BNT. AVLT = WHO-UCLA Auditory Verbal Learning Test; AVLT Delay = 20 min delayed recall; Rey-O Memory = Rey Osterrieth Complex Figure Test, 10 min delayed recall; Digit Span, Digit Symbol, and Block Design are from the Escala de Inteligencia Wechsler para Adultos (EIWA); Raven's SPM = Raven's Standard Progressive Matrices. Spanish instructions and related materials are available from *cognaid.com*.

the child or adolescent has only had exposure to English and the caregiver's acculturation is high or conversely, if the child or adolescent has only had exposure to Spanish and the caregiver's acculturation is low, then testing will proceed in the appropriate language.

If the child or adolescent has had significant exposure to both English and Spanish, based on history and caregiver acculturation levels, then a language dominance screening is required prior to proceeding with the standard battery of tests. "Significant exposure" can be conceptualized as the proportion of time the child or adolescent has spent in environments where Spanish and/or English have been utilized; the clinician must go beyond traditional oral assessment of language and must also consider the impact of nonverbal, receptive, and cultural aspects of language and cognitive processing.

A language dominance screening is conducted to determine the primary language in which the child or adolescent should be evaluated; however, bilingual responses and prompting should not be ruled out. It is also important to consider the language screening data to differentiate between neurocognitive deficits and environmental/cultural factors in the interpretation process. Additionally, the clinician should consider the impact of the secondary language on the primary language (Gonzalez, 2001). As a matter of competent practice, it is unacceptable to ignore language proficiency when assessing a child who has had significant bilingual exposure in his or her environment.

The language dominance screening includes both formal and informal assessment of English and Spanish language skills. Formal assessment of language proficiency is completed via use of standardized tests, which are administered in English and Spanish (see Table 15.3 for examples of tests). Examples of suggested domains for bilingual language assessment include

TABLE 15.3
List of Pediatric Tests Available in Spanish

Language Test	Age Group	Reference
Woodcock Language Proficiency Battery—Revised, Spanish Form	2 yrs to 90 yrs	Woodcock & Muñoz-Sandoval (1993)
Test de Vocabulario en Imagenes Peabody (Spanish adaptation of the Peabody Picture Vocabulary Test—Revised)	2½ yrs to 18 yrs	Dunn, Padilla, Lugo, & Dunn (1996)
Prueba del Desarrollo Inicial del Lenguaje (translated from the Test of Early Language Development)	3 yrs to 7 yrs	Hresko, Reid, & Hammill (1982)
Spanish Version of the Test for Auditory Comprehension of Language (TACL)	4 yrs to 4½ yrs, 6 yrs to 6½ yrs, 8 yrs 6 mo to 8 yrs 11 mo	Wilcox & McGuinn-Aasby (1988)
Clinical Evaluation of Language Fundamentals (4th ed.; CELF-4 Spanish)	6 yrs to 21 yrs 11 mo	Wiig, Secord, & Semel (2006)
Dos Amigos: Verbal Language Scales	5 yrs to 13½ yrs	Crithchlow, 1996
Preschool Language Scale (PLS-4; Spanish ed.)	Birth to 6 yrs 11 mo	Zimmerman, Steiner, & Pond (2002)
Primer PASO "First STEP"	2 yrs 9 mo to 6 yrs 2 mo	Miller (2003)

Cognitive Tests	Age Group	Reference
WISC-IV Spanish	6 yrs to 16 yrs, 11 mo	Wechsler (2004)
Escala de Inteligencia Wechsler para Niños—Revisada (WISC-RM): norming sample from Mexico City	6 yrs to 16 yrs	Padilla, Roll, & Gomez-Palacio (1982)
Escala de Inteligencia Wechsler para Niños—Revisada de Puerto Rico (EIWN-R): norming sample from Puerto Rico	6 yrs to 17yrs, 11 mo	Herrans & Rodriguez (1992)
Escala de Inteligencia Wechsler para Niños—Revisada (EIWN-R): norming sample from New York	6 to 17 yrs, 11 mo	OREA (1991)
Bateria III Woodcock-Muñoz:	2 yrs to 90 yrs	Woodcock & Muñoz-Sandoval (2005)
The Leiter International Performance Scale—Revised	2 yrs to 40 yrs	Roid (1997)

Kaufman Assessment Battery for Children (K-ABC) (Bateria Kaufman de Evaluacion para Niños)	2½ yrs to 12½ yrs	Kaufman, Kaufman, & Padilla (1984)
McCarthy Scales of Children's Abilities	2½ yrs to 8½ yrs	McCarthy (1972)
Academic Performance Tests	*Age Group*	*Reference*
Bateria III Woodcock-Muñoz	2 yrs to 90 yrs	Woodcock & Muñoz-Sandoval (2005)
Spanish-Language Aprenda Achievement Test (3rd ed.)	K–12	Harcourt Assessment, Inc. (2005)

receptive & expressive vocabulary, formulation, production/fluency, recall (e.g., sentences/stories), processing (e.g., oral commands/instructions), comprehension, and reasoning. Informal assessment of language proficiency occurs during the interview process and/or during initial play interactions; at this time, the clinician assesses conversational/spontaneous communication skills (e.g., sentence structure, grammar, semantics, syntax, pronunciation, articulation) and overall familiarity and comfort with the language. Informal assessment of language proficiency may also include observation of the child/adolescent while interacting with others (e.g., caregivers, siblings, children/adolescents) or direct interviews with other primary adult figures (e.g., teachers). It is highly recommended that data from the language dominance screening be reported in a separate section in the neuropsychological test report.

The following decision tree (Gonzalez, 2001) provides a useful approach to assessing the language in which the bilingual child should be evaluated.

If the child/adolescent needs to be evaluated in Spanish, Table 15.3 provides a list of available Spanish language tests for assessment of pediatric patients. The list is not meant to be exhaustive. For extended discussion of tests used to assess Hispanic children, the reader is referred to Gonzalez (2001).

SUMMARY

Neuropsychological assessment across cultures is perhaps the most challenging field of work for clinicians in the years to come. It is a nascent and vastly unexplored field that must go beyond the mere exercise of translating tests and developing norms for existing tests into a discipline all its own. Critical issues for future research and development in this field involve multiple areas ranging from the standard of practice to the impact of moderator variables on test performance (e.g., culture, acculturation, education, level of bilingualism, etc.) to the operationalization of "Spanglish," as a form of bilin-

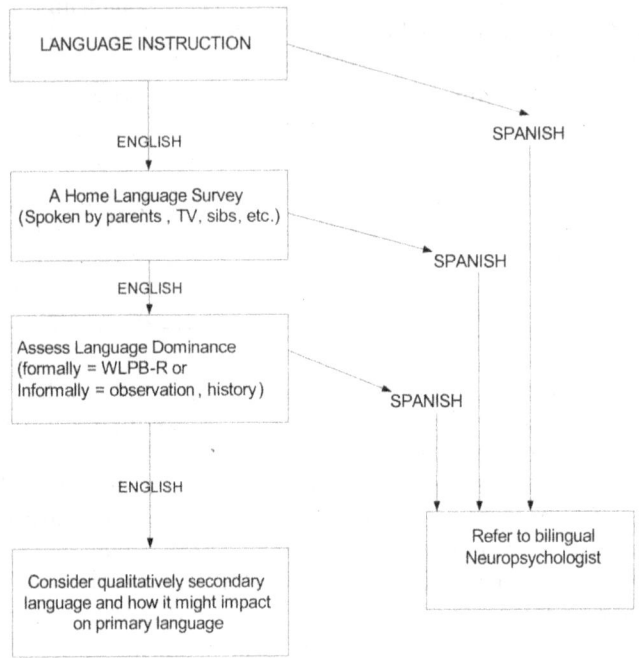

FIG. 15.2. From "Pediatric Assessment" by J. J. Gonzalez (2001), in *Neuropsychology and the Hispanic Patient: A Clinical Handbook*, p. 108. Copyright by Lawrence Erlbaum Associates. Reprinted by permission.

gualism. The degree of bilingualism an individual professes to have and actually possesses also requires further assessment, particularly as it relates to cognitive functioning. Interesting developments in the field include large normative efforts by main test publishers of known tests. Many more efforts are ongoing and will soon cross the "research-clinical" barrier. At a minimum, new developments in this field of assessment must take into account acculturation and variations in language use. This chapter attempts to provide an overview of the issues involved in the assessment of this population, offering guidelines for practice, identifying areas for future research, and providing relevant references for available measures. Because this is a fluid and evolving field, and because there are multiple measures that are developed informally, the current review does not pretend to be exhaustive. Organizations such as the Hispanic Neuropsychological Society (hnps.org) can be consulted as a resource in this nascent field.

REFERENCES

American Psychological Association. (1992). Ethical principles of psychologists and code of conduct. *American Psychologist, 12,* 1597–1611.

15. ASSESSMENT OF THE HISPANIC PATIENT

American Psychological Association. (2002). Ethical principles of psychologists and code of conduct. *American Psychologist, 57*(12), 1060–1073.
American Psychological Association. (2003). Guidelines on multicultural education, training, research, practice, and organizational change for psychologists. *American Psychologist, 58*(5), 377–402.
Ardila, A. (1995). Directions of research in cross-cultural neuropsychology. *Journal of Clinical and Experimental Neuropsychology, 17*(1), 143–150.
Arnold, B. R., Cuellar, I., & Guzman, N. (1998). Statistical and clinical evaluation of the Mattis Dementia Rating Scale—Spanish adaptation: An initial investigation. *Journals of Gerontology: Series B. Psychological Sciences & Social Sciences, 53B*(6), P364–P369.
Artiola i Fortuny, L. (2000). *Manual de Normas y Procedimientos para la Batería Neuropsicológica en Español.* The Netherlands: Swets & Zeitlinger.
Artiola i Fortuny, L., & Mullaney, H. A. (1997). Neuropsychology with Spanish speakers: Language use and proficiency issues for test development. *Journal of Clinical & Experimental Neuropsychology, 19*(4), 615–622.
Artiola i Fortuny, L., & Mullaney, H. A. (1998). Assessing patients whose language you do not know: Can the absurd be ethical? *Clinical Neuropsychologist, 12*(1), 113–126.
Bialystok, E. (1986). Factors in the growth of linguistic awareness. *Child Development, 57,* 498–510.
Bialystok, E. (1988). Levels of bilingualism and levels of linguistic awareness. *Developmental Psychology, 24*(4), 560–567.
Bialystok, E. (1999). Cognitive complexity and attentional control in the bilingual mind. *Cognitive Development, 70*(3), 636–644.
Cervantes, R. C., & Acosta, F. X. (1992). Psychological testing for Hispanic Americans. *Applied & Preventive Psychology, 1,* 209–219.
Corona-LoMonaco, M. E.(2000). *Impact of language and culture on a neuropsychological screening battery for Hispanics.* Unpublished doctoral dissertation, University of Southern California, UMI Dissertation Services, Ann Arbor, MI.
Crithchlow, D. E. (1996). *Dos amigos: Verbal language scales (An English-Spanish aptitude test).* Novato, CA: Academic Therapy Publications.
Cummins, J. (1989). Language and literacy acquisition in bilingual contexts. *Journal of Multilingual and Mulicultural Development 19,* 17–31.
De Bleser, R., Dupont, P., Postler, J., Bormans, G., Speelman, D., Mortelmans, L., & Debrock, M. (2003). The organisation of the bilingual lexicon: A PET study. *Journal of Neurolinguistics, 16*(4–5), 439–456.
Diaz, R. M. (1985). Bilingual cognitive development: Addressing three gaps current research. *Child Development, 56,* 1376–1388.
Dunn, L. M., Padilla, E. R., Lugo, D. E., & Dunn, L. M. (1986). *Test de vocabulario en imagenes Peabody: Adaptacion Hispanoamericana* [Peabody Picture Vocabulary Test: Hispanic American Adaptation]. Circle Pines, MN: American Guidance Service.
Felix-Ortiz, M., Newcomb, M. D., Myers, H. (1994). A multidimensional measure of cultural identity for Latino and Latina adolescents. *Hispanic Journal of Behavioral Sciences, 16*(2), 99–115.
Garcia, E. E. (1986). Bilingual development and the education of bilingual children during early childhood. *Special Issue: The Education of Hispanic Americans: A Challenge for the Future, 95*(1), 96–121.
Genesee, F., Nicoladis, E., & Paradis, J. (1995). Language differentiation in early bilingual development. *Journal of Child Language, 22*(3), 611–631.
Gollan, T. H., Montoya, R. I., & Werner, G. A. (2002). Semantic and letter fluency in Spanish-English bilinguals. *Neuropsychology, 16*(4), 562–576.

Gonzalez, J. (2001). Pediatric assessment. In M. O. Pontón & J. Leon-Carrion (Eds.), *Neuropsychology and the Hispanic patient: A clinical handbook* (pp. 105–136). Mahwah, NJ: Lawrence Erlbaum Associates.

Grigsby, J., Kaye, K., Shetterly, S. M., Baxter, J., Morgenstern, N. E., & Hamman, R. F. (2002). Prevalence of disorders of executive cognitive functioning among the elderly: Findings from the San Luis Valley Health and Aging Study. *Neuroepidemiology, 21*(5), 213–220.

Harcourt Assessment Inc. (2005). *Spanish-language Aprenda Achievement Test* (3rd ed.). San Antonio, TX: Author.

Harris, J. G., Cullum, C. M., & Puente, A. E. (1995). Effects of bilingualism on verbal learning and memory in Hispanic adults. *Journal of the International Neuropsychological Society, 1*(1) 10–16.

Herrans, L. L., & Rodriguez, J. M. (1992). *Escala de Inteligencia Wechsler para Ninos-Revisada* [Wechsler Intelligence Scale for Children—Revised]. San Diego, CA: The Psychological Corporation.

Hresko, W. P., Reid, D. K., & Hammill, D. D. (1982). Test review: Prueba del desarrollo inicial del lenguaje [Test of Early Language Development]. *The Reading Teacher, 428–431.*

Kaufman, A. S., Kaufman, N. L., & Padilla, E. R. (1984). *Bateria Kaufman de Evaluacion para Ninos: Manual para el examinador* [Kaufman Assessment Battery for Children: Examiner's Manual]. Circle Pines, MN: American Guidance Service.

Kiernan, R. J., Mueller, J., & Langston, W. (1998). Cognistat (Neurobehavioral Cognitive Status Examination. López, E. Versión Español). Fairfax, CA: The Northern California Neurobehavioral Group.

Leon-Carrion, J. (1997). Rehabilitation and assessment: Old task revisited for computerized neuropsychological assessment. In J. Leon-Carrion (Ed.), *Neuropsychological rehabilitation: Fundamentals, innovations, and directions* (pp. 47–61). Del Ray Beach, FL: St. Lucie Press.

Leon-Carrion, J. (1998a). Neurologically-related changes in personality inventory (NECHAPI): A clinical tool addressed to neurorehabilitation planning and monitoring effects of personality treatment. *Neurorehabilitation, 11,* 129–139.

Manly, J J., Miller, S. W., Heaton, R. K., Byrd, D., Reilly, J., Velasquez, R J., Saccuzzo, D. P., Grant, I., & The HIV Neurobehavioral Research Ctr Group (1998). The effect of African-American acculturation on neuropsychological test performance in normal and HIV-positive individuals. *Journal of the International Neuropsychological Society, 4*(3), 291–302

Marin, G., Sabogal, F., Marin, B. V., Otero-Sabogal, R., & Perez-Stable, E. J. (1987). Development of a short acculturation scale for Hispanics. *Hispanic Journal of Behavioral Sciences, 9*(2), 183–205.

Marin, G., & Marin, B. V. (1991). *Research with Hispanic populations.* Newbury Park, CA: Sage.

Marrero, M. Z., Golden, C. J., & Espe-Pfeifer, P. (2002). Bilingualism, brain injury, and recovery: Implications for understanding the bilingual and for therapy. *Clinical Psychology Review, 22*(3), 463–478.

Melendez, F. (2001). Forensic assessment of Hispanics. In M. O. Pontón & J. Leon-Carrion (Eds.), *Neuropsychology and the Hispanic patient: A clinical handbook* (pp. 321–340). Mahwah, NJ: Lawrence Erlbaum Associates.

McCarthy, D. (1972). *Manual for the McCarthy Scales of Children's Abilities.* Cleveland, OH: The Psychological Corporation.

Miller, L. J. (2003). *Primer PASO.* San Antonio, TX: The Psychological Corporation Harcourt Brace and Company.

OREA. (1991). *New York City norms for the Escala de Inteligencia Wechsler para Ninos-Revisada*. New York: NYC Board of Education.
Ostrosky-Solís, F., Ardila, A., & Rosselli, M. (1997). *NEUROPSI: Evaluació neuropsicológica breve en Español. Manual, instructivo y protocolo de aplicación* [NEUROPSI: A brief neuropsychological evaluation in Spanish. Manual, Instructions, and application protocol]. Mexico, DF: Bayer de México.
Padilla, E. R., Roll, S., & Gomez-Palacio, M. G. (1982). The performance of Mexican children and adolescents on the WISC-R. *Interamerican Journal of Psychology*, *16*(2), 122–128.
Paradis, M. (1996). Selective deficit in one language is not a demonstration of different anatomical representation: Comments on Gomez-Tortosa et al. (1995). *Brain & Language*, *54*(1), 170–173.
Paradis, M. (2000). Cerebral representation of bilingual concepts. *Bilingualism: Language & Cognition*, *3*(1), 22–24.
Paradis, M. (2001). The need for awareness of aphasia symptoms in different languages. *Journal of Neurolinguistics*, *14*(2–4), 85–91.
Pialorsi, F. (1981). A pilot test to measure basic English pattern proficiency among bilingual children. *International Review of Applied Second Language*, *19*(1), 45–64.
Pontón, M. O. (2001a). Hispanic culture in the United States. In M. O. Pontón and J. Leon-Carrion (Eds), *Neuropsychology and the Hispanic patient: A clinical handbook* (pp. 15–38). Mahwah, NJ: Lawrence Erlbaum Associates.
Pontón, M. O. (2001b). Research and assessment issues with Hispanic populations. In M. O. Pontón & J. Leon-Carrion (Eds), *Neuropsychology and the Hispanic patient: A clinical handbook* (pp. 39–58). Mahwah, NJ: Lawrence Erlbaum Associates.
Pontón, M. O., & Ardila, A. (1999). The future of neuropsychology with Hispanic populations. *Archives of Clinical Neuropsychology*, *14*(7), 565–580.
Pontón, M. O., Gonzalez, J. J., Hernández, I., & Igareda, J. (2000). Factor analysis of the Neuropsychological Screening Battery for Hispanics (NeSBHIS). *Applied Neuropsychology*, *7*(1), 32–39.
Pontón, M. O., & Leon-Carrion, J. (2001a). *Neuropsychology and the Hispanic patient: A clinical handbook*. Mahwah, NJ: Lawrence Erlbaum Associates.
Pontón, M. O., & Leon-Carrion, J. (2001b). The Hispanic population in the United States: An overview of sociocultural and demographic variables. In M. O. Pontón & J. Leon-Carrion (Eds.), *Neuropsychology and the Hispanic patient: A clinical handbook* (pp. 1–13). Mahwah, NJ: Lawrence Erlbaum Associates.
Pontón, M. O., Satz, P., Herrera, L., Ortiz, F., Urrutia, C. P., Young, R., et al. (1996). Normative data stratified by age and education for the neuropsychological screening battery for Hispanics (NeSBHis): Initial report. *Journal of the international Neuropsychological Society*, *2*, 96–104.
Ricciardelli, L. A. (1992). Bilingualism and cognitive development in relation to threshold theory. *Journal of Psycholinguistic Research*, *21*(4), 301–316.
Roberts, P. M. (1998). Bilingual aphasia: Some answers and more questions. *Aphasiology*, *12*(2), 141–146.
Roid, G. H. (1997). *Leiter International Performance Scale—Revised*. Wood Dale, IL: Stoelting Co.
Rosselli, M., & Ardila, A. (2003). The impact of culture and education on non-verbal neuropsychological measurements: A critical review. *Brain & Cognition*, *52*(3), 326–333.
Selby, M. J., Jeffrey, A., & Laver, G. D. (2001). The effects of cultural experience on neuropsychological performance in a forensic population. *American Journal of Forensic Psychology*, *19*(4), 75–86.
Taussig, I. M., Henderson, V., & Mack, W. (1992). Spanish translation and validation of a neuropsychological battery: Performance of Spanish and English speaking

Alzheimer's disease patients and normal comparison subjects. *Clinical Gerontologist, 11*(3–4), 95–108.

Taussig, M., & Pontón, M. O. (1996). Issues in neuropsychological assessment of Hispanic older adults: Cultural and linguistic factors. In G. Yeo & D. Gallagher-Thompson (Eds.), *Ethnicity and the dementias* (pp. 47–58). San Francisco: Taylor & Francis.

Teng, E. L. (2002). Cultural and educational factors in the diagnosis of dementia. *Alzheimer Disease & Associated Disorders, 16*(2), S77–S79.

Touradji, P., Manly, J. J., Jacobs, D. M., & Stern, Y. (2001). Neuropsychological test performance: A study of non-Hispanic White elderly. *Journal of Clinical & Experimental Neuropsychology, 23*(5), 643–649.

U.S. Census Bureau. (2003a, September 22). *Hispanic Heritage Month: September 15–October 15* (Public Information Office, Release Bulletin CB03-FF.14). Retrieved July 2004 from http://www.census.gov/Press-Release/www/2003/cb03-100.html http://www.census.gov/Press-Release/www/2002/cb02-168.html

U.S. Census Bureau. (2003b, October 8). *Language use and English-speaking ability: 2000* (Public Information Office, Release Bulletin CB03-157). Washington, DC: Author.

U.S. Census Bureau. (2006, May 10). U.S. Census Bureau News, Bulletin, CB06-72. Retrieved September 3, 2006 from http://www.census.gov/Press-Release/www/releases/archives/population/006808.html

U.S. Census Bureau. (2006). 2005 American Community Survey Data Profile Highlights. Retrieved August 31, 2006, from http://factfinder.census.gov/servlet/DataSetMainPageServlet?_program=ACS&_submenuId=&_lang=en&_ts=

van de Vijver, F. J. R. (2002). Cross-cultural assessment: Value for money? *Applied Psychology: An International Review, 51*(4), 545–566.

Vygotsky, L. S. (1978). *Mind in society: The development of higher psychological processes.* Cambridge, MA: Harvard University Press.

Wechsler, D. (2004). *Wechsler Intelligence Scale for Children* (4th ed., Spanish). San Antonio, TX: Harcourt Assessment.

Westwood, R., & Low, D. R. (2003). The Multicultural muse: Culture, creativity and innovation. *International Journal of Cross Cultural Management, 3*(2), 235–259.

Wiig, E. H., Secord, W. A., & Semel, E. (2006). *Clinical evaluation of language fundamentals* (4th ed., Spanish). San Antonio, TX: Harcourt Assessment.

Wilcox, K. A., & McGuinn-Aasby, S. (1988). The performance of monolingual and bilingual Mexican children on the TACL. *Language, Speech, and Hearing Services in the Schools, 19,* 34–40.

Woodcock, R. W. (1982) *Bateria Woodcock Psycho-educativa en Espanol* [Woodcock-Johnson Psychoeducational Battery]. Chicago: Riverside.

Woodcock, R. W. (1991). *Woodcock Language Proficiency Battery—Revised.* Chicago: Riverside.

Woodcock, R. W., & Muñoz-Sandoval, A. F.(1993). *Woodcock Language Proficiency Battery—Revised, Spanish Form* (Suppl. manual). Chicago: Riverside.

Woodcock, R. W., & Muñoz-Sandoval, A. F.(1996). *Bateria Woodcock-Muñoz: Pruebas de aprovechamiento—Revisada* [Woodcock-Johnson III Tests of Achievement]. Chicago: Riverside.

Woodcock, R. W., & Muñoz-Sandoval, A. F.(1996). *Bateria Woodcock-Muñoz: Pruebas de Habilidad Cognitiva—Revisada* [Woodcock-Johnson Tests of Cognitive Ability—Revised]. Chicago: Riverside.

Woodcock, R. W., & Muñz-Sandoval, A. F. (2005). *Bateria III.* Itasca, IL: Riverside.

Zimmerman, I. L., Steiner, V. G., & Pond, R. E. (2002). *Preschool Language Scale* (PLS—4; Spanish ed.) San Antonio, TX: The Psychological Corporation Harcourt Brace & Company.

Chapter 16

Clinical Neuropsychology of Spanish Speakers: The Challenge and Pitfalls of a Neuropsychology of a Heterogeneous Population

Gabriel D. Salazar
University of North Carolina Wilmington

Miguel Perez Garcia
Universidad de Granada (Spain)

Antonio E. Puente
University of North Carolina Wilmington

Clinical neuropsychology has been an active and growing specialty within psychology. The interface with cultural issues, often seen in other areas of psychology, has occurred only relatively recently. Ardila (1995) stated that within the specialty of clinical neuropsychology, there have been few studies addressing cultural variables, thus our understanding of the influences that cultural differences have on assessment is acutely limited. The development of cross-cultural neuropsychology owes itself to the growth of neuropsychology in general as well as to the concerns of society regarding those individuals who live in the United States who are culturally different (Puente & McCaffrey, 1992). According to Puente and Perez-Garcia (2000), cross-cultural neuropsychology describes the differences in performances and treatment of individuals in different cultures, expands the concepts of traditional cross-cultural psychology to compare and contrast the issues of how one group, a minority group, compares and contrasts to a larger group (presumably in position of power and control), and factors the role of culture and minority status in understanding brain function and dysfunction. The goal then, is to be able to assess while at the same time limiting potential bias. If we can understand the role of culture, then perhaps we can be closer to understanding the role of brain function. In an example of this attention to cross-cultural psychology, Hall (1997) stated that there has been a major increase in the psychological literature over the past 10 years regarding this issue. If this statement is true, then where is the proof? PsycLit and PsycInfo produce relatively few articles involving the interface between culture and clinical neuropsychology.

Of particular interest is the interface between cultural and neuropsychological studies involving Hispanics considering that this subgroup of the American population represents the fastest growing ethnic minority group. In the world, Spanish speakers represent one of the largest cohesive language groups. However, a review of the literature reveals even less when Hispanics and cross-cultural neuropsychology (or psychology for that matter) are considered. In fact, one of the most highly regarded neuropsychological assessment books entitled *Neuropsychological Assessment* (3rd ed.) edited by Lezak (1995) contains no references to Hispanics and the term "culture" is briefly discussed in one paragraph. The purpose of this chapter is to address the issues of neuropsychological assessment as it applies to Spanish-speaking populations, both in the United States as well as in Spain.

In choosing not only to address how neuropsychology applies to Hispanics in North America, but to Spanish speakers living in the Iberian peninsula, some overlap for a more universal understanding of the clinical neuropsychology of Spanish speakers should be obtained.

DEFINING THE PROBLEM

For the purpose of addressing the issue of clinical neuropsychological assessment of Spanish speakers, the primary focus is to take, even with all its apparent limitations, an American perspective. As a consequence, the concept of culture, majority group, and Hispanic will have an American-centric perspective. To provide a contrast, however, this approach is then compared with how clinical neuropsychological assessment has been addressed in Spain as the country of origin of the Spanish language.

Culture Defined

For the purpose of this chapter, it is important to operationally define "culture." This term, however, has many possible definitions. Taussig and

Ponton (1996) have defined culture rather easily, stating "it is a way of the people." Others have defined culture as similar thoughts, feelings, behaviors including but not limited to traditions, customs, and ways of life (Padilla, 1999) whereas some define it as the way in which a group survives and adapts (Ardila & Moreno, 2001). Handwerker (2002) has stated that culture is an arrangement of cognition, emotion, and behavior. Culture could easily be considered a term for any subgroup, whether it be the hippies of the 1960s or southerners living in North Carolina.

What Does Hispanic Mean?

More specific than culture is that of Hispanic culture. However, a definition of Hispanic must first be addressed. According to Puente and Ardila (2000), Hispanic is usually defined in the United States as a person whose primary (or, in some cases, secondary) language is Spanish. The U.S. Census (2003) reports that about 66% of Hispanics living in the United States are of Mexican origin, 14.4% are of Central or South American origin, 10.6% are Puerto Rican, 4.2% Cuban, and 7.4% are classified as being of "other origin."

Heterogeneity

As the preceding information suggests, Hispanics are a heterogeneous group. Each group (e.g., Mexican, Cuban, Puerto Rican) has its own distinct cultural characteristics, heritage, and behavioral patterns. Further, Hispanics living in the United States and Canada are more likely to know some English and the American way of life. This could include an understanding of standardized testing, the importance of time and time-based productivity, and competition in academic situations (Puente & Ardila, 2000). It is also noted by these authors that Hispanics from the United States are more likely to appear similar to North Americans on standardized tests than would Hispanics from Mexico, Central or South America, and so forth, although there is very little data in this area. Padilla (1999) concurred and suggested that within-group comparisons should be considered due to the fact that Hispanics are often considered unidimensional.

Acculturation

The role of acculturation provides a critical variable in the neuropsychological evaluation of Hispanics. Berry (1997) defined acculturation as the individual's ability to understand and maneuver outside of the culture in which they were raised and with which they are most familiar. Berry further stated that acculturation is a process in which both psychological and behavioral changes occur as a result of long-term contact with another culture. If this is the case, how can acculturation be measured? As culture can be considered dynamic in nature, this task is difficult. Zea, Asner-Self, Birman, and Buki (2003) have suggested that many individuals are affected by several cultures at once, and the mix and interactions are always changing. Although there are many tests of acculturation, it is difficult to isolate highly specific variables that address all subgroups of Hispanics. However, one example would be to give a Hispanic a timed test. If the patient understands the value of time, then they should be able to perform the task. However, if they do not understand that that they must respond as quickly as possible (this is the case with many Hispanics as the concept of time may be different for them), they will not perform as well and possibly present themselves as brain damaged (Ardila, Rosselli, & Puente, 1994). According to Shorris (1992), the degree of acculturation among Hispanics varies. As time goes by, patterns of behavior, beliefs, and values become similar to those of Americans. Thus, as a rule, Hispanics living in the United States eventually integrate their values with American values.

Demographics

As of the year 2001, the U.S. Census reported that Hispanics comprise about 12.5% of the entire U.S. population. This figure does not include the high number of Hispanics who are in the United States illegally. In California alone, Hispanics account for 32.4% of the population. The Bureau of the Census (2003) has recently reported that Hispanics have surpassed African-Americans as the largest minority in the United States. Further, by the year 2050, Hispanics will comprise 25% of the entire population in the United States (54 million). In fact, the nation's Hispanic population continues to grow at a much faster rate than the population as a whole. Additionally, the population of Hispanics (who may be of any race) reached 39.9 million on July 1, 2003, accounting for about one-half of the 9.4 million residents added to the nation's population since 2000 Census. Its growth rate of 13.0% over the last 3 years was almost four times that of the total population (3.3%).

TRANSLATING NEUROPSYCHOLOGICAL CONCEPTS AND TESTS INTO SPANISH

Although there are many issues in the translation process of a test from Spanish to English, the topics of copyright, literal versus cognitive equivalence, norms, education, and the use of translators are the focus of this section.

Many tests are translated from English into Spanish without the permission of the company producing the tests (Puente, 2000). This presents a copyright infringement. Not only are there legal ramifications but also questions regarding the integrity of the "translated" test. Often the items are translated literally with no cognitive (or emotional) equivalence in mind. For example, a person in the United States may know who Martin

Luther King was, but a Hispanic may not. Further, these tests have limited validity, yet in many cases are being used to determine a patients' status.

The issue of norms is perhaps the most important issue plaguing the neuropsychologist in assessing Spanish speakers (Puente, 2000). Even if a test is properly translated using the correct statistical methods, it means little without an appropriate normative sample. A test normed according to U.S. census figures may be of limited value in Spain or Latin America. In addition, some of the tests that are normed in one country (e.g., Ardila et al., 1994) only present one segment of the Spanish-speaking population. An example would be a test that is given to a Cuban that was normed on Mexicans. Tests such as these do not take into full consideration the heterogeneity of Hispanics. This creates problems of generalizability. Of course, the alternative may mean less applicability. That is, would it better to use a test appropriately translated into Spanish and normed in a Latin country different than the country of origin of the patient (e.g., Mexican norms and Honduran patient) or to use a test appropriately translated and normed in the United States (e.g., U.S. norms and Honduran patient)?

Education is also an important issue because of the differences in equivalence from country to country (Ardila et al., 1994). The educational systems in the United States vary from those in Latin American countries in that 12 years of education may or may not be the equivalent of a high school diploma in the United States. There may also be variance from country to country such as Mexico and Chile, and so forth.

The use of translators (Puente & Perez-Garcia, 2000) may also be problematic for a neuropsychologist who is not fluent in Spanish language or culture. Often a family member, usually a child, serves as the interpreter. Untrained staff members or even trained interpreters are often used as well. The problem with any of these methods to gather data is that increased error is implicitly introduced into the evaluation process.

Samples of Neuropsychological Tests Available in Spanish

In order to obtain a more comprehensive understanding of what tests are available, the following is a sample of neuropsychological tests available in Spanish (Puente, Puente, & Salazar, 2004; Table 16.1). The list was compiled using test catalogs as well as a PsychInfo literature review. The list is not meant to be exhaustive; however it should provide the reader with a basis for what is currently available with regard to Spanish speaking assessment.

The Case of Measuring Intelligence

A salient method of illustrating the issues heretofore addressed in this chapter is the measurement of intelligence. This construct is one of the most widely measured concepts both in clinical psychology and clinical neuropsychology (Camara, Nathan, & Puente, 2000). The most common way to measure intelligence has been to administer an intelligence test, the most common being the Wechsler Scales (Camara et al, 2000). Nonverbal intelligence scales have also been widely used for their simplicity to administer and time-saving qualities as well as their applicability for individuals with limited language and educational attainment.

Over the years, there have been several versions of the Wechsler Adult Intelligence Scale (WAIS) intended for Spanish speakers. Three of these are discussed: The Puerto Rican version called the EIWA, the Spanish version made by TEA, and most recently the Mexican version translated by Manual Moderno. The EIWA (Escala de inteligencia para adultos) was normed in Puerto Rico during the 1960s. The Spanish edition made by TEA was produced in 1998. More recently, Manual Moderno released the WAIS-III with Mexican norms ini 2004.

The WISC (Wechsler Intelligence Scale for Children) has gone through a similar history with a Puerto Rican version appearing first (1992). However, The Psychological Corporation finally released a version (WISC-IV) based on the current Hispanic norms in the United States in 2004. This version took 10 years to be developed, with one of the authors' (Puente) as the first external project director.

There are also alternative methods for assessing intelligence, most notably nonverbal intelligence tests. These tests in many cases require minimal instruction, time, and little or no writing by the patient. The most common are the BETA-III (The Psychological Corporation, 1999), the TONI-3 (Western Psychological Services, 1997), the UNIT (Riverside, 1998), and the GAMA (Pearson, 1997).

The Beta-III includes instructions in Spanish and new norms, and may also be administered in a group setting. There is no reading required by the patient. The TONI-3 (Test of Non-Verbal Intelligence, 3rd ed.) is also language free and has a very large sample size (3,000). The TONI-3 is the quickest of the four to administer at 15 min. The UNIT, or Universal Non-Verbal Intelligence test, is for use with children from the ages of 5 to 15 and takes about 30 min to complete. Finally, the GAMA (General Abilities Scale for Adults) may also be administered to more than one individual at a time, and takes 25 min to complete. The GAMA is also normed according to U.S. Census figures and is applicable to adults over the age of 18 with a reading level of the third grade or higher. The GAMA also has Spanish instructions available.

Although the issue of assessing Spanish speakers in clinical neuropsychology has been addressed over the past decade, the issues are still complex especially when it comes to intellectual assessment. Assessment is difficult enough in English, where many tests are deemed acceptable. When assessing a Spanish speaker, one should take into account the heterogeneity of Hispanics, the lack of widely acceptable tests, and the limited normative samples available. Even if adequate tests are used, there is still the question of adaptive abilities, which are difficult to measure in Spanish-speaking patients. However, all things being equal, there is both an interest in the field as well as an indication that tests are becoming available to measure intellectual functions in Spanish speakers.

Clinical Neuropsychology in Spain

Although Spain has never produced studies such as Sweet, Moberg, and Westergaard (1996) or Camara et al. (2000) that analyzed the practice of neuropsychology, it follows this paradigm with regard to practice and administration of test batteries. Research on appropriate administration of test batteries (Hamsher, 1990) and testing with deprived populations (Bauer, 1994) has been reviewed extensively. It is important to note that this viewpoint is not necessarily Spanish in nature; it is correspondent with the current major views of neuropsychology.

At the present time, there is a great disparity between the development of the science and the practice of clinical neuropsychology. Although both are a large part of the curriculum and the importance of clinical neuropsychology is stressed, there are, in general, a lack of neuropsychologists in hospitals as well as in private practice settings. Health care in Spain is universal, and is given at a reduced cost. In addition, the Spanish government has not acknowledged the new clinical specialty that is clinical neuropsychology, thus making it difficult to establish a following. Despite this lack of foresight by the government, neuropsychologists in Spain continue to work with neurosurgeons and neurologists regularly in both scientific and clinical endeavors.

Historically, the focus on neuropsychology in Spain has been limited to theoretical and academic development, with little or no attention paid to practice. The international focus, much like Spain's, needs to provide more development in this area as well as in the areas of evaluation and rehabilitation. A review of current practices in clinical neuropsychology in Spain follows.

Neuropsychological Evaluation

As indicated earlier, in light of past research on other populations, there is not a widely recognized clinical protocol in Spain. Thus, current research dictates what would be most appropriate in a clinical evaluation.

The clinical evaluation is most often pursued in three phases.

(1) clinical interview, (2) neuropsychological testing, (3) follow-up interview with test results and treatment plan, if necessary.

Clinical Interview. Following Lezak's (1995) recommendations, the clinical interview should consist of the following:

1. Understanding the patients' current state;
2. Understanding the problem;
3. Establishing a hypothesis regarding the problem; and
4. Using the previous findings as a guide for deciding on a test battery.

The interview should be conducted with the patient alone, if possible (this is sometimes difficult depending on the state of the patient). The neuropsychologist should establish rapport with the patient in such a way to elicit as much information as possible. In order to accomplish this, Lezak (1995) suggested the following tactics:

1. Explain the objectives of the interview.
2. Explain what the evaluation will consist of (citing memory, attention, etc).
3. Explain how the test results will be used, who will get copies, and so forth.
4. Explain that results will be kept confidential unless stated otherwise on informed consent.
5. Information regarding who will get the results and when should be discussed.
6. Describe neuropsychological testing in such a manner that is understandable to the patient.
7. Explain that the evaluation is a partnership that can be good or bad, depending on the patient's outlook.

Once rapport has been established, the interview should be conducted compiling information regarding family history, school history, job history, and any other relevant issues (medical problems) prior to the head injury.

The end result of the interview should be a thorough description of the patient and the presenting problem. This information can come from various sources: self-report, records, family members, medical charts, and/or other medical records. Cognitive affect as well as emotional state should be considered as well in addition to the sequalae.

Of importance is how the patient's daily life has been affected by the injury with regard to their job, social and familial life. This information will be a valuable contributor in the establishment of limitations as well as in rehabilitation for the patient.

The information obtained during the interview should be used as a basis for a hypothesis regarding the patients' current neuropsychological strengths and deficits. Inasmuch, the information should also guide the clinician in the selection of appropriate testing instruments. Consideration when choosing a test battery should not be limited to instruments that show impairment, however.

Neuropsychological Testing. As noted previously, testing follows the interview. It is important to note that information obtained in the interview may be tainted, so it is wise to choose a thorough test battery consisting of instruments that will paint a complete picture of the individual's strengths and weaknesses.

When choosing the tests, it is noteworthy to include tests specific to the individuals suspected deficiencies as well as strengths. For example, a patient with hemiplegia of the dominant hemisphere would be administered the Benton Visual Retention Test (BVRT), whereas a patient who has suffered a transient ischemic attack without motor difficulty would be given the RCFT. In both cases, visual memory is explored but through different methods.

Test selection according to Vanderploeg (1994) should be as follows: 1) The tests chosen should reflect the referral question as well as the hypothesis; 2) Both high-level tests such as memory and low-level tests such as sensory-perceptual tests should be administered; 3) If quantitative tests are to be used, make sure they are normed appropriately; 4) Utilize tests that can be adjusted to the patients level of ability; 5) Avoid tests that are not neuropsychologically based. "Tests for brain injury almost always measure cognitive ability, but tests of cognitive ability hardly measure brain injury" (Vanderploeg, 1994, p. 18); and 6) If multiple tests measuring a similar dimension (i.e., memory) are to be used, try not to administer tests in that area that would produce redundancy.

Lezak (1995) offered the following suggestions regarding the order in which the tests should be administered: 1) Administer difficult tests at the beginning while the patient is fresh. Be careful not to give a test that may be too hard and demoralize the patient; 2) Combine difficult and easy tests; 3) Combine verbal and nonverbal tests; and finally, 4) Take into account how long each test may last, and administer appropriately. The average session is about 50 minutes. White and Rose (1997) have suggested that patients should be taken to their limit in order to analyze their capacity. The clinician should also be aware of the types of errors the patient is making.

Compared to other countries such as the United States, Spain has not addressed the issue regarding the use of technicians in neuropsychology, although as the discipline grows it may too become a topic of much discussion. Once testing has been accomplished, it is necessary to confirm the hypothesis and rule out any differential diagnosis. The next step is sharing the results with the patient.

Follow-Up Interview With Test Results. The follow-up interview is the final phase of the evaluation and should never be omitted (Walsh, 1999) even if the evaluation has been ordered by another professional. The follow-up can be divided into two parts: the final interview and written report. The follow-up interview is conducted after all testing, scoring, and interpretation have been done. The information presented to the patient should reflect strengths and weaknesses, and how these strengths and weaknesses will affect their functioning and/or their rehabilitation. All of the information discussed with the patient should also be conveyed in the written report.

The written report is fundamental not only in communicating results to the patient but also to the relevant individuals with whom this patient is working with (Walsh, 1999). Although there are a variety of ways this information can be conveyed, it is important to be succinct yet thorough. The report should be well written and understandable by other professionals. At the minimum, the written report should consist of the referral question, family, social, work, and medical histories. Any neuropsychological damage should be noted regarding the clinical process (testing, results, and interpretation).

In sum, the typical neuropsychological evaluation in Spain consists of interviews to determine pre and postinjury functions, to decide on a test battery, and to establish an hypothesis regarding neuropsychological sequelae. The battery given will surely depend on the background of the clinician, and the results of the testing should be conveyed through a written report both to the patient and to those who are involved in the case. With testing being such a fundamental part of the clinical process, it is necessary to include a list of instruments at the disposal of the neuropsychologist.

Neuropsychological Instruments

In comparison with the Anglo population, the quantity of tests available to Spanish neuropsychologists is quite limited. Two companies, TEA and PSYMTEC, offer neuropsychological tests. Of those tests, most of those are in English. In addition, some of these tests do not include Spanish norms, therefore it is difficult to interpret them without caution.

In Spain, there has been a trend in utilizing tests that were made for other activities, ranging from personnel selection to clinical psychology. As in most countries, there are many tests oriented toward deficits in general but not very many regarding verbal deficits (Perez, Godoy, Laserna, Vera, & Puente, 1998) although more functional tests have demonstrated the same utility as ones used for deficits in general.

Table 16.1 presents a list, (although not exhaustive) of neuropsychological tests commonly used in Spain. There is no frequency distribution for their usage, as that exceeds the scope of this chapter. It is also important to

Table 16.1

Test	Publisher	Test Type	Norms	Instructions	Items in Spanish or English	Age Range	Author	Yr. Published
Adaptive Behavior Assessment System	The Psychological Corporation	TEST	DSM-IV	ENGLISH	ENGLISH	5-89 YRS.	Harrison, P., & Oakland, T.	
Advanced Progressive Matrices (AFM)	H. K. Lewis & Co. Ltd.	NVIQ	NO	PANTOMIME	NONVERBAL	ADOLESCENT & ADULT	Raven, J.C.	1987
Bateria-R	Riverside Publishing	COGNITIVE ABILITY/ACHIEVEMENT	YES	SPANISH	SPANISH	2-90+	Woodcock, R. & Munoz-Sandoval, A.	
Beck Anxiety Inventory	The Psychological Corporation	Anxiety	NO	ENGLISH	ENGLISH	17-80	Beck, A.	1993
Beck Depression Inventory-II	The Psychological Corporation	DEPRESSION	NO	ENGLISH	ENGLISH	13-80	Beck, A., Brown, G. & Steer, R.	1996
Beck Hopelessness Scale	The Psychological Corporation	HOPELESSNESS	NO	ENGLISH	ENGLISH	17-80 YRS.	Beck, A.	1993
Beck Scale for Suicidal Ideation	The Psychological Corporation	Suicide	NO	ENGLISH	ENGLISH	17-OLDER	Beck, A.	1991
BETA III	The Psychological Corporation	NVIQ	NO	ENGLISH	ENGLISH	16-89	Kellog, C., & Morton, N.	
Bilingual Verbal Ability Tests	Riverside Publishing	INTELLIGENCE	yes; Puerto Rican & Mexican	BOTH	BOTH	5+	Munoz-Sandoval, A. M., Cummins, J., Alvarado C. G., & Ruef, M. L.	1998
BVAT (Bilingual Verbal Ability)	Riverside Publishing	BILINGUAL ABILITY	YES	BOTH	BOTH	5-ADULT	Munoz-Sandoval, A. M., Cummins, et. Al.	
Cattell Infant Intelligence Scale	The Psychological Corporation	NVIQ	NO	PANTOMIME	NONVERBAL	3-30 MONTHS	Psyche, C.	1998
Clinical Evaluation of Language Fundamentals (CELF-3)	The Psychological Corporation	Language	NO	ENGLISH	ENGLISH	6-21 YRS.	Semel, E., Wiig, F. & Second, W.	
Congitive Diagnostic Battery (CDB)	Psychological Assessment Resources, Inc.	NVIQ	NO	PANTOMIME	NONVERBAL	ALL AGES	Kay, S. R.	

continued

TABLE 16.1 (continued)

Test	Publisher	Test Type	Norms	Instructions	Items in Spanish or English	Age Range	Author	Yr. Published
Congitive Linguistic Quick Test	The Psychological Corporation	Screening for Impairment	NO	ENGLISH	ENGLISH	18-89	Helm-Estabrooks, N.	
Compound Series Test (CST)	Educational and Industrial Test Services, Ltd.	NVIQ	NO	PANTOMIME	NONVERBAL	6-ADULT	Horrisby, J. R.	
The Culture Fair Series: Scales 1, 2, 3	Insitute for Personality & Ability Testing, Inc.	NVIQ	NO	PANTOMIME	BOTH	4+	Catell, R. B. & Catell, A.K.S.	
Das-Naglieri Cognitive Assessment System	Riverside Publishing	INTELLIGENCE	Yes	BOTH	BOTH	5-17.11	Trahan, D. E., A & Larrabee, G. J.	1997
EIWN-R PR	The Psychological Corporation	INTELLIGENCE	Yes, Puerto Rican	SPANISH	SPANISH	6-16.11		1993
EIWN-R	The Psychological Corporation	INTELLIGENCE	Yes, Chicano, Puerto Rican, Cuban	SPANISH	SPANISH	6-16.11		1983
EIWA	The Psychological Corporation	INTELLIGENCE	Yes, Puerto Rican	SPANISH	SPANISH	17-ADULT		1997
General Ability Measure for Adults	NCS (Minnetonka)	NVIQ	Yes	BOTH	NONVERBAL	18-96	Naglieri, J. A., & Bardos, A. N.	1997
Goodenough-Harris Drawing Test	The Psychological Corporation	NVIQ	NO	PANTOMIME	NONVERBAL	3-15 YRS.	Goodenough, F. L. & Harris, D.B.	1988
Gordon Personal Profile Inventory	The Psychological Corporation	Personality	NO	ENGLISH	ENGLISH	ADOLESCENT & ADULT	Godon, L.	1993
Haptic Intelligence Scale	Stoelting Co.	INTELLIGENCE	NO	PANTOMIME	NONVERBAL	ADULT (BLIND)	Shorrager, H. C., & Shorrager P. S.	
Kahn Intelligence Test (KIT: Exp): A cultural-Minimized Experience	The Psychological Corporation	NVIQ	NO	PANTOMIME	NONVERBAL	all ages	Kahn, T. C.	

Test	Publisher	Construct	?	Instructions	Response	Age	Author	Year
Kasanin-Hanfmann Concept formation Test (Vygotsky Test) & Modified Vygotsky Concept Formation Test	Stoelting Co.	NVIQ	NO	PANTOMIME	NONVERBAL	all ages	Wang, P. L.	
Kaufman Assessment Battery for Children (K-ABC)	Stoelting Co.	NVIQ	NO	PANTOMIME	NONVERBAL	all ages	Kahn, T. C.	
Knox's Cube Test (KCT)	Stoelting Co.	NVIQ	NO	PANTOMIME	NONVERBAL	all ages	Wang, P. L.	
Kohs Block Test	American Guidance Services	INTELLIGENCE	NO	BOTH	ENGLISH	2.5-12.5 YRS.	Kaufman, A. S., & Kaufman, N. L.	
Leiter International Performance Scale (Revised)	Stoelting Co.	NVIQ	NO	PANTOMIME	NONVERBAL	child-adolescent	Stone, M., & Wright, B.	
Leiter International Performance Scale (arthor adaption)	Stoelting Co.	NVIQ	NO	PANTOMIME	ENGLISH	ages 3-19 mentally	Kohs, S. C.	1999
Leiter International Performance Scale (LIPS)	Stoelting Co.	NVIQ	NO	PANTOMIME	NONVERBAL	2-12 YRS.	Leiter, R. G.	
Multilingual Aphasia Exam	PAR	Assessment of Aphasics	YES	SPANISH	SPANISH	K-6, 16-69	Benton, A. Hamshen, K. & Sivan, A.	
Naglieri Nonverbal Ability Test	Stoelting Co.	NVIQ	NO	PANTOMIME	NONVERBAL	2-18 YRS.	Leiter, R. G.	1998
Neuropsi	Stoelting Co.	INTELLIGENCE	YES	PANTOMIME	NONVERBAL	2.0-20.11; adults	Roid, G. H., & Miller, L. J.	1987
Non-language Learning Test	Associated Services for the Blind	NVIQ	NO	PANTOMIME	NONVERBAL	8-12 years (Blind)	Chatterji, S. & Mukerjee, M.	1997
Non-verbal ability tests (NAT)	Riverside Publishing	INTELLIGENCE	NO	BOTH	BOTH	5-17.11 YRS.	Trahan, D. E. A., & Larrabee G. J.	1997
Non-Verbal Reasoning Test Series	Ardila & Roselli	Congnitive Functions	YES	SPANISH	SPANISH	16-86	Ardila & Roselli	1997
Nonverbal Test of Cognitive Skills (NTCS)	Associated Services for the Blind	NVIQ	NO	PANTOMIME	NVIQ	8-12 YRS. (BLIND)	Chatterji, S. & Mukerjee, M.	
Ohio Classification Test	The Australian Council for Educational Research Limited	NVIQ	NO	PANTOMIME	NVIQ	8-adult	Rowe, H. A. H.	
Personality Assessment Inventory (PAI)	The Psychological Corporation	Personality	NO	ENGLISH	ENGLISH	18-OLDER	Morey, L.	

continued

TABLE 16.1 (continued)

Test	Publisher			Language		Age	Author	Year
Pictorial Test of Intelligence (2nd Edition)	Nelson Publishing Company Ltd.	NVIQ	NO	PANTOMIME	NVIQ	7-15 YRS.	Johnson, G. O., & Boyd, H. F.	
Porteus Mazes	The Psychological Corporation	NVIQ	NO	PANTOMIME	NVIQ	GRADES K-7	Johnson, G. O., & Boyd, H. F.	
Preschool Language Scale (PLS-3)	The Psychological Affiliates	INTELLIGENCE	NO	ENGLISH	NONVERBAL	adult	Sell, D. E., Scollay R. W., & Vernon, L. N.	
Quick Test (QT)	PRO-ED	INTELLIGENCE	YES	BOTH	BOTH	HIGH SCHOOL AND ADULTS	Jackson, D. N.	1998
Silver Drawing Test of Cognition & Emotion (3rd Edition Revised)	Ablin Press Distributors	NVIQ	NO	ENGLISH	ENGLISH	5 + (Hearing Impaired)	Silver, R.	1998
Spanish Language Assessment Procedures (SLAP)	WPS	Communication in Disorders	YES	SPANISH	SPANISH	3-9 YRS.	Matts, L. J.	
Stoelting Brief Nonverbal Intelligence Test	The Psychological Corporation	NVIQ	NO	PANTOMIME	NVIQ	all ages	Porteus, S. D.	
System of Multicultural Pluralistic Assessment (SOMPA)	The Psychological Corporation	Language	No	ENGLISH	ENGLISH	BIRTH-6	ZIMMERMAN, I., Heiner, V., & Pond, R.	
TARPS	The Psychological Test Specialists	NVIQ	NO	PANTOMIME	NVIQ	2-ADULT	Ammons, R. B. & Ammons, C. H.	
The Standard Progressive Matrices (SPM-1956)	Ablin Press Distributors	NVIQ	NO	ENGLISH	ENGLISH	5 &.> (Hearing Impaired)	Silver, R.	1998
Spanish Language Assessment Procedures (SLAP)	Stoelting Co.	NVIQ	YES	PANTOMIME	NONVERBAL	6.0 -20.11	Roid, G. H., & Miller, L. J.	1999

Test	Publisher	Measures	Normed on Hispanics	Instructions	Language	Ages	Author	Year
The Test of Nonverbal Intelligence-2 (TONI-2)	The Psychological Corporation	NVIQ	Yes	BOTH	NONVERBAL FOR STUDENTS & Both lang. For parent interview	5-11 YRS.	Mercer, J. R. & Lewis, J. F.	1988
UNIT	Wide Range	Reasoning & Processing				5-14 YRS.	Gardner, M.	
The Wiesen Test of Mechanical Aptitude	PRO-ED	NVIQ	NO	PANTOMIME	NONVERBAL	ALL AGES	Kahn, T. C.	
Wechsler Scales: Wechsler Adult Intelligence Scale (WAIS)	Manual Moderno	INTELLIGENCE	Mexican	SPANISH	SPANISH	16+	Wechsler, D.	2004
Wechsler Scales: Wechsler Intelligence Scale for Children (WISC-IV)	The Psychological Corporation	INTELLIGENCE	Yes	BOTH	BOTH	5-16YRS.	Wechsler, D.	2004
Wechsler Scales: Wechsler Intelligence Scale for Children Revised (WISC-R)	The Psychological Corporation	INTELLIGENCE	Puerto Rican	SPANISH	SPANISH	5-16 YRS.	Wechsler, D.	1992
Wonderlic Personnel Test and Scholastic Level Exam	Stoelting Co.	INTELLIGENCE	NO	BOTH	ENGLISH	2.5-12.5 YRS.	Kaufman, A. S. & Kaufman, N. L.	
Woodcock Language Proficiency	Stoelting Co.	NVIQ	NO	PANTOMIME	NONVERBAL	CHILD-ADOLESCENT	Stone, M., & Wright, B.	
Woodcock-Munoz	Stoelting Co.	NVIQ	NO	PANTOMIME	ENGLISH	AGES 3-19 (MENTALLY)	Kohs, S. C.	

note that this table presents a general idea; it does not offer the actual purpose of each test, nor does it include all areas of neuropsychological testing for each test. Any given test may represent more than one area. Thus, it is apparent that there are a number of tests available to Spanish psychologists; however, more tests are needed in order to be able to effectively evaluate those with neuropsychological deficits.

Neuropsychological Rehabilitation

As noted earlier, the area on neuropsychological rehabilitation is much less developed than the evaluation area; however there is a growing interest in this field.

Rehabilitation services for the government offer the majority of clinical opportunities in Spain. It is a public system consisting of medical doctors, occupational and physical therapists, and very rarely, neuropsychologists and psychologists. A brain injury center named el Centro Estatal de Atencion al Dano Cerebral (loosely translated means Center for Brain Damage) has been recently established. For this reason, a rise in neuropsychological rehabilitation has come from private hospitals such as the Aitamenni Hospital, who contract psychiatrists, psychologists, neuropsychologists, and rehabilitation doctors in order to treat individuals with brain injury.

Although there is some debate, most of the neuropsychological rehabilitation done in Spain is holistic and multidisciplinary (Fernandez-Guinea, 2001; Junqué, Bruna, Mataró, & Puyuelo, 1998; León-Carrión, Machuca, Murga, & Dominguez, 2001; Muñoz-Céspedes & Tirapu, 2001). A therapeutic environment is then created in order for the patient to feel comfortable. Also typical of these programs is the contact they maintain with the patients' families. This is done in order to provide support for the patient as well as for facilitation of rehabilitation.

As with most of the world, cognitive rehabilitation is an important part of the rehabilitation process. The principle areas focused on during this process are memory, attention, and executive function (Muñoz-Céspedes & Tirapu, 2001). Wilson (1997) defines "cognitive rehabilitation" as a combination of learning, cognitive psychology, and neuropsychology. Using this paradigm, the patients' deficiency, intervention strategies, and the efficacy of treatment are explored. These principles underlie cognitive psychology and neuropsychology. The principles of learning used in cognitive rehabilitation include memory tests, problem solving, and attention. It is important to note that patients' functioning as a result of this treatment may or may not improve over the course of rehabilitation (Wilson, 1997).

In order to facilitate cognitive rehabilitation, programs such as Rehacom (TEA) and Gradior (INTRAS foundation) have been established. Rehacon consists of a module type rehabilitation that taps into attention, memory, visual-perceptual, motor, and spatial abilities. Gradior contains modules regarding attention, orientation, calculating, psychomotor, memory, perception, and verbal learning abilities. Both companies offer the modules as programs or independently.

In addition to rehabilitation, there are programs designed for modification of behavior, specifically behavior that is considered maladaptive (i.e. aggression). These programs are often combined with programs used to assist the individual in gaining more autonomy. This could include making shopping lists, and so forth. In reality, there is little known about the effectiveness of these programs (Léon-Carrión et al., 2001).

In sum, neuropsychological rehabilitation in Spain is a holistic and multidisciplinary enterprise. Although not quite on par with evaluation, it is garnering more attention, and is a topic worthy of future consideration.

SUMMARY

Hispanics continue to represent an ever-growing segment of the American population as well as an important segment of the world's population. As clinical neuropsychology continues expanding, it would appear that simultaneous expansion of knowledge and clinical services in our field should occur. Unfortunately, intellectual and clinical growth, in both North America and Spain, has been slow, and, at times, uneven, even contentious. There are patterns in the assessment of Spanish speakers and, for better or worse, they have been largely set by American, rather than European traditions. As a consequence, the typical clinical scenario, including both interviewing and testing of Spanish speakers on either side of the Atlantic, appear similar. However, problems abound.

A major problem is determining the concept of culture, acculturation, and the criterion validity in clinical neuropsychology. Puente and Agranovich (2002) have recently proposed that clinical neuropsychology assessment may be nothing more than testing of cultural knowledge. In other words, our field may be measuring no more than culture knowledge and, hence, neuropsychological performance, may be nothing more than appreciation and execution of cultural competence.

Even if this was true, the problem lies in the availability of adequate instruments, services, and personnel to carry out this critical task. At present, there are few tests currently available, on either side of the Atlantic. Often, tests are simply translated or adapted as best as possible. And, more frequently than that, is the difficulty associated with normative information. If normative problems could be resolved (e.g., is there subgroup heterogeneity?), the problems still persist that adequate comparison samples rarely exist.

We find ourselves with a major task of understanding and serving large segments of the population of both North America and the world but we are not in a position, with information, theory, and/or personnel to address this formidable situation. The decade of the brain has come and gone and, unfortunately, Spanish speakers have been left behind.

REFERENCES

Ardila, A. (1995). Directions of research in cross-cultural neuropsychology. *Journal of Clinical and Experimental Neuropsychology, 17,* 143–150.

Ardila, A., & Moreno, S. (2001). Neuropsychological test performance on Aruaco Indians: An exploratory study. *Journal of the International Neuropsychological Society, 7*(4) 510–515.

Ardila, A., Rosselli, M., & Puente, A. E. (1994). *Neuropsychological assessment of the Spanish speaker.* New York: Plenum.

Artiola, L., Hermosillo, D., Heaton, R. K., & Pardee, R. E. (1998). *Manual de Normas y Procedimientos para la Batería Neuropsicológica en Español* [Norms and procedures manual for the neuropsychological battery in Spanish]. Lisse, The Netherlands: Swets & Zeitlinger.

Bauer, R. M. (1994). The flexible battery approach to neuropsychological assessment. In R. D. Vanderploeg (Ed.), *Clinician's guide to neuropsychological assessment* (pp. 419–482). Hove, England: Lawrence Erlbaum Associates.

Berry, J. W. (1997). Immigration, acculturation, and adaptation. *Applied Psychology, 46,* 5–68.

Camara, W. J., Nathan, J. S., & Puente, A. E. (2000). Psychological test usage: Implications in professional psychology. *Professional Psychology: Research and Practice, 31,* 141–154.

Fernández-Guinea, S. (2001). Estrategias a seguir en el diseño de los programas de rehabilitación neuropsicológica para personas con daño cerebral [Strategies to follow in implementing neuropsychological rehabilitation programs in persons with brain injury]. *Revista de Neurología, 33,* 373–379.

González-Montalvo, J. I. (1991). *Creación y validación de un test de lectura para el diagnóstico del deterioro mental en el anciano* [Validation of a lecture test for diagnosing mental deterioration in the elderly]. Unpublished doctoral dissertation, Granada, Spain.

Hall, C. C. (1997). Cultural malpractice: The growing obsolescence of psychology. *American Psychologist, 52,* 642–651.

Hamsher, K. (1990). Specialized neuropsychological assessment methods. In G. Goldstein & M. Hersen (Eds.), *Handbook of psychological assessment* (2nd ed., pp. 256–279). New York: Pergamon.

Handwerker, W. P. (2002). *Quick ethnography.* Walnut Creek, CA: Altamira.

Junqué, C., Bruna, O., Mataró, M., & Puyuelo, M. (1998). *Traumatismo cráneo-encefálico: Un enfoque desde la Neuropsicología y la Logopedia.* Barcelona, Spain: Masson.

León-Carrión, J., Machuca, F., Murga, M., & Domínguez, R. (2001). Eficacia de un programa de tratamiento intensivo, integral y multidisciplinar de pacientes con traumatismo cráneo-encefálico. *Revista de Neurología, 33,* 377–383.

Lezak, M. D. (1995). *Neuropsychological assessment* (3rd ed.). London: Oxford University Press.

Muñoz-Céspedes, J. M., & Tirapu, J. (2001). *Rehabilitación neuropsicológica* [Neuropsychological rehabilitation]. Madrid, Spain: Síntesis.

Muñoz-Céspedes, J. M., Tobal, M., & Cano, A. (2000). Evaluacion de las alteraciones emocionales en personas con traumatismo craneo-encefalico. *Psicothema, 12,* 99–106.
Padilla, A. M. (1999). Hispanic psychology: A 25-year retrospective look. In D. Dinnel & W. J. Lonner (Eds.), *Merging past, present, and future in cross-cultural psychology: Selected papers from the Fourteenth International Congress of the International Association for Cross-Cultural Psychology* (pp.73–81). Netherlands: Swets.
Pearson Assessments. (2005). Catalog.
Pérez, M., Godoy, J. F., Vera, M. N., Laserna, J. A., & Puente, A. E. (1998). Neuropsychological evaluation of everyday memory. *Neuropsychology Review, 8,* 203–227.
Pérez, M., & Godoy, J. F. (1998). A comparison between a "traditional" memory test and a "behavioral" memory battery in spanish patients. *Journal of Clinical and Experimental Neuropsychology, 20,* 496–502.
Puente, A. E. (2000, September). *Does culture affect brain function? Questions and answers from clinical neuropsychology.* Paper presented at Grand Rounds, Duke University.
Puente, A. E., & Agranovich, A. (2003). The cross in cross-cultural neuropsychology. In G. Goldstein & S. Beers (Eds.), *Comprehensive handbook of psychological assessment: In??? and neuropsychological assessment.* Hoboken, NJ: Wiley.
Puente, A. E., & Ardila, A. (2000). Neuropsychological assessment of Hispanics. In E. Fletcher-Janzen, T. L. Strickland, & C. R. Reynolds (Eds.), *Handbook of cross-cultural neuropsychology* (pp. 87–104). New York: Kluwer/Plenum Academic Publishers.
Puente, A. E., & McCaffrey, R. J. (Eds.). (1992). *Handbook of neuropsychological assessment.* New York: Plenum.
Puente, A. E., & Perez-Garcia, M. P. (2000). Psychological assessment of ethnic-minorities. In G. Goldstein & M. Hersen (Eds.), *Handbook of psychological assessment* (pp. 527–551). Boston: Allyn & Bacon.
Puente, A. E., Puente, K. P., & Salazar, G. D. (2004). *Intellectual assessment of Hispanics.*
Reitan, R., & Wolfson, D. (1995). *The Halstead-Reitan Neuropsychological Battery* (2nd ed). Tucson, AZ: Neuropsychology Press.
Riverside Publishing. (2005). Catalog.
Sedo, M. (2000a). *Instrucciones y procedimiento de administración del Oral Trails* [Instructions and procedures of administering the Oral Trails]. Retrieved from www.sedo.net
Sedo, M. (2000b). *Instrucciones y procedimiento de administración del Five Digits Test* [Instructions and procedures of administering the Five Digits test]. Retrieved from www.sedo.net
Shorris, E. (1992). *Latinos.* New York: Norton
Sweet, J. J., Moberg, P., & Westergaard, C. K. (1996). Five-year follow-up survey of practices and beliefs of clinical neuropsychologists. *The Clinical Neuropsychologist, 10,* 202–221.
Taussig, M. I., & Ponton, M. P. (1996). Issues in neuropsychological assessment for Hispanic older adults: Cultural and linguistic factors. In G. Yeo & D. Gallagher-Thompson (Eds.), *Ethnicity and the dementias* (pp. 000–000). Washington, DC: Taylor & Francis.
TEA Ediciones. (2005). [Catalog]. Retrieved from: www.teaediciones.es
The Psychological Corporation.
U.S. Bureau of the Census (1999). *United States population.* Washington, DC: Author.
U.S. Bureau of the Census (2001). *United States population.* Washington, DC: Author.
U.S. Bureau of the Census (2003). *United States population.* Washington, DC: Author.

Vanderploeg, R. D. (1994). Interview and testing: The data-collection phase of neuropsychological evaluations. En R. D. Vanderploeg (Ed.), *Clinician's guide to neuropsychological assessment* (pp. 000–000). Hove, England: Lawrence Erlbaum Associates.

Walsch, K. W. (1999). Neuropsychological assessment. In K. W. Walsch & D. Darby (Eds.), *Neuropsychology: A clinical approach* (pp. 000–000). Toronto, Canada: Churchill Livingstone.

White, R. F., & Rose, F. E. (1997). The Boston process approach: A brief history and current practice. In G. Goldstein & T. M. Incagnoli (Eds.), *Contemporary approaches to neuropsycological assessment* (pp. 000–000). New York: Plenum.

Wilson, B. A. (1997). Cognitive rehabilitation: How it is and how it might be. *Journal of the International Neuropsychological Society, 3,* 487–496.

Wechsler, D. (1991). *Manual for the Wechsler Adult Intelligence Scale* (3rd ed.). San Antonio, TX: The Psychological Corporation.

Western Psychological Services. (2005). Catalog.

Zea, M. C., Asner-Self, K. K., Birman, D., & Buki, L. P. The Abbreviated Multi-Dimensional Acculturation Scale: Empirical validation with two Latino/Latina samples. *Cultural Diversity and Ethnic Minority Psychology, 9*(2), 107–126.

Chapter **17**

Cultural Issues in Clinical Context With Asian Indian Patients: Guidelines for the Health Care Team

Amee P. Shah
Cleveland State University

The 1980 U.S. Census Bureau officially recognized the term "Asian Indians," a subcategory of "Asian and Pacific Islander Americans" (Dutta, 1980, 1982). The term, "Asian Indian", refers to people of the Indian subcontinent and is used to distinguish people of India from other "Indian" groups, such as Native Americans and people of the West Indies.

Many Asian Indians have been immigrating to countries around the world, including the United States, England, and Africa. Since 1900, an estimated 10 to 15 million Asian Indians have immigrated to other countries. In 1980, the U.S. Census Bureau reported the population of Asian Indians in the United States to be 382,000. By 1990, this population had increased to 815,000. In that period, a 200 % increase in the influx of Asian Indians was reported. An average of 20,000 Asian Indians enter the United States annually, according to the U.S. Census Bureau's 1992 report. As the influx of these immigrants increases, so does the likelihood that they will need health care services. This becomes relevant to health care workers. It is imperative that mainstream health care workers gain a general understanding of the Asian Indian culture, and in particular, the issues that affect their ability to receive health care services.

The health care team, which consists of physicians, neuropsychologists, nurses, psychologists, speech-language pathologists, social workers, and so on, must be made aware of the cultural nuances within this group of patients so that they can better interact with them and treat them in a more effective manner.

BRIEF HISTORICAL AND GEOGRAPHICAL BACKGROUND

A brief orientation to the country, India, as a whole is useful in order to understand the cultural background of the Asian Indians.

Cultural Diversity of India

Multilingualism. India is a multilingual country with 18 official languages and myriad dialects. English is the official Lingua Franca, and Hindi is the national language common to most people in the North and Central parts of the country (primary language of 30% of the people). In addition, each of the 25 regional states has one official language that is spoken by most residents of that state. Therefore, in general, most Indians speak at least two to three languages, some of them as many as six to eight languages. Each of these languages may share some vocabulary and grammar characteristics, but for the most part, they are not mutually intelligible. Most languages have a different phonetic (speech sound) system, as well as a different orthography (alphabet).

Multiculturalism. India is a multicultural country, with a diverse array of customs, beliefs, daily practices, foods, clothing, and occupations. The diversity can be categorized by religion as well as by the regional states. Hinduism, which originated in India, was historically the foremost religion and still bears the highest representation within the country (80% of Asian Indians). Other predominant religions that originated in India are Buddhism (0.7%), Jainism (0.5%), and Sikhism (2%). All other religions became part of the Indian culture by way of foreign invasions as well as settlements of people from other countries (Mandelbaum, 1972; Williams, 1988). These were the later religions that have, over the years, become an officially recognized part of the country's system. Among these "newer" religions are the larger minority groups, such as Muslim/Islam (14%) and Christianity (2.4%), and other smaller groups, such as Parsee/Zoroastrianism, Judaism, and others (adding up to 0.4%).

With the above background information, we can picture the considerable range in diversity that characterizes the Asian Indian culture. This variety in cultural diversity continues to play a vital role even after Asian Indians relocate to a different country. Indeed, shared cultural values yield a comparable picture across immigrant Asian Indians, regardless of the country to which they have relocated, as can be seen in the following section.

Immigration Issues

Education. Education is not only highly valued, but expected within the Asian Indian community. Asian Indians receive an average of 16 years of education compared with U.S.-born individuals, who receive an average of 12 years or more of education. Duleep (1988) reported that 90% of new Asian Indian immigrants to the United States held professional degrees, compared to 75% Korean, 67% Filipino, and 46% Chinese immigrants.

Vocation. Among all immigrant groups to the United States, Asian Indians are the highest represented group in professional occupations. The largest number of foreign health professionals, a large number of engineers, and scientist groups holding academic positions are composed of Indians (Sheth, 1995). Most Indian immigrants abroad are more functional in English than the rest of the immigrants, as most spoke English in India as a result of prior influence of British colonization in India (Sheth, 1995). This lack of a serious language barrier in the Indian population enables more Indians—compared with other immigrant groups—to find professional vocations, and to maintain and even improve upon their pre-immigration professional occupations. Those Indians not able to find professional employment for various reasons (such as acculturation difficulties or illegal immigration status that prevents them from finding legal jobs) still manage to find a channel to be self-employed. In this case, a mismatch in employment type can be noted from pre- to post-immigration status. For example, many science and engineering degree holders maintain careers that are unrelated to their prior professional degrees; for example, driving a taxi; running hotels, motels, travel agencies, or newsstands; or being self-employed in real estate brokerage or with major insurance companies.

Model Minority—A Myth? Before 1980, Asian Indian immigrants to the United States held very high educational and vocational status. Moreover, these immigrants exhibited fewer social problems compared to the rest of the community in United States (Sandhu & Malik, 2001). Therefore, the earlier Asian Indians were known as a "model minority" within the United States. However, due to the recent passing of the Family Unification Act, the newer waves of Asian Indian immigrants do not live up to that image. Sandhu and Malik (2001) reported that recent immigrants generally come from rural areas, are less educated and less fluent in English than their predecessors, and work as taxi drivers, small motel operators, and convenience store clerks. These immigrants have exhibited a higher incidence of alcohol and drug problems due to lower educational and vocational functioning (Joe, 1996; Yen, 1992). Therefore, the "model minority" image appears to be more of an anachronism, and, according to Sandhu

(1997), this early image needs to be reassessed. Crucially, health care providers need to be aware of the increased social and medical problems in this population.

Characteristics of Indians (Both in India and Abroad)

Belief System

As mentioned, the major religion practiced in India is Hinduism. Therefore, the overall Indian philosophy and belief system rests on principles of Hinduism. The notion of fate, or karma, is fundamental to the Indian belief system (Almeida, 1996). This principle maintains that all actions during one's lifetime have consequences, and determine one's destiny in this life, as well as in the afterlife. Hinduism also includes the notion of rebirth and new life. Present misfortunes are taken as punishments for sins of the past or previous birth. The religion advocates graceful acceptance of all misfortunes and hardships. In the context of health care and health-related issues, the health care provider may mistake this attitude as passivity or fatalism.

Role of Family

Many Asian Indians live in extended or joint families, with several generations of family members living under the same roof (Nishio & Bilmes, 1997). As is true of other Asian groups, Asian Indians, too, consider family to be the central focus of their lives. Every family member serves a specific role, and the actions of every individual have an impact on the entire family. Each person's problems, handicap, or misfortune affects the family as a whole. Together, the whole family is involved in the decision-making process, as well as in offering moral support to the individual patient.

Gender Differences

Asian Indians, like other groups of Asians, discriminate between males and females within the family. Males receive preferential treatment. They enjoy increased privileges, material comfort, distribution of resources (Root, 1986), higher education, and more leeway in disciplinary issues. Traditionally, males serve the role of breadwinners and providers for the family and women take care of domestic responsibilities. Males also act as the decision makers in all the important issues outside of, and within the home. A definite "pecking-order" exists within the family that distinguishes male and female roles. The head of the household is the oldest male in the family, and the rest of the males (sons or brothers) submit to the oldest male. The women and children submit to the rest of the males.

Role of Women

Asian Indian women are socialized from very early on to take care of the family at the cost of giving up their needs and ambitions. Asian Indian women are expected to get married, raise children well, take care of all domestic responsibilities, and serve as the link that keeps the whole extended family together. Most of the time, they are expected to be full-time homemakers. An Asian Indian woman whose family has immigrated to another country may also take on a job, in addition to the domestic responsibilities, in order to supplement her spouse's income (Nandan & Eames, 1980; True, 1990). Among the daughters of immigrant families, the gender gap in education and income is reported to have been closed, yet they continue to maintain traditional roles at home (Sheth, 1995). They also continue to be considered inferior, and are expected to be deferential to all the male family members.

Notions of Guilt and Shame

Asian Indian families use the notions of guilt and shame to inculcate discipline and "keep the family together." Actions of any family member bear implications on the "good name" of the entire family. Therefore, children refrain from doing anything that might displease the family. A handicap, or disability, might be borne by the Asian Indian patient with feelings of guilt, shame, and disgrace for having let the entire family down. The patient may feel too ashamed to seek professional help, and may not want to involve the family or burden everyone with the treatment process (Root, 1990).

Asian Indians try to solve family problems, including health-related issues, in the privacy of their home, out of fear of stigma, shame, and ridicule from the rest of the Indian community. They avoid seeking assistance for "invisible" problems like those of speech, cognition, and language issues following strokes or other neurological conditions. Parents may shy away from seeking professional help for their child's physical or mental difficulty because they fear being perceived as unfit to raise a child. In the extreme cases when they are relegated to using outside help, they prefer to use the services of agencies or private practitioners, located some distance away from their immediate community to avoid gossip or exposure within the community.

Communication Styles

The Indian communication style has been described as indirect, with frequent use of innuendo, hinting, reading-between-the-lines, suggestions, and examples through metaphors and stories (Sandhu & Malik, 2001). A question may be answered using cliches and metaphors and an event described with vivid (albeit redundant) details.

ISSUES DURING INTERVIEW OR EVALUATION OF THE MEDICAL PROBLEM

Initial Approach

The belief in karma or destiny on the part of the traditional Asian Indian patient may prevent him or her from seeking professional intervention for a medical condition. The patient may feel that he or she has been "punished" with this affliction due to past sins and, therefore, has to do penance to get cured. He or she may opt not to seek any intervention to alleviate the suffering. Alternately, he or she may alleviate the health problem by practicing superstitious/alternative forms of treatment that do not involve medication, therapy, or surgery. Even among more acculturated immigrants, the fear of social stigma and sense of guilt and shame may prevent the patient or family from seeking professional intervention. Public suppression of both physical, as well as mental problems has been documented (Sue & Sue, 1990). Therefore, when these patients or their families approach the clinician, they may not be as forthcoming or open because they may be weighed down by feelings of guilt and shame. The clinician may have to encourage them and ask direct questions rather than open-ended questions such as, "Tell me about your problem" (Paniagua, 1994).

On the flip side, traditional Asian Indians lack faith in contemporary medicine, allopathy, or health care, and believe in more natural and traditional treatment approaches. Further, the "invisible" problems of speech, language, communication, or cognition, which fall under the domains of neuropsychology, psychology, speech pathology, and so on, are not recognized by Asian Indians as "real" problems. They tend to scoff at professions, such as speech-language pathology and psychology. For example, many label speech-language pathologists as, "glorified teachers." Therefore, health care professionals may be viewed with cynicism and lack of attention until patients or their families are convinced of progress in therapy. The clinician may have to "prove" his or her expertise to the patients or their families. Paniagua (1994) recommended that the clinician demonstrate two important qualities—expertise and authority—to elicit the attention of the patients and their families, as well as to ensure that they return for subsequent sessions.

Once the expertise has been established, the assumed experts in health care professions, like all doctors, are looked up to with deference and intimidation. Asian Indians have been socialized to regard experts, especially doctors, as authority figures and to show respect by not challenging their recommendations. The same attitude may translate toward the other health care providers, as well. The patients or their families may not question the diagnosis, treatment approach, or any other recommendations. In fact, they may not even seek elaboration or clarification if they do not know the nature of their affliction. Therefore, the health care provider should not anticipate questions. Rather, he or she should *overtly volunteer* information that both alerts and informs the patient and his or her family. This volunteered information can address diverse matters; provide an explanation of the diagnosis, prognosis, and recommendations; and inform patients or their family that they have a general right to question, request a second opinion, and/or refuse treatment. This approach may inspire increased confidence in, and a better rapport with the health care professional and thereby, resulting in shared responsibility in the recovery process.

ETHNICITY-, GENDER-, AND AGE-MATCH

Asian Indian families find a certain comfort in working with a health care professional of the same ethnicity and gender as the patient. However, due to the many intra-group differences of language and religion, a sufficient enough ethnic match with shared cultural identity between the patient and clinician might not be possible, even if the clinician were to be Asian Indian. For example, despite both being Asian Indians, the clinician and the patient may differ in age and degree of acculturation and assimilation. Gender may also differ between the patient and clinician. Such differences produce an ethnic mismatch, which can, in turn, give rise to certain issues that can detract from the clinical effort. For example, in light of the fixed notions of gender roles, many male patients may feel that a female clinician is not important or powerful enough to be useful to them. Conversely, many female patients may become shy or intimidated by a male clinician, and may not confide sufficiently in him to build the necessary rapport for therapy to be successful. Thus, if possible, it is recommended that the clinician and patient be of the same gender for a better rapport (Nishio, 1982).

Age is also an important variable in the interaction between the clinician and the patient. The elderly patients may have a bias against accepting recommendations or counseling tips from a young clinician. The younger the clinician, the less seriously he or she will be taken. Therefore, in this situation, the younger clinician may benefit from appearing to be somewhat deferential to the older patient by addressing the patient with a formality (e.g., using "Mr." or "Mrs."), being careful to not sound patronizing, patiently listening to all responses, and displaying confidence and expertise.

Pragmatics

The Asian Indian culture expects formality in all professional interactions. Therefore, the clinician should avoid levity or jokes and overly friendly behavior, yet show caring, concern, and a general empathy. The clinician need not take it as a sign of failure to build rapport if they initially find the patient to be distant and formal. Over time, with increased interaction and by gaining confidence in the clinician, the patient may be more responsive.

Non-verbal behavior also differs between Asian Indians and people from the Western cultures. As with verbal formality, non-verbal behavior in the Asian Indian culture also requires a certain physical distance and reserve. The patient, especially if he or she is of the opposite gender than the clinician, may be uncomfortable if the clinician initiates any physical contact, such as shaking hands, or squeezing the patient's arm to indicate support or sympathy. The initial greeting varies among the Asian Indians, and ranges from a joining of hands and saying "namaste" for the Hindus, to a salute and saying "salaam valeykum" for the Muslims. To avoid making a social faux pas, the clinician could simply say, "Hello, how are you?" without a handshake. Conversely, depending on the assimilation level of the patient, if the patient initiates a handshake, the clinician should, of course, shake hands.

Eye contact is also different in this culture (Paniagua, 1994). Asian Indians are socialized to show respect by keeping their eyes lowered and not looking directly into the eyes while speaking to an older person or to someone of authority. Likewise, women are expected to avoid eye contact with males out of modesty. A female clinician, for example, who makes direct eye contact with a male patient, may be considered rude or may be disconcerting to that patient. Conversely, the mainstream clinician must be aware of this cultural difference and understand that a lack of eye contact does not necessarily signify a lack of attention, interest, or pragmatic difficulties on the patient's part.

Further, during the interview process, the clinician may find the patient to be quiet and seemingly passive. This behavior is also a culturally acceptable norm, as Asian Indians are socialized to be polite and show respect by talking less, not arguing or talking back to people of authority. Sometimes, they may even go to the extent of answering all questions affirmatively to be polite, even when they do not understand the clinician's question (Chung, 1992; Root, Ho, & Sue, 1986). Sometimes silence is also used to express anger, disagreement with, or disapproval of the clinician's behavior without direct confrontation (Root, 1997).

Another non-verbal behavior likely to be misinterpreted by the mainstream clinician is head-nodding on the part of Asian Indian clients (Root, 1997). The Western culture has distinct head movements to indicate "yes" and "no," with a vertical up-and-down head movement indicating agreement, and a side-to-side or horizontal movement indicating a negative. In contrast, there are several intra-group differences in head movements among Asian Indians. Rotary, tilting, or angular movements can indicate different purposes, such as affirming, negating, encouraging the speaker to continue speaking, and so on. However, this may confuse the mainstream clinician, who may take a side-to-side, tilting movement of the head to be a "no" or disagreement, when instead, the patient may be affirming what the clinician is saying. Therefore, it is advisable to elicit a verbal response from the patient and not just assume a response based on head-nodding.

As mentioned previously, Asian Indians tend to speak with an indirect style. The clinician's question may be answered with many preliminaries and hedging. The mainstream evaluator may mistake this for tangential, circumlocutory, or evasive behavior, leading to misdiagnosis in differential diagnosis of aphasia or right hemisphere brain lesions. It sometimes may even be mistaken for some types of psychoses. The evaluator needs to be aware that this pragmatic style is not pathological, but rather a common part of the culture (Root, 1997). This style may also be frustrating to the mainstream clinician who is pressed for time and used to more direct responses. The clinician, in turn, may respond by becoming rushed and abrupt, thus appearing patronizing or brusque to the patient, who may get more upset by the clinician's attitude, setting off a negative cycle.

Modesty of clothing is another culturally accepted norm among the Asian Indian culture. The people of this culture wear clothes that cover them from head to toe. Sometimes an extra measure of modesty is present, such as the wearing of a veil or "purdah" among the Muslim women or covering the sari over their heads, among the Hindu women. They may find it uncomfortable to be part of the interview or evaluation if they consider the clinician to be dressed immodestly. Examples of modest dress code for professional women outside the culture are long skirts below the knees, long dresses, and closed-neck or high-collar blouses. The Asian Indian culture frowns upon wearing shorts, cut-offs, revealing clothes, and sleeveless shirts or blouses in the professional milieu. Moreover, light-colored clothing is preferred, and flashy colors and designs are not considered professional.

Source of Information: Whom to Address?

As mentioned, the patriarchal nature of the Indian family has a distinct "pecking order." Even though the patient may be a woman or child, it is important for the evaluator or clinician to address the husband or father first. If the entire family is present during the initial interview, it is preferable to first address the oldest male member, as a means of recognizing the patriarchic system (Root, 1997).

Stimuli and Task Selection

During assessment, the stimuli, task, and topic of discussion need to relate to the cultural background of the patient. There exists a large heterogeneity within the group of Asian Indians. This diversity can be noted in the kinds of foods eaten, clothes worn, and festivals celebrated. The mainstream can avoid the likelihood of offending the patient by not mentioning the cultural markers of one subgroup in the context of interacting with another. For example, it would be offensive to talk about chicken or goat curry to a Hindu, vegetarian patient, even though he is Asian Indian and eats curry. Similarly, it would not be appropriate to talk about "Diwali," the Hindu festival of Lights, to an Asian Indian Muslim patient.

Language of Testing

During evaluation of basic communication functioning, as well as in the course of detailed speech-language assessment, it becomes imperative to enquire about the patient's premorbid language skills in each of the languages known to him or her. After a brain stroke or onset of aphasia, for example, the patient may show relative difference in degree of preservation (or loss) of speech, language, cognitive, as well as general communicative functioning in one or the other languages known. Various theories of aphasia and language loss in bilingual patients have indicated differential preservation and loss before and after the stroke. The most fluent language, for example, may be the first one to show a breakdown. Another pattern seen in multilingual patients is for the least familiar language, usually third- or fourth-known language, to be impaired, with the first two languages remaining intact. Therefore, the speech and language clinician needs to ascertain the premorbid language skills in each of the languages known to the patient and, subsequently, test the patient in each of those languages as part of the aphasia assessment.

Interlanguage Issues

As mentioned, many Asian Indian patients may know at least two, if not more, languages. Behaviors typically seen in this culture are code switching, code mixing, and lexical borrowing between the different languages known to them. The interviewer needs to exercise caution in over interpreting this behavior and mislabeling it as a sign of reduced functioning in any one language. The interviewer needs to be sensitive to this interlanguage issue in the bilingual/multilingual client, and not penalize him or her for this socially acceptable norm.

Use of Translators

Translators or interpreters are often used during evaluations when the clinician is of a different language and/or ethnicity background from the patient. A word of caution: Certain concepts or emotional topics may not translate across languages or cultures. Translators may edit or truncate information and just convey the overall message of the patient, without interpreting the finer clinical nuances of language or thought. Moreover, using family members or acquaintances of the patient is not advisable, as they may be internally biased and may modify responses, over interpret information, or extend the responses out of the clinical context. Many Asian Indian patients and their families may decline the need for translators out of pride or desire to not inconvenience the clinician, as they may be familiar with English themselves. However, if later they face communication difficulties, in absence of a translator, they may lose interest in returning to therapy (Pine et al., 1990).

Reporting Results and End of Evaluation Counseling

Clinicians should follow certain guidelines with Asian Indian clients to conclude the interview and the evaluation process (Root, Ho, & Sue, 1986; Sue & Sue, 1990). To prevent overwhelming the patient and the family, it is recommended that the clinician clearly explain the findings and diagnosis, the prognosis, the implications of the medical condition in everyday functioning, and the recommendations. Also, the clinician needs to provide tangible and concrete advice with suitable examples and demonstrations of the activities the patient and family can do for the recovery process. Ambiguous and indirect suggestions are to be avoided. Prolonged verbal exchanges between the patient and the clinician are contraindicated, as they may confuse or overwhelm the patient. The clinician needs to avoid overusing professional jargon, abbreviations, or pedantic explanations. The clinician may need to show overtly active participation and expect fewer questions from the Asian Indian patients or the family than most mainstream patients.

ISSUES DURING THERAPY OR TREATMENT OF THE MEDICAL CONDITION

Expectations From the First Session

After overcoming the barrier of shame and stigma, when the Asian Indian patient and/or family finally approach the health care worker for help, it is usually at an advanced stage of the problem. At this point they are likely to seek quick answers and immediate relief (Root, 1997). The concept and experience of "therapy" of any kind is unfamiliar to them. This places the onus of information dissemination and providing an overview of the entire intervention process on the clinician. The clinician is recommended (Root, 1997) to take the lead and explain goals, a reasonable timeline, and the sequence of progress expected. The first session can also be used to explain the medical condition and its probable causes and solutions. In cases of conditions, such as dementia, aphasia, autism, and mental retardation, the clinician can affirm that the patient is indeed not "crazy" or weak, and explain the specific limitations and strengths of the patient's communicative and learning skills. The clinician can also empathize with the patient and family and demonstrate that he or she understands that the patient or family may be embarrassed to seek help from a health care professional. Finally, any confusion as to how therapy can help change the patient's condition can be cleared in this session. All of this will help ensure adequate understanding on the part of the patient and the family, which will further encourage the patient's optimal involvement and regular attendance in future sessions.

Role of Family

The extended family plays a critical role in the patient's life. This family network can be tapped into during the recovery process. The family needs to be debriefed regarding the individual's strengths and limitations. Further, the clinician needs to explain and demonstrate to the family the specific activities that can be done at home to supplement the therapy process in the clinical setting. The family's moral support, encouragement, and understanding will optimize the recovery process.

Conversely, some of the principles recommended for success in treatment may go against the Asian Indian patient's notion of the role of family (Root, 1997). For example, the need for separating the individual's needs, exerting one's independence, and claiming time and attention for the individual patient's needs, may all be difficult to implement and may be frowned upon by the family. This is especially true for female patients, who may find it difficult to claim attention for themselves over the needs of the family and children. For male patients, a source of conflict in their value system may be admitting their handicap and that they need help, both of which go against the image of the male being the strong, dependable, provider of the family.

Age Differences

The patient's age and generation level plays an important role in the therapy process. The elderly patients may be more traditional and have an "old school approach," in which their beliefs and coping strategies may be colored by superstitions, faith in God, and the previously mentioned fatalistic attitude. They may, therefore, refuse contemporary treatment approaches, such as medications, surgery, alternate modes of feeding, biopsies, and speech, language and cognitive therapy. Younger patients and second-generation individuals may be less inclined to hold on to traditional approaches, and may be more open to recent forms of treatment. They may also exhibit higher motivation and perseverance to succeed in the recovery process compared to their older counterparts.

Religious Issues

The older subgroup of patients may participate in religious practices that may interfere in the recovery process. For example, many Hindu, Jain, and Muslim people observe religious fasting, sometimes of the very stringent kind, forfeiting food and water for several days. This may prevent these patients from meeting their nutritional and dietary requirements, especially for patients admitted to hospitals and nursing homes. Many religious Hindus and Jains tend to be strict vegetarians, and may refuse to eat food cooked in hospital or nursing home kitchens, as it is cooked in the same place that meat was prepared. This may require the family members' involvement in bringing food from home that meets the dietary restrictions for patients with diabetes, swallowing issues, and other feeding problems. The speech pathologist and dietitian may need to pay attention to ensure the family adheres to the food type and consistency recommendations when they bring food from home for the dysphagic patient.

Selecting Topics and Tasks Appropriately

Pais (1991) reported a career mismatch for many Indians in immigrant countries. Many taxi drivers and owners in the United States have college and professional degrees from India in fields such as engineering, science, and business administration. This needs to be considered in the selection of a suitably motivating topic, task, and stimuli in the therapy setting. For example, the patient may feel more passionate and interested in discussing his vocation or field of study in India as opposed to discussing the non-professional work or menial jobs he undertakes in the immigrant country. Identifying a topic of conversation that is close to the patient's heart and structuring therapy activities around that area may increase his or her motivation and, thereby, the chances of progress.

Gift-Giving

Asian Indian patients often enjoy returning the favor of receiving treatment from the clinician. They may show their gratitude by offering small gifts (snacks or tea during home-based visits, for example). Refusing a gift may be offensive to the patient and family. Root (1990) recommended accepting these gifts with sincere appreciation, but also recommended ensuring that the patient understands that the clinician does not expect to receive gifts.

CONCLUSION

This chapter highlights the cultural issues among the Asian Indian community that may impact their interaction with various health care professionals. The cultural guidelines offered here may be used only to gain a preliminary understanding of the culture for health care providers unfamiliar with the Asian Indian culture. Health care professionals should not use these guidelines to build stereotypes about Asian Indians, nor should they consider them to be a homogenous group. These guidelines are aimed at helping smooth out the initial interaction with a patient group that differs from mainstream health care professionals. Each individual patient and his or her family needs to be recognized as unique, and not simply fitted into the general profile described in this chapter.

Although Asian Indian immigrants may show several cultural similarities, there may be marked differences among different families, depending on how long they have lived in the foreign country, their acculturation and assimilation levels, experiences in the foreign country, and their cultural background in the home country. If health care professionals use the cultural information offered here with sufficient consideration, it is expected that their professional interaction with this group of patients will be optimized.

REFERENCES

Almeida, R. (1996). Hindu, Christian, and Muslim families. In M. McGoldrick & J. Giordino (Eds.), *Ethnicity and family therapy* (2nd ed., pp. 395–423). New York: Guilford.

Chung, D. K. (1992). Asian cultural commonalities: A comparison with mainstream American culture. In D. K. Chung, K. Murase, & F. Ross-Sheriff (Eds.), *Social work practice with Asian Americans* (pp. 27–44). Newbury Park, CA: Sage.

Duleep, H. O. (1988). *Economic status of Americans of Asian descent.* Washington, DC: U.S. Commission on Civil Rights.

Dutta, M. (1980). Asian and Pacific American employment profile: Myth and Reality. In *Civil rights issues of Asian and Pacific Americans: Myths and realities* (pp. 445–494). Washington, DC: U.S. Government Printing Office.

Dutta, M. (1982). Asian Indian Americans: Search for an economic profile. In S. Chandrashekhar (Ed.), *From India to America: A brief history of immigration, problems of discrimination, admission, and assimilation* (pp. 76–79). La Jolla, CA: Population Review.

Joe, K. A. (1996). The lives and times of Asian-Pacific American women drug users: An ethnographic study of their methamphetamine use. *Journal of Drug Issues, 26*(1), 199–218.

Mandelbaum, D. G. (1972). *Society in India: Vol. 2. Change and continuity.* Berkeley: University of California Press.

Nandan, Y., & Eames, E. (1980). Typology and analysis of the Asian Indian family. In P. Saran

& E. Eames (Eds.), *The new ethics: Asian Indians in the United States* (pp. 000–000). New York: Praeger.
Nishio, K. (1982). *Southeast Asian refugee mental health project.* Unpublished manuscript.
Nishio, K., & Bilmes, M. (1997). Psychotherapy with Southeast Asian American clients. In D. R Atkinson, G. Morten, & D. W. Sue (Eds.), *Counseling American minorities* (pp. 000–000). Boston: McGraw-Hill.
Pais, A. (1991, July 12). Lure of the taxi business. *India Abroad.*
Paniagua, F. A. (1994). *Assessing and treating culturally diverse clients: A practical guide* (Series 4). Thousand Oaks, CA: Sage.
Pine, J. P., Cervantes, J., Cheung, F., Hall, C. C., I., Holroyd, J., LaDue, et al. (1990). *Guidelines for providers of psychological services to ethnic, linguistic, and culturally diverse populations.* Washington, DC: American Psychological Association.
Root, M. P. (1986). Facilitating psychotherapy with Asian American clients. In D. R. Atkinson, G. Morten, & D. W. Sue (Eds.), *Counseling American minorities* (pp. 000–000). Boston: McGraw-Hill.
Root, M., Ho, C., & Sue, S. (1986). Issues in the training of counselors for Asian Americans. In H. P. Lefley & P. B. Pedersen (Eds.), *Cross-cultural training for mental health professionals* (pp. 199–209). Springfield, IL: Thomas.
Sandhu, D. S. (1997). Psychocultural profiles of Asian and Pacific Islander Americans: Implications for counseling and psychotherapy. *Journal of Multicultural Counseling and Development, 25,* 7–22.
Sandhu, D. S., & Malik, R. (2001). Ethnocultural background and substance abuse treatment of Asian Indian Americans. In S. L. A. Straussner (Ed.), *Ethnocultural factors in substance abuse treatment* (pp. 368–392). New York: Guilford.
Sheth, M. (1995). Asian Indian Americans. In P. G. Min (Ed.), *Asian Americans: Contemporary trends and issues* (pp. 169–198). Thousand Oaks, CA: Sage.
Sue, D. W., & Sue, D. (1990). *Counseling the culturally different: Theory and practice* (2nd ed.). New York: Wiley.
True, R. H. (1990). Psychotherapeutic issues with Asian American women. *Sex Roles, 22*(7–8), 477–486.
Williams, R. B. (1988). *Religions of immigrants from India and Pakistan: New threads in the American tapestry.* Cambridge, England: Cambridge University Press.
Yen, S. (1992). Cultural competence for evaluators working with Asian/Pacific Island communities: Some common themes and important implications. In M. A. Orlandi, R. Weston, & L. G. Epstein (Eds.), *Cultural competence for evaluators: A guide for alcohol and other drug abuse prevention practitioners working with ethnic/racial communities* (pp. 261–291). Rockville, MD: U.S. Department of Health and Human Services.

Chapter **18**

Epidemiological, Social, and Cultural Aspects of Illness: A Case Study of Brain Injuries, Stroke, and HIV/AIDS in South Africa

Leah Gilbert
Stephen Tollman
*University of The Witwatersrand, Johannesburg
South Africa*

> *In most cases genetic endowment and racial origin play only a small role in determining the types and severity of disease most prevalent in a particular region or a social group. Whether they be African, American Indian, European or Oriental origin, and whatever complexity of their racial mixtures—human populations usually acquire the burden of diseases characteristic of the geographical area and the social group in which they are born and live.*
>
> —*Dubos (1968, p. 94).*

Although due recognition is given to the role of biological and genetic factors, there is wide acceptance of the importance of social factors in the etiology, development, and treatment of disease. This is mainly due to the fact that many scholars, based on numerous studies in the last 30 years, have confirmed this (Curtis & Taket, 1996; Desjarlais, Eisenberg, Good, & Kleinman, 1995; Jones & Moon, 1987; Wilkinson, 1996), and in the process developed theoretical paradigms in order to further explain the social nature of health determinants (Albrecht, Fitzpatrick, & Scrimshaw, 1999; Annandale, 1998; Davey, Gray, & Seale, 1995). Changing patterns of disease, reflected in the rise of chronic and life-style related conditions and the multifactorial nature of their causation, accompanied by a demographic transition affecting the age structure of populations (Fitzpatrick,1996; Moon,1995), have contributed to a shift in thinking about health, disease, and disability. This has been the shift from an emphasis on the so called "bio-medical model" to a more comprehensive "psychosocioenvironmental model" (Hart, 1996; Nettleton, 1995). The latter emphasizes the role of people's behavior—what work they do and how and where they live their lives—in determining their health status and disease outcome (Gilbert, Selikow, & Walker, 2002). However, it goes beyond that: Whereas the bio-medical model essentially keeps health, disease, and disability within a biological context, the psychosocioenvironmental model places it in a social context, advocates a multidisciplinary approach, and thus contributes an additional dimension to the understanding of the onset of disease and disability as well as of treatment and rehabilitation.

Needless to say, the propagators and major contributors to this approach are social scientists. Nevertheless, the health professions have acknowledged this paradigm and include it in their training programs. Thus, throughout the world, a new generation of health workers is being trained along these lines (Gilbert et al., 2002; Lee & Greene, 1999; Moon & Gillespie, 1995) with the hope that this broader understanding will contribute toward the promotion of health, enhance treatment modalities, and improve the rehabilitation process. Recognizing the complementarity of the two models has the potential to extend our understanding of health, disease, and disability in society, as well as the role of health professionals in it.

The emergence of Neuropsychology as a discipline, is a prime example of this complementarity because it rests on an integration of the previously separate disciplines of neurology and psychology, is concerned with cross-cultural attributes (Watts, 1999), and is often practiced in multidisciplinary teams (Nelson & Adams, 1997). Social factors have been identified as important in the assessment as well as rehabilitation of patients treated by neuropsychologists (Nell, 1999; Nelson & Adams, 1997). For this reason, it is necessary to be aware of and engage with the social components of disease and disability in the practice of neuropsychology. Examples of social variables include geographic location, age, gender, class, race, and culture. It is beyond the scope of this chapter to fully engage with all of them,[1] however, an attempt is made to elucidate

---

[1] It is hoped that the list of references provided will assist the reader in obtaining further information.

some of these aspects and their relevance in the context of the epidemiological data presented in the case studies that follow later in this chapter.

As noted, among the social factors recognized as most significant in the practice of neuropsychology is the cultural dimension in the assessment, treatment, and rehabilitation of patients. Cultural background directly affects people's life experiences, their assumptions about the world as well as their understanding of "reality"(Lee & Greene, 1999). "Cultural interpretations" involve a continuous process of making sense of, and giving meaning to what people see and what happens to them (Wolffers, 1997).

Health, disease, and disability feature prominently in this context—the ideas people hold about them are a product of wider structural and cultural forces operating in society at large (Gilbert et al., 2002; McElroy, & Jezewski, 1999). All communities have these concepts integrated into their culture. What is experienced as health, disease, or disability represents a complex intimate and cultural understanding in a particular social context (Airhihenbuwa, 1995; Preston-Whyte, 1999; Richter & Griesel, 1999), and not only a set of neurological, physiological, and biochemical findings (Gilbert et al., 2002). This "social construction" (Lee & Greene, 1999) extends beyond the stage of understanding of symptoms and signs to the realm of "illness behavior" (McElroy, & Jezewski, 1999; Senior & Viveash, 1998). This includes the recognition of symptoms as abnormal and the response to symptoms such as pain, which are all socially and culturally influenced (Gilbert et al., 2002; Moon & Gillespie, 1995; Morris, 1998; Senior et al., 1998).

Once symptoms have been recognized as abnormal and needing attention, the activities that follow will be governed by the "way things are usually done" or the dominant mode of operation in a particular culture. In most communities "help-seeking behavior" includes consultations with family, friends, and neighbors, or what is referred to as the "lay referral system" (Blaxter, 2004). This means that the decision to act on symptoms is not only taken by the person experiencing them, but is also based on the advice of networks within a particular social and cultural milieu.

Increasing cultural complexity is one of the features of modern society, reflected in many different cultures and subcultures coexisting with one another (Gilbert et al., 2002). This gives rise to a number of different healing systems, or ways of diagnosing and treating illness, which are rooted in the cultural differences and linked to the dominant value system of a particular culture (Cant & Sharma, 1999). This "co-existence and availability of different ways of perceiving, explaining and treating illness" is often referred to as "medical pluralism" (Gilbert et al., 2002, p.49).

It is essential that health workers take cognizance of this, especially if they work within diverse, multicultural settings. Because culture influences all aspects of a person's life, there cannot be a "culture-free" encounter. This is particularly true in the context of patient–health worker encounters into which both bring, in addition to their lay-professional differences, their diverse cultural legacies. For this reason, there are frequent references in the literature to problematic "inter-cultural encounters" or "cross-cultural difficulties." Dissimilarities between health worker and patient can result in miscommunication and misunderstanding. It is thus essential that health workers familiarize themselves with the cultural context of the people they treat, and develop an enhanced "cultural sensitivity" as well as techniques that are "culture specific" (Lee & Greene, 1999). Not only can this increase their understanding of "where their patients are coming from," it can also greatly enhance the therapeutic relationship (Allen-Meares & Burman, 1999) and contribute to the effectiveness of their professional role by improving their diagnostic as well as therapeutic skills, thus benefiting the patient (Airhihenbuwa,1995; Gopaul-McNicol & Brice-Baker, 1998; Pierrepointe, Navas, Bragin, & Diaz, 1999).

Following this introduction, we would argue that in addition to the common understanding that the onset of certain diseases is linked to their social and geographical context, the way ill-health is perceived, interpreted, and treated is also socially and culturally bound. This significantly influences the establishment of a therapeutic relationship with health workers, as well as the outcomes of treatment and rehabilitation efforts. For all health professionals, and neuropsychologists in particular, such understanding can be pivotal in the assessment as well as the rehabilitation of patients.

South Africa presents a fitting example, as well as a significant challenge to the discussion thus far. In the next section, three case studies are presented in an effort to illustrate some of the issues that have been raised.

SELECTED SOUTH AFRICAN CASE STUDIES

South African society—like many other developing societies—is a society in transition. This is reflected in its disease and disability profiles. During the last century, both child and adult mortality declined dramatically due to improved income, food, and living conditions, and access to medical care (Health Systems Trust, 1996). This was accompanied by declining fertility rates and an increase in the aging population. However, due to the unique social and political structure in South Africa, the pace of this transition in different sectors of the population varies markedly. Apartheid policies have resulted in a close correlation between socioeconomic status and population group.[2] South African society is characterized by gross inequalities that

---

[2]According to the Population Registration Act of 1950, all South Africans were classified into a "population group" at birth, and assigned a status as White, Indian, Coloured, and Black (African). This "status" was fundamental in determining access to employment, social services, educational opportunity, property ownership, and place of residence. Although the Act was repealed in 1991, its social impact will continue for a long time to come. For this reason, certain statistics in this chapter are presented using this classification.

manifest mainly along racial lines. The morbidity and mortality profiles of whites and Indians are characteristic of more industrialized societies as chronic and degenerative diseases gain prominence, whereas the disease and death profiles of Africans and Coloreds also reflect the situation of less developed societies, with a prominence of "social diseases" of deprivation (Health Systems Trust, 1995). As in many other middle income countries, South Africa is experiencing a coexistence of poverty related diseases with the diseases associated with social development and economic affluence. This is apparent in morbidity and mortality patterns where diseases of the rich and poor coexist and can be correlated with the so-called "population groups." In addition, because South Africa's social transition has been accompanied by high unemployment and crime/violence rates, it is evident that injury is making a disproportionately large contribution to the burden of disease and disability in the country. The rapid growth of the HIV/AIDS epidemic in South Africa (Benatar, 2004; Health Systems Trust, 1997) adds a further dimension to the patterns outlined, as well as to the challenges facing the health professions and society as a whole.

The previous discussion is of some poignancy when considering the health care available to the various population groups. This was captured by Barron (1998, p.1) when he stated: "South Africa, in 1998, remains a land of stark contrasts, between those that have and those who have not. A land where some people have amongst the best standards of living, and good health and access to health services and care, and where some have very poor living standards, a great deal of ill health and poor access to health care."

The following case studies have been chosen due to their relevance to the practice of neuropsychology.

Brain Injuries

According to Nelson and Adams (1997), neuropsychologists are important members of the multidisciplinary rehabilitation team managing the consequences of traumatic brain injury (TBI). Two categories dominate the South African injury profile: violence, which has consistently been shown to account for between 45–55% of all injuries, and transport-related causes that account for between 20–25% of injuries. Most of the remaining 20% result from unintentional causes occurring, for the most part in the home where injuries to children are of critical concern (Butchart & Peden, 1997).

> In the transformation from apartheid to democracy, there was the belief that because the motives for violence in South Africa were political, democratisation would bring a cessation in violence, and a reduction in violence related injuries. However, while the ultimate causes of violence may lie in factors produced by political strategies of repression, most violence is an outcome of

largely unpremeditated interpersonal attacks. (Butchart & Peden, 1997, p. 213)

Violence plays a significant role in health in South Africa and its outcomes are of great concern to all health professionals (Gilbert, 1996). Consequently, trauma is the major cause of lost years of life (PYLL)[3] owing to premature deaths between 1 and 65 years (Health Systems Trust, 1995). However, the analysis of mortality data provides an inadequate view of the impact of trauma on society. Temporary and permanent disability in nonfatally injured victims play a considerable role in the final analysis of the impact of trauma on health professionals as well as on society and the economy.

The Harvard Burden of Disease Unit (Murray & Lopez, 1996) estimated that, in 1990, injuries contributed 14% of all DALYs[4] lost to sub-Saharan Africa. In South Africa, application of the DALY to 1994 mortality data show that external causes (i.e., injuries) account for 32% of the overall disease burden (Butchart & Peden, 1997)—more than double the figure for the subcontinent.

Injury surveillance in South Africa is incomplete and fragmented (Gilbert, 1996). The data presented later is based on the research conducted by the South African Medical Research Council, Cape Metropolitan Study (CMS), which has been collecting detailed information on head injuries (Medical Research Council, 1999). These data show that the brain injury profile is a reflection of the social structure and that it is important for health professionals in order to consider it in this context.

An examination of the data (Table 18.1) clearly shows that the rate of injuries is highest among the Colored population. This data is consistent with similar data from other studies in Cape Town (Gilbert, 1996).

As can be seen in Fig. 18.1, more than 37% of head injury occurs in the 15–29 age group and 19.6% in the 30–44 age group. Alarmingly, close to one third (29.7%) of head injuries occurs in the 0–14 age group. More than two thirds occurs between ages 15–60.

Males constitute 70.3% of sufferers of head injury; a finding that resembles the general trauma profile reported elsewhere (Gilbert, 1996) and casts a light on the gender differences associated with violent behavior.

It is most striking that 84.1% of traumatic head injuries occurred among families with a very low monthly income (less than R1000—less than $200). These and additional data point toward association between class (or poverty in this case) and head injuries. Eighty-one percent of people with head injuries had no medical insurance, 29.2% were unskilled/semiskilled laborers, 19.6% were unemployed, and 21.0% were preschool children; 31.2% had no education, whereas 33.2% had only primary school level education.

---

[3] Potential Years of Life Lost.
[4] DALY: "Disability Adjusted Life Years" is a recently developed composite index used to measure the "burden of disease" due both to mortality and morbidity.

TABLE 18.1
Cape Metropolitan Study Head Injury and Population Profile

Population Groups	% of Total Study Population	% of Head Injuries
Colored	21:36	59.6
Black/African	21:36	24.9
White	4:48	15.3
Asian	< 1	0.2

Source: Medical Research Council, 1999.

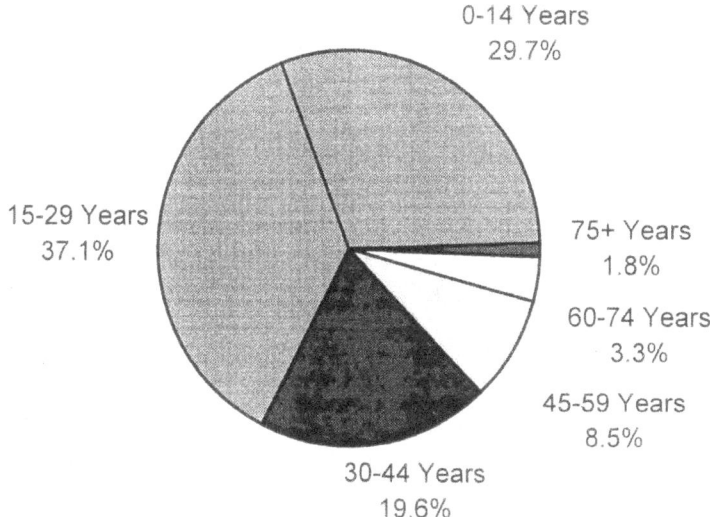

FIG. 18.1. Cape metropolitan study head injury: Age Groups. *Note.* $N = 18,504$. From *Cape Metropolitan Study*, by Medical Research Council, 1999.

These variables can be seen as social class indicators, illustrating the powerful effect of social context on head injury profiles.

Virtually half (49%) of the injuries took place in the road or on the street and 33.0% at home, mostly on the weekend—15.9% on Friday, 25.4% on Saturday, and 17.7% on Sunday. Significantly more than half (57.5%) occurred during the evening. These findings, and the fact that a substantial percentage (37.2 %) was related to alcohol intake, suggest a strong association with lifestyle patterns.

Although the data presented here are from a single local study, the patterns revealed are consistent with other work conducted in South Africa (Butchart & Peden, 1997; Gilbert, 1996). Considering the data in the con-

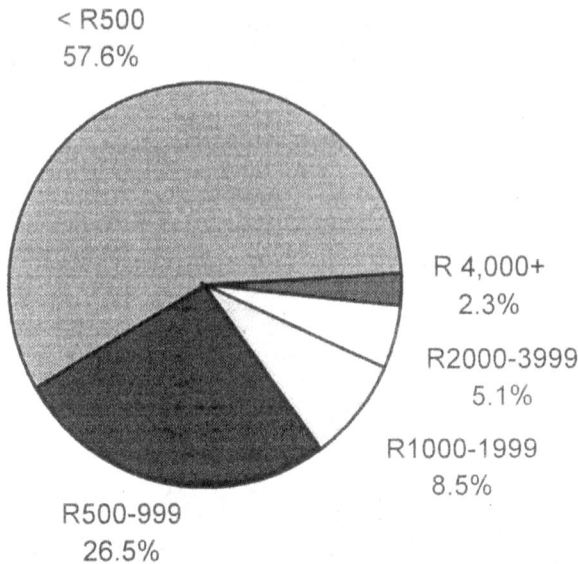

FIG. 18.2. Cape metropolitan study head injury: Family income/month. Note. N= 12,514. From *Cape Metropolitan Study*, by Medical Research Council, 1999.

text of the South African society and its health profile should help to provide the health team with a greater understanding of their brain-injured patients and the social reality from which they come.

Stroke in Rural South Africa

The "epidemiological transition" refers to the changing disease profile as diseases of poverty and underdevelopment (infections and malnutrition) give way to predominantly chronic conditions, often characterized as the "diseases of lifestyle" (commonly, circulatory diseases and a spectrum of malignant conditions; Omran, 1971). This evolution tends to be associated with the so-called "demographic transition"—the progression from high fertility, high mortality populations to communities where mortality has fallen significantly and where, over time, this is paralleled by a marked reduction in pregnancies and childbirth.

This somewhat linear picture has for some time reflected our general understanding of health development, and was thought to hold true for most populations and societies. Moreover, economic development was assumed to produce a development path that would inevitably result in positive social—and thus health—development. Recent research in developing settings, however, contradicts this common (and too-tidy) interpretation. A number of middle-income countries, such as Mexico and Brazil, have provided examples of "epidemiological polarization," the persistence of poverty-related diseases among the poorer social groups, whereas the lifestyle diseases emerge among the more affluent.

This transitional theme is evident in the Agincourt subdistrict of rural South Africa, an area adjacent to the country's border with Mozambique. As shown in Table 18.2, the Agincourt disease profile reflects the coexistence of poverty and lifestyle related diseases *within the same community* (Kahn, Tollman, Garenne, & Gear, 1999). Put differently, an "unfinished agenda" of infectious disease and nutritional problems is coexisting with an "emerging agenda" of circulatory disease, cancers, and related conditions.

A Summary of Age and Sex Patterns. The Agincourt subdistrict comprises some 11,500 households with a population of 70,000 people (approx) living in 21 discrete villages. The area is dry with a sandy soil, better suited to game and cattle farming than to subsistence agriculture. Reasonably typical of much of rural South Africa, particularly the former bantustan areas (or "homelands"), Agincourt is home to some of the country's poorest citizens. Lack of formal sector employment leads most men (and increasing numbers of women) to seek employment as migrant workers on adjacent farms, in distant towns, or in the mining sector (Tollman, Herbst, Garenne, Gear, & Kahn, 1999).

In common with much of sub-Saharan Africa, the area lacks a functioning system of vital registration. To address this, the University of the Witwatersrand introduced, in 1992, a "demographic and health surveillance system" (DHSS) involving repeated annual censuses that are serially linked: The DHSS is a unique source of trend data on all births, deaths, and migration events that occur within the population of the Agincourt subdistrict.

Every death is the subject of a "verbal autopsy." In outline, this consists of an in-depth interview—conducted in the vernacular by a well-trained local fieldworker—with the primary caregiver of the recently deceased during their terminal illness. The verbal autopsy is scrutinized by three physician reviewers who, blind to each others' findings, use a system of consensus criteria to reach a diagnosis (Kahn et al, 1999). The cause of death profile detailed in Table 18.2 was derived in this way.

A notable finding was the prominence of circulatory disease, in particular stroke and heart failure in the older age groups. Little is known about stroke in rural African populations, and the few studies of stroke in sub-Saharan Africa have concentrated on hospitalized urban cases (Joubert 1999; Matenga, Kitai, & Levy, 1986; Rosman, 1986).

TABLE 18.2
Leading Causes of Death, by Age Groups. Agincourt 1992–1995

Rank	0–4	5–14	15–49	Age Groups (Years) 50–74	75+	Total
1	Diarrhoea	Motor vehicle accident	Assault	CVA*	CCF*	Diarrhoea
2	Kwashiokor	Unintentional injury	Motor vehicle accident	CCF*	CVA*	Assault
3	Unintentional injury	Diarrhoea	AIDS	Pulmonary tuberculosis	Pulmonary tuberculosis	CVA*
4	ARI*, incl. pneumonia	Epilepsy	Pulmonary tuberculosis	Genito-urinary cancer	Diarrhoea	CCF*
5	Prematurity	Congenital defect	Suicide	Liver disease	Gastrointestinal cancer	Pulmonary tuberculosis

*ARI, acute respiratory infection; CVA, cerebrovascular accident; CCF congestive cardiac failure.
Note. Source: Kahn, Tollman, Garenne, & Gear (1999). From "Who Dies From What? Determining Cause of Death in South Africa's Rural North-East," by K. Kahn, S. M. Tollman, M. Garenne, and J. S. S. Gear, 1999, *Tropical Medicine and International Health, 4*, p. 438.

TABLE 18.3
Stroke Mortality Rate per 100,000 by Age and Sex. Agincourt 1992–1995

	Age (Yrs)		
	35–64	> 65	Total (> 35)
Men	100 (16)	315 (10)	135 (26)
95% CI			83–187
Women	62 (12)	354 (17)	120 (29)
95% CI			76–163
Total	80 (28)	338 (27)	127 (55)
95% CI	50–108	211–466	93–160

*Number of deaths in parentheses.
Note. From "Stroke in Rural South Africa—Contributing to the Little Known About a Big Problem," by K. Kahn and S. M. Tollman, 1999, *South African Medical Journal, 89*, p. 64.

Not only was stroke the most important cause of death among the older middle aged, contributing 11% of deaths among those 55–74 years; it was the second most common cause of death among adults 35–54 years, contributing 8% of deaths in this age group, these lying between assault (10% of deaths), and motor vehicle accidents (7% of deaths). The proportion of deaths occurring in this younger adult age group (with a modest preponderance of men over women) is of particular concern because of the social and economic consequences of premature death (Kahn & Tollman, 1999).

Age-specific stroke mortality rates for both sexes rose with age, and were higher among men than women; 135/100,000 compared with 120/100,000 in the population aged over 35 years (Table 18.3). This is comparable to findings from Tanzania where a census of stroke-related disability found an age-standardized prevalence of 154/100,000 men and 114/100,000 women over 15 years of age (Walker, 2000). The Agincourt trend holds over all 10-year age strata above 35 years, with the exception of the 65–74 year stratum. Stroke mortality for men in this age group was lower than that for women (and lower than that for men aged 55–64 years; Kahn & Tollman, 1999).

Perceptions of Stroke: Organic Pathology or Bewitchment? In developing populations like Agincourt, the emergence of stroke as a common cause of death can be expected to become more pronounced as life expectancy improves and the number of adults reaching middle age increases (Reddy & Yusuf, 1998).[5] Clearly, the ability to provide reliable and robust estimates of

---

[5]In South Africa, as with much of Southern and East Africa, the still-rising prevalence of HIV/AIDS is having a profound impact on mortality patterns. Although serving to delay manifestation of a full stroke/cardiovascular epidemic, recent findings from Agincourt demonstrate resoundingly high levels of cardiovascular risk factors among adults—blood pressure and body mass in particular.

the age–sex prevalence of stroke-related mortality in African settings is an important step forward. However, without a sociocultural understanding of stroke in its local setting, community-based efforts at stroke prevention and management will face potentially insurmountable obstacles.

Shangaan-speaking communities, forced northward from the east coast of South Africa during the mid to late 19th century by the territorially expansive Zulu (Ritchkin, 1995) took root in parts of what is now southern Mozambique and northeastern South Africa. The Agincourt subdistrict falls squarely into this roughly contiguous region.

Preliminary anthropological research (Chalmers & Edwards, 1998) revealed that, although western understanding of stroke is recognized in this population, and associated with the problem of "high blood" (hypertension), there is another condition—"*Xifulana*" (pronounced shifulana)—with essentially identical symptoms, but that is believed to be caused by bewitchment and is thus not amenable to preventive health strategies.

As expressed by Patience, a young female student, "… I would go to a traditional healer if I had *Xifulana* … this is where loss of movement is experienced in the limbs. It is caused by witchcraft and the sprinkling of dust so the traditional healer is the only person who can cure a person suffering from *Xifulana*. It is like someone inside your body—a doctor cannot find this" (Chalmers & Edwards, 1998).

In contrast, another informant comments, "… I would go straight to the hospital, for a doctor to measure my blood flow [i.e., blood pressure]; a traditional healer would be a secondary measure as they do not have the machine for measuring blood flow" (Chalmers & Edwards, 1998).

The association of dual explanations (*Xifulana* and stroke) with a single symptom complex (single-sided hemiplegia), together with the view among the Shangaan that stroke and *Xifulana* exist independently of each other, accentuates the acute preventive, diagnostic, and management challenge facing western-trained practitioners. If the purpose of stroke care is not only to treat sick individuals but also to diminish the burden of stroke among communities, it is clear that this will require the strengths of a multidisciplined team, further social science research into local systems of disease causation, an understanding of traditional health practices along with clients' help-seeking behaviors, and an ability on the part of physicians, nurses and other practitioners to suspend personal judgement, if effective health care provision is to result.

HIV/AIDS

There is no doubt that the HIV/AIDS epidemic—a social as much as a biological phenomenon—represents one of the greatest threats to public health at the end of the 20th century and beyond (Benatar, 2004; Ford, 1994).

HIV/AIDS is essentially a new sexually transmitted disease (STD); such diseases, associated with the most intimate sexual behavior, have for centuries of human history been subject to the taboo and social stigma through which societies have sought to regulate and control patterns of sexual behavior (Selvin, 1984). This sexual dimension, coupled with the absence of a cure for AIDS and the fears associated with its fatal consequences, have led to the widely negative responses encountered by this epidemic. A "third epidemic" of denial, blame, stigmatization, prejudice, and discrimination has accompanied the progression of the HIV/AIDS epidemic (Panos Institute, 1990). Thus, the social challenges of addressing HIV/AIDS are, on one hand, to foster social structures and patterns of behavior conducive to the prevention of transmission and, on the other, to encourage and to cultivate a compassionate, nondiscriminatory response toward those already infected from the public at large, but from health professionals in particular.

Since the start of the epidemic, some 50 million individuals worldwide have been infected with the human immunodeficiency virus (HIV), of whom over 16 million have died. A report by the Joint United Nations Program on HIV/AIDS (UNAIDS) and the World Health Organization (WHO) showed that AIDS deaths reached a record 2.6 million in 1999, and that new HIV infections continued unabated, with an estimated 5.6 million adults and children worldwide becoming infected the same year (UNAIDS, 1999). According to this report, "the overwhelming majority of people with HIV—some 95% of the global total—live in the developing world. That proportion is set to grow even further as infection rates continue to rise in countries where poverty, poor health systems and limited resources for prevention and care fuel the spread of the virus" (p. 4).

For some years it has been clear that Africa, especially south of the Sahara, is the area of the world worst affected by HIV and AIDS. Recent trends in Southern and Eastern Africa suggest a pandemic, described by UNAIDS as "explosive." Infection levels are highest, access to care is lowest, and the social and economic safety nets that might help families cope with the impact of the epidemic are badly frayed, in part because of the extent and impact of the epidemic itself (UNAIDS, 1999). Of the 23,3 million people living with HIV/AIDS in sub-Saharan Africa, most will die within the next 10 years. They will leave behind shattered families and crippled prospects for economic and social development. Life expectancy at birth, which rose from 44 years in the early 1950s to 59 years in the early 1990s, is set to drop to just 45 between 2005 and 2010 (Caelers, 1999). Although the region is home to only 10% of the world's population, it carries the burden of almost 70% of infections.

There is an immense gap in HIV infection rates and AIDS deaths between industrialized and lower income countries, and more particularly between Africa and the rest of the world (Table 18.4). This gap is likely to grow even larger in the next century (UNAIDS.org, AIDS epidemic update, 1999, p.6).

TABLE 18.4
Regional HIV/AIDS Statistics and Features, December 1999

Region	Epidemic Started	Adults & Children Living With HIV/AIDS	Adults & Children Newly Infected With HIV	Adult Prevalence Rate (*)	Percent of HIV-Positive Adults Who Are Women	Main Model(s) of Transmission (#) for Adults Living With HIV/AIDS
Sub-Saharan Africa	late '70–early '80s	23.3 million	3.8 million	8.0%	55%	Hetero
North Africa & Middle East	late '80s	220,000	19,000	0.13%	20%	IDU, Hetero
South & South-East Asia	late '80s	6 million	1.3 million	0.69%	30%	Hetero
East Asia & Pacific	late '80s	530,000	120,000	0.068%	15%	IDU, Hetero, MSM
Latin America	late '70s–early '80s	1.3 million	150,000	0.57%	20%	MSM, IDU, Hetero
Caribbean	late '70s–early '80s	360,000	57,000	1.96%	35%	Hetero, MSM
Eastern Europe & Central Asia	early '90s	360,000	95,000	0.14%	20%	IDU, MSM
Western Europe	late '70s–early '80s	520,000	30,000	0.25%	20%	MSM, IDU
North America	late '70s–early '80s	920,000	44,000	0.56%	20%	MSM, IDU, Hetero
Eastern Europe & Central Asia	early '90s	360,000	95,000	0.14%	20%	IDU, MSM
Western Europe	late '70s–early '80s	520,000	30,000	0.25%	20%	MSM, IDU
North America	late '70s–early '80s	920,000	44,000	0.56%	20%	MSM, IDU, Hetero
Australia & New Zealand	late '70s–early '80s	12,000	500	0.1%	10%	MSM, IDU
TOTAL		33.6 million	5.6 million	1.1%	46%	

*The proportion of adults (15 to 49 years of age) living with HIV/AIDS in 1999, using 1998 population numbers.
#MSM (sexual transmission among men who have sex with men), IDU (transmission through injecting drug use), Hetero (heterosexual transmission).
Note. From *AIDS Epidemic Update: December 1999*, by UNAIDS, 1999.

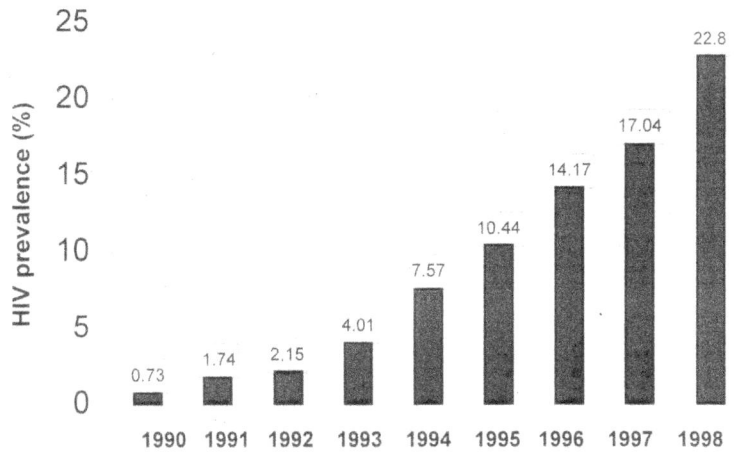

FIG. 18.3. HIV prevalence trends in South Africa 1990–1998. *Note.* From Summary Report: 2002 National HIV Sero-Prevalence Survey of Women Attending Public Antenatal Clinics in South Africa, by Department of Health, 2003.

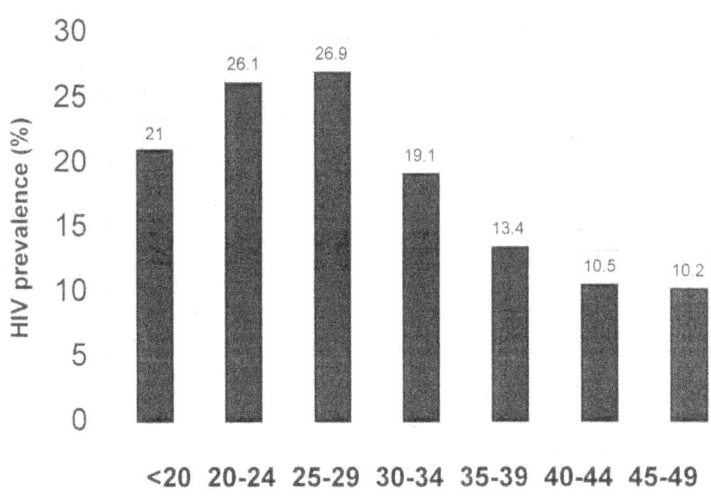

FIG. 18.4. 1998 HIV prevalence rate (90) by age in South Africa.

In South Africa, the latest antenatal survey[6] of infection rates among women attending public sector antenatal clinics confirms these trends (Department of Health, 2003).

These findings describe the growing HIV/AIDS epidemic in South Africa. Women in their 20s have the highest infection rates at 26.1% for the 20–24 age group and 26.9% for the 25–29 age group. The rate of increase by age is a notable feature and should guide the planning of preventive programs. Among teenagers (15–19 years) this was highest, being 65.4% in comparison with increases of 32.5% and 47.8% among women in the age group 20–24 and 25–29 respectively.

These findings reflect the alarming pace of the epidemic in South Africa, with the 20–29 year age group being at greatest risk, although infection is clearly evident in adolescent women as well (Department of Health, 2003). Considerable variation in HIV prevalence rates is also found in the different geographical districts (provinces), as demonstrated in Fig. 18.5.

There appear to be significantly more women than men living with HIV infection in sub-Saharan Africa. The information available suggests that between 12 and 13 African women are currently infected for every 10 African men (UNAIDS, 1999). Why this should be so is not fully understood; a combination of biological as well as social/cultural factors are clearly involved. However, the prime factor seems to be the difference in age patterns of HIV infection in men and women. Women tend to become infected at a considerably younger age than men. It is clear that older men—who often coerce girls into sex or buy their favors—are among the main sources of HIV infections in teenage girls (Wood & Jewkes, 1997).

The development of the HIV/AIDS epidemic in South Africa is an exceptional example of the additional contribution and explanatory power of the psychosocioenvironmental model of health and disease presented earlier in this chapter. The high background level of sexually transmitted infections (STIs[7]), the migrant labor system and "oscillatory" migration coupled with poverty, and the subordinate social status of women appear to be critical risk factors contributing to the rapid transmission of HIV in South Africa (Gilbert & Walker, 2002). Of particular concern in South Africa is the fact that young African women from their teens to mid to late 20s, are most at risk. Because these are the years in which women initiate and then consolidate their reproductive lives, the disastrous repercussions extend to their babies as well.[8]

---

[6]The results of the annual survey of antenatal clinics are used to estimate the overall number of South Africans infected with the virus by extrapolating the HIV levels found in antenatal clinic attendees to the total population (Floyd, 1997).

[7]It is estimated that approximately four million episodes of STIs occur each year in South Africa (USAID, 1997).

[8]Recent estimates are that nearly 90% of the 500,000 children born with HIV or infected through breast feeding in 1999, were living in sub-Saharan Africa (UNAIDS, 1999).

18. EPIDEMIOLOGICAL, SOCIAL, AND CULTURAL ASPECTS

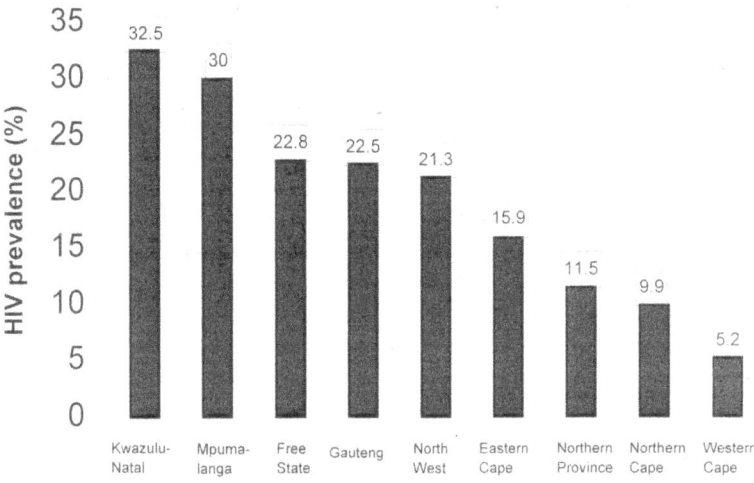

FIG. 18.5. HIV prevalence by province in South Africa, 1998.

Preston-Whyte (1999), in her opening address to the 22nd International Neuropsychology Conference, suggested that we cannot beat the repercussions of the epidemic "unless we adopt an holistic and essentially a multidisciplinary and participative approach." To do so, it becomes critical to explore the social and cultural complexities associated with the lack of success of "our best intentioned HIV/AIDS intervention programmes" (Preston-Whyte, 1999).

The use of condoms is one of the principle methods recommended for the prevention of HIV transmission. Without entering into an in-depth analysis, the primary importance of the immediate and cultural environment affecting decision making around HIV protection, for African women in particular, becomes evident. What health professionals regard as "choice" emerges as no choice at all when contextualized within their social and cultural reality (Walker & Gilbert, 2002). The historical association of condoms provided to African men in family planning clinics during the apartheid era and perceived as a means to curtail their reproduction; the high value placed on demonstrated fertility and the birth of children to sexually active couples in the African community; the subordinate status of women in a patriarchal society and the high level of violence in many conjugal relationships (Campbell, 1992) all combine to render condom usage as a formidably difficult protective option for black South African women (Preston-Whyte, 1999). Failure to appreciate these issues obstructs an understanding of the full social and interpersonal mechanisms that produce or constrain protective behavior to HIV.

It is for these reasons that widely recommended preventive and treatment interventions need to be in tune with local African culture and belief systems, rather than currently dominant western sexual and medical understandings alone. In addition, in order to maximize chances for success, HIV interventions should be based on community support and participation. As elaborated on by Preston-Whyte (1999), "... such mechanisms seek to provide a radically new social and interactional context in and through which the support of protective behaviour to counter HIV can be negotiated. A further elaboration of the same principle leads to the use of participatory methods to elicit and use locally derived 'common sense' in the development and execution of intervention programmes" (p. 3). By extension, similar principles should guide health professionals throughout the stages of illness behavior, from diagnosis to treatment and rehabilitation. This is the route necessary if we are to take cognizance of cultural impacts on individual and community understanding of disease and its treatment, and apply this to our patients' and communities' advantage (Wight, 1999). These recommendations are far from the conventional biomedically oriented paradigm that stresses so-called "scientific knowledge" and often ignores or underplays the value of indigenous cultural systems and the practices that make sense to the majority of African people (Chalmers & Edwards, 1998).

The previous discussion is as relevant to neuropsychologists as it is to health professionals in general. However, because persons infected with HIV are at greater risk of presenting with neurological dysfunction, it acquires additional significance. According to Desjarlais et al. (1995):

> the virus enters the central nervous system in most infected persons shortly after systemic infection occurs. This has been shown by antibodies and by virus isolation from cerebrospinal fluid. Although the brain infection usually remains asymptomatic for long periods (months and years), almost all patients who die from AIDS have multiple brain lesions at autopsy; many exhibit dementia before they die. In addition to the damage from direct infection by the HIV virus, the patient may contract uncommon infections (such as toxoplasmosis, cryptococcal meningitis, tuberculosis, cytomegalovirus and herpes zoster) that produce severe brain lesions. (p. 243)

CONCLUSION

In this chapter, the psychosocioenvironmental model of health and disease was introduced to highlight an additional dimension to the understanding of health, disease, and disability. Because social factors have been identified as important in the assessment, treatment, and rehabilitation of patients managed by neuropsychologists, it is essential to engage with these factors in the practice of neuropsychology.

Cultural complexity is one of the features of modern society. This can give rise to cultural incompatibilities in the perception and response to disease and treatment, often accompanied by miscommunication and misunderstanding, between patients and health workers—including neuropsychologists. To avoid adverse intercultural encounters, it is essential that health workers be familiar with the cultural context of the people they treat in order to boost their understanding of their patients' social reality, and thereby enhance the therapeutic relationship.

The South African case studies presented illustrate that certain prominent diseases are linked to their social and geographical context. Greater awareness among health practitioners has the potential to contribute to improved practice and more fruitful outcomes. In addition, this greater knowledge and insight should be applied not only to individual therapeutic encounters but also to future organization of neuropsychological services, as well as to the framing of the research agenda.

REFERENCES

Airhihenbuwa, C.O. (1995). *Health and culture*. London: Sage.
Annandale, E. (1998). *The sociology of health & medicine*. Cambridge: Polity Press.
Albrecht, G. L., Fitzpatrick, R., & Scrimshaw, S. C. (Eds.). (1999). *The handbook of social studies in health & medicine*. London: Sage.
Allen-Meares, P., & Burman, S. (1999). Cross-cultural therapeutic relationships: Entering the world of African Americans. *Journal of Social Work Practice, 1* , 49–57.
Barron, P. (1998). Equity in 1998: An overview. In *South African Health Review, 1998* (pp.1–6). Durban, South Africa: Health Systems Trust and the Henry J. Kaiser Family Foundation.
Benatar S. R. (2004). Health care reform and the crisis of HIV and AIDS in South Africa. *The New England Journal of Medicine, 351*, 81–92.
Blaxter, M. (2004). *Health: Key Concepts*. Cambridge: Polity Press.
Butchart, A., & Peden, M. (1997). Injury and trauma. In *South African Health Review, 1997* (pp. 213–221). Durban, South Africa: Health Systems Trust and the Henry J. Kaiser Family Foundation .
Caelers, D. (1999, November 25). Women bear the brunt of the AIDS Epidemic. *The Star.*
Campbell, C. (1992). Learning to kill: Masculinity, the family and violence in Natal. *Journal of Southern African Studies, 18*, 614–628.
Cant, S., & Sharma, U. (1999). *A new medical pluralism*. New York: UCL Press.
Chalmers, J., & Edwards, H. J. (1998). *Blood and bewitchment in the Bushveld: Community perceptions of the chronic illnesses of lifestyle* [A Preliminary Assessment of the subdistrict of Agincourt in the Bushbuckridge District, Northern Province, South Africa].
Curtis, S., & Taket, A. (1996). *Health & societies: Changing perspectives*. London: Arnold.
Davey, B., Gray, A., & Seale, C. (Eds.). (1995). *Health and disease—A reader* (2nd ed.). Buckingham, England: Open University Press.
Department of Health. (2003). *Summary report: 2002 national HIV sero-prevalence survey of women attending public antenatal clinics in South Africa*. Pretoria: Health Systems Research & Epidemiology, Department of Health.

Desjarlais, R., Eisenberg, L., Good, B., & Kleinman, A. (1995). *World mental health: Problems and priorities in low-income countries*. Oxford University Press.
Dubos, R. (1968). *Man, medicine and environment*. Harmondsworth, Middlesex, England: Penguin Books.
Fitzpatrick, R. M. (1996). Social and changing patterns of disease. In L. Gilbert, T. A. Selikow, & L. Walker (Eds.), *Society, health and disease* (pp.13–18). Johannesburg: Ravan Press.
Floyd, L. (1997). HIV/AIDS. In *South African Health Review, 1997* (pp. 187–196). Durban, South Africa: Health Systems Trust and the Henry J. Kaiser Family Foundation.
Ford, N. (1994). Cultural and developmental factors underlying the global pattern of the transmission of HIV/AIDS. In D. R. Phillips & Y. Verhasselt (Eds.), *Health and development* (pp. 153–164).
Gilbert, L. (1996). Urban violence and health—South Africa 1995. *Social Science & Medicine, 43*, 873–886.
Gilbert, L., Selikow, T. A., & Walker, L. (Eds.). (2002). *Society, health and disease*. Johannesburg: Ravan Press.
Gilbert, L., & Walker, L. (2002). Treading the path of least resistance: HIV/AIDS and social inequalities—A South African case study. *Social Science & Medicine, 54*, 1093–1110.
Gopaul-McNicol, S. A., & Brice-Baker, J. (1998). *Cross-cultural practice: assessment, treatment, and training*. New York: Wiley.
Hart, N. (1996). Health and mythology of medicine. In L. Gilbert, T. A. Selikow, & L. Walker (Eds.), *Society, health and disease* (pp. 19–29). Johannesburg: Ravan Press.
Health Systems Trust and the Henry J. Kaiser Family Foundation. (1995). *South African Health Review, 1995*. Durban, South Africa: Author.
Health Systems Trust and the Henry J. Kaiser Family Foundation. (1996). *South African Health Review, 1996*. Durban, South Africa: Author.
Health Systems Trust and the Henry J. Kaiser Family Foundation. (1997). *South African Health Review, 1997*. Durban, South Africa: Author.
Health Systems Trust and the Henry J. Kaiser Family Foundation. (1998). *South African Health Review, 1998*. Durban, South Africa: Author.
Helfrich, H. (1999). Beyond the dilemma of cross-cultural psychology: Resolving the tension between etic and emic approaches. *Culture & Psychology, 5*, 131–153.
Ingman, K. A., Ollendick, T. H., & Akande, A. (1999). Cross-cultural aspects of fears in African children and adolescents. *Behaviour Research and Therapy, 37*, 337–345.
Joubert, J. (1991). The MEDUNSA stroke data bank. *South African Medical Journal, 80*, 567–571.
Jones, K., & Moon, G. (1987). *Health, disease & society*. New York: Routledge
Kahn, K., & Tollman, S. M. (1999). Stroke in rural South Africa—Contributing to the little known about a big problem. *South African Medical Journal, 89*, 63–65.
Kahn, K., Tollman, S. M., Garenne, M., & Gear, J. S. S. (1999). Who dies from what? Determining cause of death in South Africa's rural north-east. *Tropical Medicine and International Health, 4*, 433–441.
Lee, M. Y., & Greene, G. J. (1999). A social constructivist framework for integrating cross-cultural issues in teaching clinical social work. *Journal of Social Work Education, 35*, 21–37.
Matenga, J., Kitai, I., & Levy, L. (1986). Strokes among black people in Harare, Zimbabwe: Results of computerized tomography and associated risk factors. *British Medical Journal, 292*, 1649–1650.
McElroy, A., & Jezewski, M.A. (1999). Cultural variation in the experience of health and illness. In G. L Albrecht, R. Fitzpatrick, & S. C. Scrimshaw (Eds.), *The handbook of social studies in health & medicine* (pp. 192–209). London: Sage.

Medical Research Council. (1999). *Cape metropolitan study.* Cape-Town: National Trauma Research Programme, Medical Research Council.
Moon, G. (1995). Demographic and epidemiological change. In G. Moon & R. Gillespie (Eds.), *Society & health* (pp. 9–30). London: Routledge.
Moon, G., & Gillespie, R. (Eds.). (1995). *Society & health: An introduction to social science for health professionals.* London: Routledge.
Morris, D. B., (1998). *Illness and culture in the postmodern age.* Berkeley: University of California Press.
Murray, C. J. L., & Lopez, A. D. (1996). *The global burden of disease.* Geneva, Switzerland: World Health Organization.
Nell, V. (1999). *Cross-cultural neurological assessment: Theory and practice.* Mahwah, NJ: Lawrence Erlbaum Associates.
Nelson, L. D., & Adams, K. M. (1997). Challenges for neuropsychology in the treatment and rehabilitation of brain-injured patients. *Psychological Assessment, 9,* 368–373.
Nettleton, S. (1995). *The sociology of health & illness.* Cambridge, England: Polity Press.
Omran, A. R. (1971). The epidemiological transition: A theory of the epidemiology of population change. *Milbank Quarterly 49,* 509–538.
Panos Institute. (1990). *The third epidemic.* London: Panos Institute.
Phillips, D. R., & Verhasselt, Y. (Eds). (1994). *Health and development.* Routledge.
Pierrepointe, M., Navas, M., Bragin, M., & Diaz, A., (1999). Style and substance: Examining the space between patient and therapist in the cross-cultural clinical encounter. *Journal of Social Work Practice, 13,* 39–47.
Preston-Whyte, E. (1999). *HIV/AIDS and the new millennium: Institutional and professional challenges.* Opening address to the "Neuropsychology: Towards the Millennium" 22nd International Conference, Durban, South Africa.
Reddy, K. S., & Yusuf, S. (1998). Emerging epidemic of cardiovascular disease in developing countries. *Circulation , 97,* 596–601.
Ritchkin, E. (1995) *Leadership and conflict in Bushbuckridge: Struggles to define moral economies within the context of rapidly transforming political economies.* Unpublished doctoral dissertation, University of the Witwatersrand, Johannesburg.
Richter, L. M., & Griesel, R. D. (1999). Breast feeding and infant care in the context of HIV/AIDS. *Psychology in Society. 24,* 40-56.
Rosman, K. D. (1986). The epidemiology of stroke in an urban black population. *Stroke , 17,* 667–669.
Selvin, M. (1984).Changing medical and societal attitudes towards sexually transmitted diseases: An historical overview. In K. K. Holmes (Ed.), *Sexually transmitted diseases* (pp. 3–19). London: MacGraw-Hill.
Senior, M., & Viveash, B. (1998). *Health and illness.* London: Macmillan.
Tollman, S., Herbst, K., Garenne, M., Gear, J. S. S., & Kahn, K. (1999). The Agincourt demographic and health study: Site description, baseline findings and implications. *South African Medical Journal, 89,* 858–864.
UNAIDS.org. (1999). *AIDS epidemic update: December 1999.* UNAIDS (Joint United Nations Programme on HIV/AIDS).
USAID. (1997). *USAID responds to HIV/AIDS: A report on the fiscal years 1995 and 1996 HIV/AIDS prevention programs of the United States Agency for International Development.* Washington, DC: Author.
Walker L., & Gilbert, L. (2002), Women at risk: HIV/AIDS—A South African case study. *African Journal of AIDS Research, 1,* 77–86.
Walker, R. (2000). Age-specific prevalence of impairment and disability relating to hemiplegic stroke in the Hai district of northern Tanzania. *Journal of Neurology, Neurosurgery and Psychiatry, 68,* 744–749.

Watts, A. (1999). *Clinical neuropsychology in South Africa: Times past, times present and times future*. Paper presented at the SACNA Presidential Address, INS/SACNA 22nd Mid-Year Conference, Durban, South Africa.

Wight, D. (1999). Cultural factors in young heterosexual men's perception pf HIV risk. *Sociology of Health & Illness, 21,* 735–758.

Wilkinson, R. G. (1996). *Unhealthy societies: The afflictions of inequality.* London: Routledge.

Wood, K., & Jewkes, R. (1997). Violence, rape and sexual coercion: Everyday love in a South African township. *Gender and Development, 5,* 41–46.

Wolffers, I. (1997). Culture, media and HIV/AIDS in Asia. *The Lancet, 349,* 52–54.

Chapter 19

Natural Recovery: An Ecological Approach to Neuropsychological Recuperation

Tedd Judd and Roberta DeBoard

Pepe was a 13-year-old boy who had never walked because he had had polio as a baby. David, a health care worker, visited Pepe in his rural Mexican mountain home at his father's invitation. David asked if they had tried crutches. The father replied that they could not afford to travel to the city to get some. David borrowed a machete, cut branches, and made crude crutches. The father protested they would not work, and, sure enough, when Pepe tried them, they broke under his weight. The father then took the machete and cut a more appropriate species of wood. Following David's example, he skillfully fashioned functional crutches. Within half a day Pepe was proudly walking for the first time in his life (Werner, 1990).

This episode illustrates a collaboration between a professional with specialized knowledge and a peasant with the knowledge and the skills to adapt that knowledge to local conditions. The intervention would have been unsuccessful without the knowledge from both parties.

Beginning an academic chapter with storytelling illustrates the type of break in convention that is often needed to apply clinical knowledge successfully in the developing world. In a sense, this chapter will be only one hand clapping, presenting the clinical side of the knowledge needed for success. The other hand needed for clapping is the knowledge of local resources and culture that comes from the individuals, families, and communities affected by brain disabilities.

About 7% of the world's population is disabled (Mitchell, 1999b). Worldwide, only about 1-2% (Johnston & Tjandrakusuma, 1982; World Health Organization, 1981) or possibly as much as 3% (Mitchell, 1999b) of people with chronic disabilities receive medical rehabilitation in their lifetimes. Within the population of disabled, the number of individuals affected by brain disorders is large. For example, Ardila and Rosselli (1992) have estimated that 3–5% of the population of Colombia is affected by some type of brain disorder, amounting to some 1 million people. Even in many developed countries many people with brain illnesses do not receive services that have been developed. For example, in many medical systems, traumatic brain injuries (TBIs) have a high profile and receive higher priority than do strokes, dementias, toxicities, encephalitis, and so on, yet only about 10% of individuals with TBI in the United States receive adequate diagnosis and rehabilitation (Kreutzer, Gordon, & Wehman, 1989). Care for the other conditions is probably even less adequate.

One reason for this inadequate treatment is the high cost of professional rehabilitation. For example, costs for recommended on-going rehabilitation and care (after initial medical and rehabilitation costs) in the United States for a 41-year-old man with a severe TBI were estimated to be $90,000/year ("The Tough Case," 1993). Other reasons include limited rehabilitation resources, uneven distribution of those resources, and cultural limitations of the dominant rehabilitation model. Extending the model of professional, hospital- or clinic-based neurorehabilitation, currently predominant in developed countries, to cover all those in need throughout the world would be a formidable, expensive, and possibly unwise undertaking. This is especially true for the neuropsychological aspects of rehabilitation. Clearly, if neurorehabilitation is to be of benefit to any but an elite few, alternative models of care are needed.

CULTURAL CONTRASTS RELEVANT TO NEUROPSYCHOLOGICAL REHABILITATION

Neuropsychological rehabilitation is heavily dependent on its cultural and ecological contexts. Those contexts are substantially different in the developing world as contrasted with the developed world where most neuropsychological rehabilitation has originated. Although there are many exceptions to these generalizations, the contexts of developing regions usually have fewer rehabilitation resources; less transportation, communication, and information infrastructure; less-educated populations; more myths and less understanding about brain conditions; less legal protection of the disabled; greater family protection of the disabled; less cognitively demanding environments; less valuing of speed and efficiency; more informal employment; greater family support; less valuing of personal independence; and less reliance on professionals (Table 19.1). These and other contrasts suggest the need for a distinctive approach to neuropsychological rehabilitation for developing regions, with some implications for the predominant model in developed regions.

TABLE 19.1
Cultural Contrasts Relevant to Neurorehabilitation

Developed World	*Developing World*
Personal independence valued	Personal interdependence valued
Small, nuclear and subnuclear families	Large, extended families
Marginalization of elderly	Respect for elderly
Faith in professionals, technology, law	Faith in family, religion
Formal and legal acceptance and protection of people with disabilities	Limited formal and legal acceptance and protection of people with disabilities
Variable social acceptance of people with disabilities	Social acceptance of people with disabilities within the family, but with overprotection. Marginalization within society at large
Well-developed infrastructure for people with disabilities	Poorly developed infrastructure for people with disabilities
Infrastructure is technological and oriented toward personal independence	Infrastructure is low tech and oriented toward personal interdependence
Most adults have secondary education	Educational levels are very variable
Public is well informed about health and disabilities	Public is not well informed about health and disabilities, many myths
Employment is mostly formal, institutional, technological, and specialized	Much employment is informal, via personal connections, less technological, and less specialized
Punctuality, speed, efficiency, and the task are valued	Interpersonal relations are valued
Health care is specialized, technological, highly documented, expensive, well funded	Health care is less specialized, less technological, with limited documentation and exchange of information, financially very limited
Alternative medicine has a professional and corporate base	Alternative medicine is traditionally based

The Cultural Contexts of Neuropsychological Rehabilitation

The past decade has seen a great increase in attention to an economic and cultural phenomenon that has been termed "globalization." Fueled by economic policy and improvements in communication technology, there is a homogenization and standardization of both terminology and approaches to certain problems. Although certainly transnational, this phenomenon is far from global, and might better be termed cosmopolitan because it is focused predominantly in cities. The cultural context of cosmopolitan rehabilitation is predominantly a scientific/medical model involving professional services. But it is by no means the only way people recover from or cope with brain disabilities.

Within this cosmopolitan framework, cognitive rehabilitation and neuropsychological rehabilitation are often defined in terms of a professional service offered to brain-injured patients to facilitate their recovery of cognitive and other abilities (e.g., Gordon, Hibbard, & Kreutzer, 1989). This type of definition is a reflection of the economic and social realities and power structures within which some activities favoring brain injury recovery do take place. Yet it is a definition that not only identifies the type of activity that the definers wish to promote as the most authoritative route to recuperation, but also sets the social roles of the participants. Such definitions can be seen as carrying with them a hidden agenda of legitimizing and marketing the services of the definers, while delegitimizing and disempowering the poor "victims." There is almost an implication that in-clinic, expensive training sessions under the control of and at the convenience of the professionals should be the norm, and that to deny or refuse such services would be cruel, unethical, or irrational.

Many brain injury rehabilitation programs find such a worldview shaken, however, when some of their participants are not very willing recipients of these services. An easy way to accommodate to this resistance is to see it as part of denial or of lack of awareness of deficits on the part of the brain-injured participants. It is sometimes harder to consider that the very organization of the program may not speak to the needs of those it would serve. This can be particularly telling with individuals whose cultural, social, educational, and/or religious (Yamey & Greenwood, 2004) backgrounds do not match well with those of the providers, or with such a model of service.

A bolder way of coping with rejection of services is to reorient the program. "Empowerment" models have done much in this direction (O'Hara & Harrell, 1991; Parente & Stapleton, 1993), while staying within a professional service model. Another direction has come from a social psychology perspective that has moved away from a service model toward a community model. The movement toward "Circles of Support" (Willer, Allen, Anthony, & Cowlan, 1993) is a prominent example. Yet another movement in this direction, the independent living movement, comes from a consumer-oriented community of people with disabilities, rather than from professionals, and is characterized by support groups and political movements (cf. Boschen & Krane, 1992; Lysack & Kaufert, 1994; and the newsletters, *This Brain has a Mouth,* and *Disability Rag*). The community-based rehabilitation (CBR) movement, which is mostly in developing countries, to some extent also belongs in this category (Lysack & Kaufert, 1994; Mitchell, 1999a, 1999b; Peat, 1991) and will be discussed further later.

A frequent problem related to the rejection of services is that the person recovering from a brain injury (and, often, their family, as well) may have difficulty seeing the connection between clinic tasks and home goals. For example, a person who's primary interest in rehabilitation is to return to driving may have difficulty understanding why she is continually being asked to practice vigilance for numbers on a tape recording. Such skepticism is often well founded: Generalization of cognitive retraining results to everyday functioning continues to be a challenge for rehabilitation programs (Sohlberg & Mateer, 2001).

A related problem with which rehabilitation centers sometimes struggle is the compartmentalization of the person, most often along the lines of professional specialties. A caricature of this problem, the medical butchering of the rehabilitation patient, is presented in Fig. 19.1. This problem is often most acute where interdisciplinary rivalries are most intense. The person sometimes becomes further fractionalized within disciplines, for example, into a memory problem, an attention problem, a behavior problem,

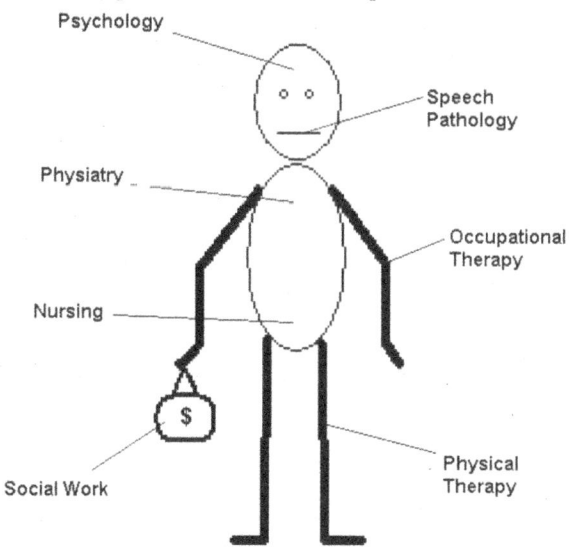

FIG. 19.1. Medical "butchering" of the rehabilitation patient.

and so forth. Although such analysis can be extremely powerful and useful, it also has its limits. Such analysis encourages modular treatments in which a single approach may be applied within a problem area (memory books for memory problems, for example), without regard to other factors that may influence the necessity or practicality of the approach (such as the client's and family's literacy abilities and habits). How to reintegrate this compartmentalized person then becomes the focus of "whole person" approaches to rehabilitation. One solution is the interdisciplinary team; a related solution is case managers.

THE NATURAL RECOVERY MODEL

The natural recovery model presented here is an attempt to integrate many of these perspectives. This model preserves a role for rehabilitation professionals as consultants to communities attempting to cope with disabilities, and, sometimes, as providers of direct treatment. However, rather than assuming that the rehabilitation center is the focal point of rehabilitation, it views the community as the focal point, supplemented by the rehabilitation center when necessary.

This model springs from experience working in rehabilitation in a number of cultures, particularly in developing countries, and from the varying needs and challenges that those cultures present to a professional service orientation. In particular, it comes from contexts of strong family ties and desires to help, but where those desires often are channeled into overprotection. Limited rehabilitation resources and a limited cognitive/academic orientation of the population were also influencing factors. The natural recovery model is congruent with the World Health Organization's (1981) appeal that rehabilitation research and development be redirected toward ways of disseminating training and information to people with limited training and to the general public (Peat, 1991; Werner, 1990; Werner & Bower, 1982).

The natural recovery model starts by expanding the definition of neuropsychological rehabilitation as follows: Neuropsychological rehabilitation is the modification of the environments and activities of recovery so as to facilitate both recovery of abilities and adaptation to target environments.

This definition assumes that there are tendencies toward healing and recovery within an injured person, family, and community, and that rehabilitation knowledge can be mobilized to facilitate those tendencies. This assumption is not unfounded. Spontaneous recovery from various forms of acute brain injury is copiously documented (Held, 1993; Selzer, 1995), and must be controlled for in any serious study of the effectiveness of rehabilitation interventions. Doubtless an important part of spontaneous recovery is due to physiological recovery of damaged brain tissue. But it is also widely accepted that the activities and experiences that take place during the time of recovery have an influence on the course of that recovery through learning and neural plasticity. Indeed, this is the main rationalization for rehabilitation efforts. Unfortunately, studies of the effects of the many variables naturally present in the environments and activities of recovering individuals are limited, especially when compared to studies of the variables associated with professional rehabilitation interventions. This bias in the focus of such research itself is so pervasive that it generally goes unrecognized in studies of environmental variables associated with recovery from brain dysfunction. For example, it is difficult to find research on the effects of family attitudes, knowledge, and availability on the recovery of their family member from brain illness.

Under the new definition of neuropsychological rehabilitation given earlier, the rehabilitation professional still has a very important role in evaluating the effects of the injury on the injured person's abilities. But this definition suggests that the rehabilitation professional then take into account all of the environments and activities of recovery (home, community, school, work, etc.), not just that portion of the environments and activities under direct professional control (typically hospital or clinic). The professional considers the adequacy of those environments and activities for facilitating recovery, as well as the potential for modifying them. Such modifications may include expanding the environment to include traditional in-clinic services, but only under certain conditions (discussed below). Fortunately, this perspective of regarding disability itself as relative to an environment has been incorporated into the World Health Organization's Classification of Functioning, Disability and Health (Schneidert, Hurst, Miller, & Üstün, 2003).

By considering neuropsychological rehabilitation as an activity aimed at facilitating adaptation to a target environment, the person with a brain injury is regarded as a person who comes from and belongs to a social context, not a malfunctioning product that has been brought in to the repair workshop to be fixed. Rather than fixing the person and then reinserting the person into an environment, finally adjusting that environment if absolutely necessary, it suggests a continuous process of readjusting the person–environment fit. It thereby puts more attention, for instance, on interventions such as family and community education and training and job coaches.

Cosmopolitan rehabilitation, congruent with its cultural context, focuses upon individual independence, so much so that it has been enshrined in the title and metric of the most widespread measure of rehabilitation outcomes, the Functional Independence Measure (Granger, 1998). In other cultural contexts, however, interdependence (Condeluci, 1995) takes greater priority, and rehabilitation goals may focus more on developing appropriate and valued roles within the family and community than on individual autonomy (Fletcher-Janzen, Strickland, & Reynolds, 2000).

The natural recovery model also emphasizes adapting the interventions to the cultural context of the person with brain dysfunction, rather than acculturating the person with brain dysfunction to the culture of the rehabilitation clinic (Table 19.2). For example, rehabilitation programs often devote considerable energy to training their patients in finding their way around the clinic, learning the names of the therapists, and the social skills appropriate for getting along with middle class professionals in an institu-

TABLE 19.2

Contrasts Between Conventional Neurorehabilitation and the Natural Recovery Model

Conventional Neurorehabilitation	*Natural Recovery Model*
What?	
A professional service offered to brain injured patients to facilitate recovery of cognition and other abilities.	The modification of the environments and activities of recovery so as to facilitate both recovery of abilities and adaptation to target environments.
Why?	
Fix the person in an affluent society that values personal independence and professional, institutional services	Fix the person–environment fit in a nonaffluent society that values interpersonal relations
Where?	
Hospital, clinic, rehabilitation center	Home, workplace, school, community
Who?	
Physiatrist, neuropsychologist, speech pathologist, occupational therapist, physical therapist, recreational therapist, vocational counselor, nurse	Family, friends, coworkers, teachers, aides, rehabilitation cooperatives (all trained by rehabilitation professionals)
When?	
Acute recovery phase	From acute recovery phase throughout life
How?	
Decontextualized exercises	Everyday activities

tional context. They rarely have the opportunity to train them in getting along with children, the proper behavior for a church or mosque, or how to avoid getting robbed in an open-air market.

Using Natural Activities to Facilitate Recovery

In many instances, what all of this translates into is home rehabilitation. But that does not mean simply a home evaluation (Starch & Falltrick, 1990), nor sending professionals to the home to provide their traditional services (Backman, 1992; Wilson & Robertson, 1992), nor taking the tasks of the clinic and sending them home on a computer disk (Gianutsos, 1992; Purdy & Neri, 1989), nor training family members to be rehabilitation paraprofessionals (Anderson & Parente, 1985) although all of these approaches have their value). Rather, it means *seeking out* the potential for facilitation of recovery in the natural activities of the person's life. After all, if someone is no longer able to do a familiar activity because of cognitive dysfunction, then that activity most likely involves a cognitive function that is impaired and it is therefore a candidate activity to be used to help retrain that function. The natural recovery model, therefore, completes the cultural adaptation of neurorehabilitation by not only taking rehabilitation into the home and community, but by also using the activities of home and the community to carry out rehabilitation, rather than imposing activities foreign to the culture.

This does not simply mean training specific activities, however. It means using specific functional activities to train more general abilities. To do this effectively, the rehabilitation specialist helps in identifying what cognitive, emotional, or self-control abilities need rehabilitation and helps in selecting functional activities and approaches that can be used to train those abilities. By using the activities of everyday life as rehabilitation experiences, the rehabilitator is freed from the constraints of clinic exercises and can do whatever it takes (Willer & Corrigan, 1994) to get the job done.

For instance, suppose Franz has had a severe TBI and is unable to cross streets alone safely or to find his way around his neighborhood, but that this is an important goal for him and his family. Suppose that he often walks around his neighborhood with various members of his family. This everyday activity can be modified to facilitate recovery by trying some of the following strategies: Walk alongside Franz, but have him point the way at each choice point. "Shadow" him; walk a few steps behind. Send him out with a responsible child, or with a dog, or on a horse that knows the way home. Make sure Franz has a note saying what to do if lost or in an emergency, and practice using the note before going out. Send Franz out alone to close destinations for short periods of time. Send him places where there will be someone to help if necessary. Have him take a cellular phone (if he knows how to answer such). Alert the neighbors en route to keep an eye out for him. Gradually increase the distance and time he travels independently, and decrease the familiarity of the route. For longer walks have him talk through the route, or find it on a map, or use written directions, checking first that he can use a map or directions accurately when walking around. In these ways, an activity Franz and his family are doing anyway can be used to facilitate his recovery of an activity they would all like him to be able to do.

This same type of approach can be applied to everyday activities in many areas, such as household chores, caring for children, managing medications, dressing, sports, games, hobbies, driving, using a bus, shopping, managing money, gardening, school, work, socializing, and even sexuality. Wilson and Robertson (1992) for instance, successfully used reading novels at home for training in attention processes.

Eight principles are presented here that facilitate the process of using natural activities to aid recovery: the zone of recovery, goals, activity analysis, environmental analysis, training natural helpers, training generalization, and incorporating cognitive strategies.

The Zone of Recovery. During the 1930s, the Russian developmental psychologist, Vygotsky (1978), developed a social-interaction approach to the understanding of child cognitive development. He argued that children develop cognitive abilities not only because their brains grow and mature, and not only because they learn by solving problems in their environment, but also because they learn particularly from other people. From his study of the kinds of interactions in which children learn he developed the concept of the zone of proximal development (ZPD). This zone is the level of difficulty of an activity that is just a little harder than the child can manage independently, that is, the kind of task the child is able to accomplish with a little help. It is in this zone, Vygotsky maintained, that the most learning takes place. This concept of the ZPD has been adapted to neuropsychological rehabilitation (Cicerone & Tupper, 1990) and is presented here as the zone of recovery.

If a given activity is too easy, the person recovering from a brain injury may become bored by it and even resentful of being given a child's task or too little responsibility (Table 19.3). If it can be done independently and easily, then it may not contribute much to recovery. Someone who is only allowed to do this kind of activity is being overprotected. If an activity is too difficult, the person may get frustrated and angry, and eventually discouraged and depressed. An activity that is just right for facilitating recovery is one that is a challenge, and that the person can do with some help (physical help, or directions, or reminders, or other cognitive strategies).

TABLE 19.3
Zone of Recovery

Too Easy	Just Right	Too Hard
Can do the task easily, independently	Can do the task with some help	Can't do the task without much help
Bored, overprotected	Challenged	Frustrated, angry, discouraged
Do it for them	Show, guide, cue	Trial-and-error
Tell, but don't involve	Person and helper are active	Guessing
Person is passive		Help is passive

Note. The concept of the Zone of Proximal Development was advanced by Vygotsky. Cicerone and Tupper took that concept and applied it to rehabilitation. Table 19.3 is a modification of the idea of applying the Zone of Proximal Development to rehabilitation.

For example, Elizabeth was a good cook before her head injury, but when she got home from the hospital and tried to cook dinner, nothing came out right. She spilled and burned things, started making things she didn't have the ingredients for and couldn't substitute, forgot to add spices or added them twice, and generally made a mess. Her husband said she had to keep trying, it was the only way. The next time she tried she got so frustrated she threw a tomato at the TV he was watching in the living room. Cooking dinner was not appropriate for her at that time; it was in her frustration zone.

Her husband switched tactics. He prohibited her from cooking anything, but made her wash all of the dishes, which she could do well. It was a large family and a big but boring job that the children usually shared. This time a sponge hit the TV. This was not an appropriate task; it was in her boredom zone.

Finally, her son offered to cook dinner with her. He asked her what she wanted to make, then guided her in checking that they had the ingredients and shopping for those that were missing. They planned what she would have to start first and when. He got her to use the recipe that she thought she had memorized, and make a pencil mark by each step as she did it. He reminded her to use a timer. When it went off and she couldn't remember what it was for, he had her look at the stove and figure it out. When dinnertime got close and not everything was ready, he pitched in to make a salad and got his father to set the table. After dinner she washed the dishes, he rinsed while they talked, and nothing hit the TV. This way of doing dinner was in her zone of recovery.

Encountering the zone of recovery is, in some respects, an art. Some people are very good at it, such as Elizabeth's son; others are not, such as her husband. Parents and teachers have often developed this skill. The rehabilitation professional can help people in developing this skill, in recognizing how to break down a task into components, how to find which components to attempt, and how and when help is needed. The rehabilitation professional can also help with the introduction of specific cognitive techniques adapted to the person, task, and circumstances.

Goals. Natural recovery activities are generally directed toward practical goals. It is often easy to see the overall goals because the activities most often consist of components of the target activity, or simplified or assisted versions of the activity. But short-term, explicit goals are also important in focusing the recovery process. In the previous example, for instance, a member of Franz's family might say, "Franz, we are two blocks from home. I am going to walk behind you. I would like you to see if you can find your way home safely without asking anyone for help." Specific goals are an important organizing tool for rehabilitation programs. The rehabilitation professional can help the recovering person and community in prioritizing goals and strategizing approaches. For recreational activities that are not intrinsically goal oriented, such as some kinds of play, being a spectator to a public event, or some nature activities, the goals may simply be participation and enjoyment for a given period of time. Secondary goals might include avoiding frustration, fatigue, embarrassment, or inconvenience to others.

In setting goals during the recovery period, it is important to distinguish for a given activity whether it is necessary to get the job done as efficiently as possible or whether there is enough time and tolerance to use the activity as a recovery exercise, because the strategies are different. Trying to be efficient usually means making full use of compensations and help, and taking frequent rests to minimize fatigue. Working on recovery may mean doing a poor job because of pushing against the limits of fatigue and, in some circumstances, because of an approach of trial and error. For example, someone with attentional difficulties who can read for 30 min before becoming fatigued may study school work in 20 min segments in order to be efficient, but read novels for 40 min at a time in order to work on cognitive stamina. That same person might minimize noise, distraction, and interruption for studying but intentionally try to read a novel on a bus in order to work on sustained and selective attention. Similarly, someone with dressing difficulty might be left alone to do the job as a recovery exercise when preparing to go for a pleasure walk, even if it takes 20 min, but when there is a hurry, a family member might direct the process and assist.

Contextual Assessment. Neuropsychologists in the developed world pride themselves in their use of standardized, normative-based, validated cognitive tests. Such tests can also play a role in the natural recovery model. However, a number of factors limit their use and applicability in the developing world:

- Appropriately standardized, normed, and validated tests may not be available for the language, culture, and educational level of the target population.
- Development of such tests is likely to be expensive and time consuming.
- Many such tests are expensive in the costs of materials, professional administration time, and level of professional skill needed to administer and interpret the tests.
- The target population for neurorehabilitation in the developing world is likely to be those individuals with fairly obvious deficits, where extensive, formal testing may not be entirely necessary to discover the nature of the problem and to develop an appropriate rehabilitation plan.

In place of or supplementary to formal cognitive assessment, the neuropsychologist or allied professional may need to develop the capacity to evaluate neuropsychological problems based primarily on direct observation; reports by the affected person, family members, and others; and by means of informal challenges and tests. The approach of dynamic assessment (Cicerone & Tupper, 1986; Lidz, 2000; Wiedl, 1999), including the concept of responsiveness to intervention (Mellard, Byrd, Johnson, Tollefson, & Boesche, 2004), can be especially useful, and appears to mitigate some of the cultural limitations of standardized tests (Peña, Iglesias, & Lidz, 2001). Formal and informal measures of adaptive behavior are likely to take a more prominent role in assessment, as well. Measures of change (Jorm, 2004; Stout, Ready, Grace, Malloy, & Paulsen, 2003) also mitigate some of the cultural limitations of standardized tests. These types of approaches may also be more readily applicable by rehabilitation workers with limited training (Jorm, 2004).

The thought of clinical neuropsychology without tests may seem an oxymoron to some, like poetry without words. This chapter is not the place to focus on the development of this idea, because the topic is rehabilitation; more about this approach can be found in manuals for CBR (Helander, Mendis, Nelson, & Goerdt, 1989; Judd, 2003; Judd & Winegardner, 1990; Werner, 1990).

Activity Analysis. Using natural activities to facilitate recovery does not mean abandoning what has been learned about cognitive abilities and their rehabilitation. Instead, it means recognizing those abilities in their natural contexts. This can be done through activity analysis. (The more common term is task analysis, but this suggests a goal directedness and an onerous quality to activities that may be neither, although they can facilitate recovery, for instance, playing with a young child or enjoying a soccer game.)

When a natural activity such as grocery shopping is no longer possible or practical, the cognitive specialist can observe and analyze the activity (Table 19.4) in light of the known limitations in the person's cognitive abilities and behavior in order to determine what might be getting in the way of success. The person can be encouraged to continue with those parts of the activity that are still possible. For the parts that are difficult or impossible, the cognitive specialist can look for ways to compensate for them and/or for strategies to relearn them.

Conventional cognitive rehabilitation might well advocate embarking on an elaborate program designed to strengthen these base cognitive skills in the clinic, then generalize them to the community. The natural recovery approach, by contrast, looks at those same impaired cognitive processes where they interfere with the shopping process and builds programs of compensation and/or restoration in the context of the shopping trip. For example, someone with visual scanning difficulties might have a goal of finding five items in 5 min in the store, with a family member cueing the area of the aisle to search, and with a left-to-right, top-to-bottom searching strategy.

Activity analysis goes beyond cognitive analysis to include attention to behavioral and emotional difficulties that might hinder an activity. Fatigue, frustration, impulsiveness, anger, discouragement, talkativeness, and similar problems along with their precipitants and consequences need to be taken into account in planning recuperative activities. For example, someone who is depressed and discouraged generally should be working closer to their zone of boredom within the zone of recovery (further to the left in Table 19.3), with activities that are only slightly challenging, so as to maximize success experiences. A shopping trip may need to include a planned rest for fatigue and a signal from a family member to interrupt talkativeness. A student may be able to learn in a small group in the morning but need individual help by afternoon.

Environmental Analysis. The natural recovery model also implies a relatively new role for rehabilitation workers evaluating the adequacy of the environment for facilitating recovery. Although this is something that rehabilitation workers have been doing informally for many years, it generally receives little attention in rehabilitation texts, research, and training. Home evaluation is well developed for related specific purposes such as wheelchair accessibility, but this is different from evaluating potential for facilitating recovery.

TABLE 19.4

Example of Activity Analysis

Functional Activity: Grocery Shopping

Functional components:

Remembering what are staples of the kitchen

Remembering or observing which staples are used up or about to be used up

Planning meals

    Remembering and taking into account the schedules of household members

    Remembering and taking into account the preferences of household members

    Remembering the ingredients required for meals planned

    Remembering if those ingredients are in the kitchen

    Remembering how long various perishables last and taking that into account in meal planning

Planning and budgeting and taking adequate money

Planning and managing transportation to and from the market

Taking appropriate security precautions throughout the excursion

Planning an efficient route in the market

Searching for and finding items

Judging price for value relative to a budget

Judging nutritional value

Arranging items so that they don't get crushed

Making appropriate judgements about possible unplanned purchases

Making appropriate substitutions for items which are unavailable, too expensive, or of poor quality

Dealing with the stimulation and social interactions of a market

Managing money at the time of purchase, and monitoring the transaction for possible errors

Storing purchases appropriately and remembering where they are stored

Cognitive components:

long-term memory

new learning

selective attention

planning

judgment

reasoning

flexibility

visual scanning

arithmetic

communication.

There are paradigms for evaluating rehabilitation centers, convalescent centers, and transitional facilities, but many of these come from an institutional perspective such as certification that does not allow for an easy judgment of whether the facility is the best place for a particular individual. Nor do they necessarily allow for comparing the facility with alternatives such as home.

Except in limited circumstances of imminent threat to life or limb, the decision of where to pursue recovery is, in theory, the consumer's decision. The rehabilitation professional can contribute to this decision by helping with a careful evaluation of the choices. In the absence of other guidelines, the outline in Table 19.5 is offered for this purpose. Although the relative weighting of various factors must be subjective in the absence of empirical data, nevertheless these guidelines may help in at least making sure that few important factors are overlooked.

Environmental analysis includes not just the physical accessibility of the environment, but also the cognitive, recreational, productivity, and social resources. The social environment is evaluated, including community access; who is available for training and assistance; and what are the attitudes, abilities, and knowledge of those in the person's social circle.

Finally, environmental analysis includes consideration of the person–environment fit. People often function substantially differently in their own kitchens, workshops, computer systems, neighborhoods, social circles, and so on, than they do in those of the clinic, and so many functional activities are best evaluated and treated in their natural contexts.

Environmental analysis then becomes a major foundation for rehabilitation planning, alongside consideration of the problems and strengths of the person to be rehabilitated.

Family and Community Training (Natural Helpers). Natural recovery exploits the presence and motivation of people in the social circle of the person with the brain dysfunction, most usually family, in structuring activities and experiences that facilitate recuperation. Family and community education and training are therefore critical components in professional intervention to facilitate natural recovery. This process goes beyond giving information about the condition and its manifestations. It involves direct training in how to structure activities and experiences, how to set goals, how to approach new activities, and how to train others who will be with the person. A repertoire of teaching and training modalities is called for (Table 19.6; Blosser & DePompei, 1995; Werner & Bower, 1982; Willer, Allen, Anthony, & Cowlan, 1993), to be matched to the needs, culture, and style of the learner and the nature of the material. Selection of trainees, materials, and teaching techniques becomes a central part of rehabilitation planning. These selections need to be individualized to the circumstances. This

TABLE 19.5

Evaluating and Modifying the Environment of Recovery

In addition to evaluating the person, the rehabilitation professional evaluates the environment of recovery (home, workplace, school, community) and plans appropriate modifications, including educating and training the social environment.

The Physical Environment

Building set-up: Wheelchair accessibility, stairs, access to outside

Emergency preparation: Escape, emergency equipment, getting help

Materials organization: Complexity, consistent location and labeling of materials, presence of distractors, noise

Memory and orientation: Calendars, appointment book, schedules, clocks, alarms, phone list, phone book

Planning/follow through: Lists for money management, transportation, shopping, home maintenance, task directions

Recreation resources: Games, sports, hobbies, TV, video, music, computer, reading, pets

Productivity resources: Kitchen, workshop, craft area, garden, animals, desk, office, computer

Community access: Alone or accompanied, availability of accompaniment, transportation, accessible community resources, barriers, access via telephone, computer, mail, etc.

Risks: Alcohol, drugs, weapons, sharp tools, vehicles, machinery, electricity, toxics, traffic

The Social Environment

Who is present?

What are their: Attitudes toward disability and teaching, skills, relationships with the person, availability to be trained, availability to provide training/guidance to the person

Who comes to visit?

Who is available in the community, and how?

Expectations of the environment: Family milieu and expectations; physical, cognitive, emotional, and social job requirements/school expectations

The Person's Functioning Within the Environment

Ability to orient to and attend to the environment and community and to their expectations

Independent living

Mobility in the environment, self-care, bathroom use, safety, meal preparation, chores

Use of time within the environment

Use of schedule, realistic scheduling, pacing of rest breaks, frustration tolerance

Communication with and ability to relate to others in the environment

Use of, interest in, and preinjury experience with each of the resources previously listed.

Note. From "The Importance of a Home Evaluation for Brain Injured Clients: A Team Approach," by S. A. Starch and E. A. Falltrick, 1990, *Cognitive Rehabilitation*, 8(6).

TABLE 19.6
Training Natural Helpers

The natural recovery model involves training natural helpers to carry out rehabilitation through everyday activities. Natural helpers are those who are in a position to help, are predisposed to, and can be trained. These may include family members, friends, hired caregivers, schoolmates, teachers, coworkers, supervisors, or members of a community rehabilitation cooperative.

Rehabilitation planning includes:

Selecting trainees

Selecting materials

Selecting teaching and training modalities matched to the needs, culture, and style of the learner and the nature of the material.

Natural helper training includes:

How to set goals

How to approach new activities

How to structure activities and experiences to facilitate recovery

How to cue and fade cues

How to cope with and manage problem emotions and behavior

How to use and train cognitive compensations

How to train others who will be with the person

Techniques of natural helper training

Answering questions

Modeling

Coaching

Mentoring

Individually written materials

Printed materials

Visual aids

Socratic dialogue

Storytelling

Metaphor

Family conferences

Support groups

Circles of support

Rehabilitation cooperatives

Group discussion

Videos

Teaching to teach others

change in perspective also implies that rehabilitation specialists need to be taught to be trainers and teachers.

Training Generalization. Neurorehabilitation programs are often limited by their recipients' difficulties in generalizing what they have learned (Sohlberg & Mateer, 2001). Skills and strategies learned in one context or task may not be readily applied in another. The rehabilitation specialist can assist the natural helpers in selecting activities that will help to generalize previously learned skills, and that will fall within the zone of recovery of the person with the brain illness. For example, in the case of Franz described earlier, his way-finding skills can be generalized by picking progressively more challenging destinations with varying means of transportation. His relearned skills in using written directions, using a cell phone, or asking for directions can be generalized by having him accomplish some errand at his destination.

Incorporating Cognitive and Emotional Strategies. Once a goal and the steps toward achieving it have been identified, there could be satisfactory progress that needs no further planning. But it could be that the process gets stuck, or does not proceed sufficiently fast. That is the point at which some cognitive (Cicerone & Tupper, 1990; Sohlberg & Mateer, 2001) or emotional (Judd, 1999, 2003) strategies may be needed. Sometimes the recovering person or the helping person, being close to the situation, may be able to come up with something that works. If not, then the cognitive rehabilitation specialist or neuropsychotherapist has a large repertoire of techniques that may be of help. The list of possibilities is long: memory books, electronic organizers, alarms, cue cards, mnemonics, study skills, rehearsal strategies, verbal mediation, tape recorders, "stop and think" strategies, errorless learning, problem-solving protocols, computer programs, relaxation techniques, cue cards, and self-talk to name but a few (Table 19.7). These techniques can be selected based on knowledge of the person's neuropsychological strengths and weaknesses.

Returning to Franz once again, suppose that his difficulty finding his way home is due to attentional difficulties. The suggestion that he try to find his way home from two blocks away without help has made it a sustained attention task, one that can be measured, repeated, and made easier or more difficult as needed to encounter his zone of recovery. The suggestion can also be modified to include explicit strategies for maintaining his attention.

Using these few principles, a natural recovery model of neuropsychological rehabilitation incorporates many of the important components that have been identified for cognitive rehabilitation (Sohlberg & Mateer, 2001). It is theory-based, goal-directed, repetitive, progressive training in impaired cognitive skills with knowledge of results and training

TABLE 19.7
Cognitive and Emotional Strategies

The natural recovery model uses the same cognitive and emotional strategies as conventional neurorehabilitation. These focus on functional goals established by the person, family, and other relevant community members.

Compensatory Strategies

Attention compensations; noise reduction, clutter reduction, interruption reduction, activity pacing, task structuring

Memory compensations; notebooks, alarms, calendars, computers, personal electronic organizers, lists, organization of space, orientation center, memory meetings, other people

Executive function compensations; written or drawn procedures, lists, organization of space, routines, schedules, other people

Restoration Strategies

Training in the use of compensations followed by reduction of use of compensation

Cueing and fading of cueing

Shadowing

Hierarchy of difficulty

Zone of recovery

Paced rehearsal

Errorless learning

Emotional Rehabilitation

Recognizing risks and warning signs

Back off, calm down, try again

Coaching and guiding

Pacing

Self-talk

Rehearsal

Cue cards

for generalization to practical situations. It goes beyond cognitive rehabilitation, however, to address emotional, interpersonal, productive, cultural, spiritual, and recreational issues, as well (Judd, 1999, 2003).

Coping With Overprotection

Although coping with overprotection is not a distinctive part of the natural recovery model, it is a common theme in rehabilitation in developing regions. Overprotection occurs when family and other caregivers do much

19. NATURAL RECOVERY 361

more than is necessary to help the injured person or do not allow that person to do things they are able to do safely. It frequently limits the experiences necessary for recovery and restricts the person's life options overall. It also frequently burdens families unnecessarily. Although overprotection of the person with the brain illness by their family (and sometimes by rehabilitation staff) is encountered from time to time in the developed world, it has not received a great deal of attention in the dominant rehabilitation literature (Croteau & Le Dorze, 1999). It appears to be a much more significant problem in many developing countries, however (A. Ardila [1996], A. M. Campos [2000], A. Dugbarty [1999], L. Gregory [1999], J. L. Henriquez [1989], F. Madrigal [1994], I. Martinez [1995], E. Sequeira [1988], U. Shah [2001], S. Tollman [1999], T. Villaseñor [1996], rehabilitation [neuro]psychologists from Colombia, Guatemala, Ghana, Zimbabwe, El Salvador, Costa Rica, Panama, Nicaragua, India, South Africa, and Mexico, respectively, personal communications). For this reason, an approach that is able to deal with this problem is very important to the natural recovery model, especially because it is often overprotective family members who will be called upon to carry out the rehabilitation. Overprotective behavior appears to have a number of different sources. Appropriate approaches to deal with this dynamic depend on which sources are responsible for the problem. Table 19.8 presents an initial attempt to address this situation.

At the same time, rehabilitation professionals need to be alert to the possibility that their perceptions of overprotection may represent cultural differences in the understanding of disability roles. For example, families that value interdependence (Condeluci, 1995) may not place high value on the cosmopolitan value of having their child move away from home by the early 20s, especially if that child has a disability. Likewise, it may be that family members are aware of dangers in the home and community that are not apparent to the rehabilitation professionals. For example, family members may know of members of the school or community who would take advantage of children who are socially disinhibited that rehabilitation professionals may not suspect. Also, family members may be culturally reluctant to communicate certain risks to professionals. For example, in some cultures it may be very difficult to talk about sexual risks, whereas in other cultures it is not proper to talk about risk of death.

Direct Neuropsychological Rehabilitation Services

Under the natural recovery model, when are direct neuropsychological rehabilitation services provided? First, they are involved in evaluation. Second, they may be involved in planning the modifications to the environment of recovery, whether that is within an institution or outside the rehabilitation system. Third, they are involved as part of the perspective

TABLE 19.8
Overprotection

Overprotection by families of people with brain dysfunction is a common problem in developing countries. Overcoming overprotection is critical for the natural recovery model. It requires understanding the multiple sources of overprotection, and having strategies for dealing with these.

General sources of overprotection

Lack of knowledge about: (1) recovery, (2) what rehabilitation is, (3) how to facilitate recovery, (4) the person's abilities, (5) community resources for people with disabilities

Acute-illness model

Passive attitude toward the medical system

Fatalism

Frustration

General strategies for dealing with overprotection (for the entire rehabilitation team)

Check the rehabilitation team's attitudes, expectations for families, modeling

Evaluate overprotection carefully first, then prioritize interventions

Educate all parties about recovery, prognosis, resources, an active model of rehabilitation

Involve the person and family in goal setting, treatment planning, treatment, record keeping

Redirect fatalism; focus on small steps, if necessary

Demonstrate the abilities of the person with the brain illness to the family

Train the family in proper care; observe them giving care and correct or adjust them.

Use support group or community to intervene and facilitate the person doing more.

Specific Sources of Overprotection and Corresponding Strategies
(for mental health professionals)

Overprotection Source	Clinical Strategy
Ill person or family member exercising control	Give other ways of exercising control, explore relationship dynamics
Caregiver fulfilled by role	Look for other ways of fulfilling role, present caregiving as helping with recovery
Expressed love and caring	Look for other ways to express love and caring, present caregiving as helping with recovery
Financial or other incentives	Make incentives for recovery more attractive, or eliminate disincentives for recovery
Guilt	Find other ways to forgive oneself
Fear	Explore fears and address them directly
Community standards	Identify and educate relevant community members
Embarrassment	Educate family and community, work on public presentation, reduce sources of embarrassment, work on attitude, use dramatization, support groups, desensitization, modeling
Following outdated discharge orders	Bring orders up to date

whenever other rehabilitation services, such as PT, OT, Speech Therapy, and so forth, are provided. Finally, the following factors may contribute to a decision to suggest supplementing home/community efforts with direct neuropsychological rehabilitation services:

1. When the person with the injury and/or family and community are unable or unwilling to provide adequate structure due to lack of time, inability, or interpersonal dynamics.
2. When it appears that motivation may be better for a professionally oriented program than a home-based and/or community-based program.
3. When the condition of the person is so complicated or difficult as to make a home-based and/or community-based approach inadequate.
4. When special circumstances suggest that a particularly intensive program is needed (for example, a deadline for recovery, an irreplaceable individual with a high level of responsibility).
5. When a home-based and/or community-based program is failing and cannot be fixed.

The main difference from prevailing models of neuropsychological rehabilitation in this regard is that the presumption is that rehabilitation should take place in the home with natural helpers unless direct professional services are necessary, rather than the presumption that rehabilitation should take place in the hospital or clinic with professionals unless circumstances do not permit it.

THE NATURAL RECOVERY MODEL IN THE CONTEXT OF COMMUNITY-BASED REHABILITATION (CBR)

The World Health Organization began supporting the model of CBR in 1978 (Mitchell, 1999a; World Health Organization, 1982) and developed a manual for community workers over the following decade (Helander et al., 1989). This model involves a three-tiered system in which lay members of the community (local supervisors), usually volunteers, are trained in basic rehabilitation techniques for common disabilities. They provide direct rehabilitation services to people with disabilities in their homes, in community centers, in schools, in community clinics, in workplaces, and so forth. They also train designated family members (family trainers) and others to continue with the training for their particular family member. They work in coordination with community institutions around issues such as transportation, childcare, social services, health services, disabled rights, community education, and other issues needing attention with respect to the needs of the people with disabilities. They refer difficult cases to specialized rehabilitation services. The local supervisors are trained by district rehabilitation professionals. The program is coordinated at a national level by the Ministry of Health (Mitchell, 1999a). In spite of initial enthusiasm, implementation of CBR remains very spotty, and formal evaluations are scarce (Mitchell, 1999b). Field reports, however, are quite promising (Mitchell, 1999b).

CBR is a particularly likely setting for implementing the natural recovery model. The principles of the natural recovery model described earlier are, for the most part, fairly simple. Communicating them adequately to local supervisors and training their implementation is not likely to be difficult. Local supervisors may even prove better than professionals at processes such as encountering the zone of recovery, environmental analysis, training family trainers, and generalization training. What continues to be lacking are simplified means of teaching neuropsychological concepts such as the components of cognition, executive functions, and altered emotions, as well as simplified means for evaluating these. It may be that such assessments will need to take place at a district level, with psychologists and other neurorehabilitation professionals providing assessments and collaborating with local supervisors and family trainers in developing treatment plans. It remains a challenge for neuropsychology to develop methods of evaluation for treatment planning purposes that could be implemented, at least in straightforward cases, by local supervisors.

CBR is based primarily on a model of identifying disabled individuals already living in the community and offering them rehabilitation. A significant part of neurorehabilitation takes place after traumatic brain injuries, cerebral vascular accidents, or similar acute brain conditions. In such instances, a natural recovery model incorporated into a CBR model might allow for a much earlier discharge from district acute in-patient rehabilitation facilities or even acute care facilities to the CBR program. Needed assessments might then come with the individual.

The application of cognitive strategies is most likely an area for collaboration between neurorehabilitation professionals and local supervisors. The professionals can bring to this process their knowledge of general principles and techniques that have served in other contexts, while the local supervisors can bring their knowledge of local resources and conditions. It is in this type of interaction where much of the cross-cultural adaptation of neurorehabilitation is likely to take place.

The Politics of Implementing the Natural Recovery Model

Any group attempting to implement a natural recovery model within a given community/rehabilitation system will first need to consider the motivations and power structure of the existing system. Much of this will be specific to local conditions, but some common themes are likely. As with CBR, the natural recovery model faces political, institutional, and attitudinal barriers. Perhaps most important, the natural recovery model disempowers rehabilitation professionals and institutions and empowers families and people with disabilities. Professionals may find it difficult to relinquish control over the rehabilitation process, and to collaborate with goals that do not fit with their priorities and/or activities with which they may not be familiar. They may fear for their jobs if lay people are able to carry out many of their functions. They may not be trained to train others. They may resist changing their usual way of operating or resist venturing into the community (Pace et al., 1999). Rehabilitation funding is often based on direct service delivery rather than on training, making it difficult to get funding for services based on a natural recovery model. Family members and people with disabilities may resist being trained, or may feel that they are getting inferior service, or that they are being asked to do for free what they are entitled to get from the rehabilitation system.

There are a number of potential ways around these barriers. In some settings, the implementation of a natural recovery model may come about through the demands of or within communities of people with brain disabilities (Lysack & Kaufert, 1994). Pilot projects with enthusiastic participants may provide models that make the possibilities more accessible to those with doubts. Training rehabilitation specialists to train others can be incorporated into the development of programs and, eventually, into the standard curricula of those disciplines. Professional identities can be restructured around new roles. There may be some reassurance about job security in being seen as the conduit for new technologies. It seems to be part of the nature of the development of many psychological technologies, for example, that they are first implemented by professionals, then by paraprofessionals, and eventually enter the popular culture. Relaxation techniques are a good example of this process. Professionals then advance to the development of new techniques and to dealing with ever more specialized circumstances.

Adjusting funding patterns presents a more formidable challenge, especially where funding is from large institutions. As with CBR, the implementation of natural recovery models may need to rely in large part on volunteer labor, community resources, and grant funding, at least in some settings. Only when cost effectiveness can be demonstrated may it become possible to seek more conventional and stable funding. The model may also come to be implemented initially in parallel with and supplementary to conventional outpatient rehabilitation services. Family members may be motivated to participate by beginning with goals that will reduce the burden of care. Their personal knowledge and cultural expertise may need to be acknowledged and valued in order for them to feel capable of offering quality assistance to their loved ones. They will also need to feel that they have support and consultation when they are uncertain about how to proceed.

Advantages and Challenges

The natural recovery model has a number of advantages over formal therapy-centered approaches. It facilitates cultural adaptation. It empowers and promotes autonomy and family unity. It deals with the problem of generalization of rehabilitation efforts. It potentially allows for greater distribution of scarce rehabilitation resources. It is often intrinsically motivating. It takes advantage of the knowledge and abilities of family and community members and may reduce inappropriate overprotection. It accomplishes all of this while getting practical things done in the life of the recovering person, family, and community. It is often less expensive. As such it may prove attractive to prepay or health maintenance financing systems.

This model also has challenges, of course. It does not fit easily into existing models of rehabilitation services, particularly fee-for-service models. It requires greater flexibility on the part of rehabilitation staff. By its nature, natural recovery must be individualized, which makes controlled measurement of its effects more problematic for the research minded. To some, the natural recovery model may seem too natural, that is, it may appear to be what everyone does anyhow. Although there certainly are many people who are very good teachers in this sense, the ability is by no means universal. And even teachers who are very good at breaking down activities and encountering the zone of recovery often are not aware of specific cognitive compensations that have been developed as part of cognitive rehabilitation technology. Furthermore, the people who are naturally good at assisting people with recovery are not necessarily the people who find themselves responsible for people with brain disabilities. So the natural recovery model faces the challenge of identifying good trainers and putting them in responsible positions or taking the people who are in responsible positions and teaching them to be good trainers.

CONCLUSIONS

In some senses, the natural recovery model is extremely old, and has only very recently begun to be supplanted, in small part, by various professional service models. But as a systematized and professionally scrutinized model, it is quite new and has barely been tried. It remains to be seen whether or not such a model can be successfully implemented within existing rehabilitation systems, and whether research can be successfully carried out on such a model without regimenting it into a caricature of itself. Meanwhile, the model itself could well skip much of the professional stage of development and enter (somewhat) popular culture by way of brain injury support groups, family groups, and foundations. Hopefully, this model can provide ways to make the knowledge of neuropsychology more practically applicable in a wide variety of cultures, thereby bringing its benefits to larger numbers of those with brain illnesses throughout the world.

REFERENCES

Anderson, J., & Parente, F. (1985). Training family members to work with the head injured patient. *Cognitive Rehabilitation, 3*(4), 12–15.

Ardila, A., & Rosselli, M. (1992). *Neuropsicología Clínica* [Clinical Neuropsychology]. Medellín, Colombia: Prensa Creativa.

Backman, L. (1992). Memory training and memory improvement in Alzheimer's disease: Rules and exceptions. *Acta Neurologica Scandinavica, 85,* 84–89.

Blosser, J. L., & DePompei, R. (1995). Fostering effective family involvement through mentoring. *Journal of Head Trauma Rehabilitation, 10*(2), 46–56.

Boschen, K., & Krane, N. (1992). A history of independent living in Canada. *Canadian Journal of Rehabilitation, 6,* 79–88.

Cicerone, K. D., & Tupper, D. E. (1986). Cognitive assessment in the neuropsychological rehabilitation of head-injured adults. In B. P. Uzzell & Y. Gross (Eds.), *Clinical neuropsychology of intervention* (pp. 59–83). Boston: Martinus Nijhoff.

Cicerone, K. D., & Tupper, D. E. (1990). Neuropsychological rehabilitation: Treatment of errors in everyday functioning. In D. E. Tupper & K. D. Cicerone (Eds.), *The neuropsychology of everyday life: Issues in development and rehabilitation* (pp. 271–292). Boston: Kluwer Academic Publishing.

Condeluci, A. (1995). *Interdependence: The route to community.* Boca Raton, FL: CRC Press.

Croteau, C., & Le Dorze, G. (1999). Overprotection in couples with aphasia. *Disability and Rehabilitation, 21,* 432–437.

Fletcher-Janzen, E., Strickland, T. L., & Reynolds, C. R. (Eds.). (2000). *Handbook of cross-cultural neuropsychology.* New York: Kluver/Plenum.

Gianutsos, R. (1992). The computer in cognitive rehabilitation: It's not just a tool anymore. *Journal of Head Trauma Rehabilitation, 7*(3), 26–35.

Gordon, W. A., Hibbard, M. R., & Kreutzer, J. S. (1989). Cognitive remediation: Issues in research and practice. *Journal of Head Trauma Rehabilitation, 4*(3), 76–84.

Granger, C. V. (1998). The emerging science of functional assessment: Our tool for outcomes analysis. *Archives of Physical Medicine and Rehabilitation, 79,* 235–240.

Helander, E., Mendis, P., Nelson, G., & Goerdt, A. (1989). *Training in the community for people with disabilities.* Geneva: World Health Organization.

Held, J. M. (1993). Recovery after damage. In H. Cohen (Ed.), *Neuroscience for rehabilitation* (pp. 388–405). Philadelphia: Lippincott.

Johnston, M., & Tjandrakusuma, H. (1982). Reaching the disabled. *World Health Forum, 3,* 307–310.

Jorm, A. F. (2004). The Informant Questionnaire on Cognitive Decline in the Elderly (IQCODE): A review. *International Psychogeriatrics, 16,* 275–293.

Judd, T. (1999). *Neuropsychotherapy and community integration: Brain illness, emotions, and behavior.* New York: Kluver/Plenum.

Judd, T. (2003). Rehabilitation of the emotional problems of brain disorders in developing countries. *Neuropsychological Rehabilitation, 13,* 307–325.

Judd, T., & Winegardner, J. (1990). Manual of practical neuropsychology (2nd ed.). Unpublished manuscript.

Kreutzer, J. S., Gordon, W. A., & Wehman, P. (1989). Cognitive remediation following traumatic brain injury. *Rehabilitation Psychology, 34,* 117–130.

Lidz, C. (Ed.). (2000). *Dynamic assessment: Prevailing models and applications.* New York: Elsevier.

Lysack, C., & Kaufert, J. (1994). Comparing the origins and ideologies of the independent living movement and community based rehabilitation. *International Journal of Rehabilitation Research, 17,* 231–240.

Mellard, D. F., Byrd, S. E., Johnson, E., Tollefson, J. M., & Boesche, L. (2004). Foundations and research on identifying model responsiveness-to-intervention sites. *Learning Disability Quarterly. 27,* 243–256.

Mitchell, R. (1999a). Community-based rehabilitation: The generalized model. *Disability and Rehabilitation, 21,* 522–528.

Mitchell, R. (1999b). The research base of community-based rehabilitation. *Disability and Rehabilitation, 21,* 459–468.

O'Hara, C. C., & Harrell, M. (1991). *Rehabilitation with brain injury survivors: An empowerment approach.* Gaithersburg, MD: Aspen.

Pace, G. M., Schlund, M. W., Hazard-Haupt, T., Christensen, J. R., Lashno, M., McIver, J., Peterson, K., & Morgan, K. A. (1999). Characteristics and outcomes of a home and community-based neurorehabilitation programme. *Brain Injury, 13,* 535–546.

Parente, R., & Stapleton, M. (1993). An empowerment model of memory training. *Applied Cognitive Psychology, 7,* 585–602.

Peat, M. (1991). Community based rehabilitation: Development and structure (Part I). *Clinical Rehabilitation, 3,* 219–227.

Peña, E., Iglesias, A., & Lidz, C. S. (2001). Reducing test bias through dynamic assessment of children's word learning ability. *American Journal of Speech-Language Pathology 10,* 138–154.

Purdy, M., & Neri, L. (1989). Computer-assisted cognitive rehabilitation in the home. *Cognitive Rehabilitation, 7*(6), 34–38.

Schneidert, M., Hurst, R., Miller, J., & Üstün, B. (2003). The role of environment in the international classification of functioning, disability and health. *Disability and Rehabilitation, 25,* 588–595.

Selzer, M. E. (1995). Mechanisms of functional recovery in traumatic brain injury. *Journal of Neurorehabilitation, 9,* 73–82.

Sohlberg, M., & Mateer, C. A. (2001). *Cognitive rehabilitation: An integrative neuropsychological approach.* New York: Guilford.

Starch, S. A., & Falltrick, E. A. (1990). The importance of a home evaluation for brain injured clients: A team approach. *Cognitive Rehabilitation, 8*(6), 28–32.

Stout, J. C., Ready, R. E., Grace, J., Malloy, P. F., & Paulsen, J. S. (2003). Factor analysis of the Frontal Systems Behavior Scale (FrSBe). *Assessment. 10,* 79–85.

The tough case: Life care plan for a behaviorally challenging patient. (1993, March/April). *Headlines, 4*(2), 18–19.

Vygotsky, L. S. (1978). *Mind in society: The development of higher psychological processes.* Cambridge, MA: Harvard University Press.

Werner, D. (1990). *Disabled village children.* Palo Alto, CA: Hesperian Foundation.

Werner, D., & Bower, B. (1982). *Helping health workers learn.* Palo Alto, CA: Hesperian Foundation.

Wiedl, K. H. (1999). Cognitive modifiability as a measure of readiness for rehabilitation. *Psychiatric Services, 50,* 1411–1413.

Willer, B. S., Allen, K., Anthony, J., & Cowlan, G. (1993). *Circles of support for individuals with acquired brain injury*. Buffalo, NY: Rehabilitation Research and Training Center on Community Integration of Persons with Traumatic Brain Injury.

Willer, B., & Corrigan, J. D. (1994). Whatever it takes: A model for community-based services. *Brain Injury, 8,* 647–659.

Wilson, C., & Robertson, I., H. (1992). A home-based intervention for attentional slips during reading following head injury: A single case study. *Neuropsychological Rehabilitation, 2,* 193–205.

World Health Organization. (1981). *Disability prevention and rehabilitation: Report of the WHO expert committee on disability prevention and rehabilitation*. Geneva, Switzerland: Author.

World Health Organization. (1982, June 28–July 3)). *Community based rehabilitation*. Report of a WHO interregional consultation, Columbo, Sri Lanka. Geneva, Switzerland: Author.

Yamey, G., & Greenwood, R. (2004). Religious views of the "medical" rehabilitation model: A pilot qualitative study. *Disability and Rehabilitation, 26,* 455–462.

Chapter 20

Emotions and Attitudes: Unbundling Sociocultural Influences

SHIRLEY G. TOLLMAN
University of KwaZulu Natal

> Umona usuka esweni utshele inhliziyo.
> Jealousy is evoked by a visual image, and
> then directs behavioural actions.
>
> —Zulu Proverb

This ancient Zulu saying encapsulates the essential wisdom of neuropsychology—that there is a network of reciprocal relationships between behavior, biological functions, and the surrounding environmental condition.

Behavioral responses are inextricably linked to each person's unique sociocultural heritage. All individuals are born into and develop within a particular sociocultural and educational milieu. It follows then that socialization within that culture will shape the way in which the individual thinks, interprets the world, and responds. Neuropsychologists therefore need to understand these influences in order to correctly interpret behavioral responses and to develop appropriate assessment and rehabilitation techniques.

Cultural factors present subtle and pervasive confounding variables. The importance of the sociohistorical context for shaping the development of children, their higher mental functions, thoughts, attitudes, activities, and goals was pointed to by Luria (1976), whereas Vygotsky (1978) emphasized the mediating role of parents, teachers, and "informed others" in the process of cultural transmission. Each culture has its own "species-specific" social organization, and so the behavior of the developing child is shaped for adaptive functioning within that society. The individual internalizes the social norms, communicatory cues, the mannerisms, the aspirations, and even the thinking mode of its own particular culture.

In sum, from the moment of birth, we are shown which of the features of the environmental stimuli need to be attended to, and which must be ignored, what information is important to process, and what information is not, what is beautiful and what is ugly, when to be fearful and when to be happy, and how to please, and how to anger. The perceptions and ideas, the beliefs and attitudes, the social mores and meanings of responses that are initially imposed by external sources, such as the ecological system, become internalized, and incorporated into the functional organisation of the brain. In turn, this unique brain connects individuals with the world, and mediates their particular responses.

PLAN: UNBUNDLING SOCIAL AND EMOTIONAL INFLUENCES

The sections that follow demonstrate the profound effects that each particular ecosystem exerts on the individual. It is argued that in order to obtain reliability and validity, an intimate knowledge not only of neuropsychology, but also of the prevailing culture, is essential.

This chapter, in demonstrating the impact of culture on social and emotional behavior, draws mainly on research with the multicultural South African community. In particular, on contrasts between the South Africans with a westernized cultural heritage and their traditional African counterparts who embrace an "ancestral-spiritual" culture with direct unity between past, present, and future lives. Notwithstanding, it must be remembered that there are universals; parallels with other multicultural societies world-wide. Lezak (1995, p. 99) used the term "species-wide performance expectations" to describe the many cognitive functions and skills that follow a common course of development that is maturational, rather than being dependent on social learning. However, the complex behaviors that characterize our emotions and attitudes, our social lives, incorporate the social mores of the society.

In demonstrating the pervasive effects of culture on social and emotional issues, the sections that follow focus on similar emotional presentations but different meanings, such as eye contact and spontaneous speech; the individual in society—different worldviews—ancestral influences, and behavioral pathology—how cultural perspectives differ regarding causation;

individual versus collective identity—nuclear and extended family system, the individual within the community, and self-awareness; data analysis—communities in flux—a rapid rural-urban drift,[1] including populations in transition, the nature–nurture issue and psychometric versus qualitative information, and psychometric tests.

SIMILAR EMOTIONAL PRESENTATIONS BUT DIFFERENT MEANINGS

Different cultures have imposed different meanings on similar responses. Even expressions of emotion are culturally determined, and unless the culture is understood, the behavior could be misinterpreted.

Eye Contact and Spontaneous Speech

Within a western framework, direct eye contact is construed as a sign of acknowledgment, an attempt to make contact, perhaps even a gesture of good faith and honesty, whereas appropriate spontaneous speech is seen as a sign of self-confidence and good adjustment. From a traditional African perspective, however, the reverse is true. Direct eye contact, and speaking without having been addressed, is seen as a sign of disrespect and insolence, especially toward an elder. Zulu children are taught to obey and uphold authority figures. As a sign of respect, the eyes are averted when talking to a "superior," and a strict hierarchy based on factors including age, ancestry, leadership, and so forth exists. In any interview situation, the clinician or therapist represents an authority figure and so eye-to-eye contact is avoided, as is a spontaneous offering of speech or behavior. Such behavior, when assessed according to a western frame of reference, could be indicative of adynamia and/or pathological inertia.

The following incident exemplifies the issue: A child from a traditional African background was brought to see the author for a medicolegal assessment because the child had been involved in a motor vehicle accident. A previous psychologist, not versed in traditional African custom, had maintained that there was nothing wrong with the child's behavior, and he was in fact well behaved. However, the father was insisting that the child's behavior had changed, and he had become unmanageable and disrespectful. When the father was asked to elaborate on his assertion, he responded, "he looks me straight in the eyes." From a western perspective, this would be a "normal" response from a child, but from a traditional African viewpoint, it indi-

---

[1] The rapid urbanization of rural communities in South Africa, and the interaction between communities, means that Africanized and westernized cultures are slowly being integrated. In addition, the new dispensation in South Africa, the poorer rural communities are at different stages of their development in terms of rural–urban; illiterate–literate; socioeconomic climate.

cated to the parents a sign of disturbance. Indeed, further probing confirmed dysinhibited behavior.

Another sign of disturbance from a traditional African perspective is the display of anger. Anger is greatly feared, and must be controlled, because if not, it will result in evil actions (Thorpe, 1991). This is in contrast to the modern western view, which views the suppression of emotions as harmful, and encourages socially appropriate (verbal) expression of negative emotions, anger included. Indeed, when emotions are successfully inhibited, the individuals are labeled emotionally shallow. There are in fact, certain occasions where traditional Africans are encouraged to bring their anger to the surface, but these are at community gatherings, where the group comes together as a whole and can neutralize the negative or evil influence of the anger.

THE INDIVIDUAL IN SOCIETY: DIFFERENT WORLDVIEWS—ANCESTRAL INFLUENCES

In contrast to the westernized existential approach that focuses on the "here and the now," our traditional African colleagues hold that there is a reciprocal relationship between the living members of the family and those who have died—the ancestors are respected and honored, and included in family functions and decision-making processes, and in turn, the living family members rely on the ancestors for protection and prosperity.

African theologians suggest that God, the Supreme Being, is never far from an African's thoughts or perceptions of the world. (Kruger, Lubbe, & Steyn, 1996). Intermediaries are needed in order to facilitate communication with the Supreme Being, and these intermediaries are the ancestral spirits, or "living dead" (amadlozi). Thus, although ancestors are not worshipped as such, they are very much revered, remembered, and form an integral part of the living family's existence. The traditional African community consists of all family members, both living and dead, and the influence of these deceased ancestors is frequently not fully appreciated by westerners. Clinicians need to be cognizant of these frames of reference, and guard against misinterpreting cultural and social mores as psychopathology.

It is essential to find out about the ancestors and work within the aura that they have provided for family members.

In a society, such as the traditional African one, in which there is a continuity between past, present, and future life, rules for proper burial customs are of vital importance. If a person dies prematurely, or of a certain illness, witchcraft or sorcery is suspected—in such a case, the deceased person could be enlisted as a spirit helper for evil purposes, rather than as an ancestor for protecting the community (Thorpe, 1991). This concept has profound effects on many aspects of life, including attitudes toward illness. Certain causes of death, such as sexually transmitted diseases, are considered to be grounds for the denial of a proper burial. If a person is not buried properly, then they cannot take their place in the ancestral hierarchy, and consequently, cannot offer guidance and protection to those still living. Worse, however, is that they can be used for evil purposes. Therefore the cause of death that is given by the family of the deceased is sometimes opposed to the medically determined cause of death. The implications of this are far-reaching, especially with a disease such as AIDS, and requires a high degree of personal responsibility and precaution in order to halt its spread.

This excerpt from an article from the Sunday *Tribune* (December 3, 2000) illustrates the devastating misconceptions that can occur if allowance for culture is ignored:

> The AIDS campaign is a joke in this area ... young people simply don't believe it. They believe that witchcraft is the reason why they are sick and dying. They will tell you that a sickness curse has been placed on them by ancestors who are angry about political violence that displaced families from 1993 to 1997.

Cultural beliefs persist. In 2006, our Minister of Health in South Africa still only embraces ARV drugs in combination with cultural beliefs.

Behavioral Pathology: Cultural Perspectives Differ Regarding Causation

One consequence of the differing religious and cultural beliefs regarding the living individual's relationship with ancestors and other forces relates to the etiology of the pathology, that is, as a disturbance of "being" due to external forces, or, to internal factors arising from the socioecological environment? In the latter situation exemplifying a westernized view of the world—responsibility for change lies within the afflicted individual, whereas in the former, the traditional African view, disablement is due to external forces, and change, therefore, is beyond the control of the individual. Thus, the family spirits are believed to be in contact with the living relatives, and it is important to keep on favorable terms with these ancestors. There are several forms of ritual, all of which have their special uses. Some are used for harmful purposes, some are curative remedies, and others are love charms. From a western perspective, some of the procedures involved in these rituals have been interpreted as hallucinations!

From a traditional African perspective, the body and the spirit are one, and when people become dysfunctional, they are treated in their entirety, as if the body, the psyche, and in fact the entire community were suffering by extension. No distinction is made between the physical, visible being, and the invisible spirit being (Thorpe, 1991). Thus the community, whether living or deceased, plays an integral role in individual sickness and restoration of health. Their interventions have been misinterpreted to be superficial, treating only the symptoms and not the cause. For example, a brain lesion would not be regarded as a cause for severe headaches, but rather as a symptom. A cause would be something like witchcraft enacted by a deceased person who had not received a proper burial. In order to remediate the problem, certain rites and rituals are performed, the specifics of which are communicated to the traditional healers from the spirit realm (ancestors). Similarly, pain is not predominantly physical and individualistic, but is psychical and has deep social influences. Pain can be felt when relationships are troubled, or when there is political, economic, or environmental unrest. This pain cannot always be readily described, thus making it difficult for western clinicians to be of assistance. Thus, many western practitioners are regarded with skepticism and suspicion, and the clinician of choice would be a traditional healer.

Zulu traditional healers, or *izangoma*, differ in many ways from western clinicians. A primary difference is that izangoma diagnose and prescribe in consultation with the ancestors, and consequently are able to look into the past, as well as the future, by asking the ancestors for the required information. A Zulu patient would go to a traditional healer and expect to be told, rather than be asked, not only what was ailing them at that particular time, but also, aspects of their past as well as of their future. A doctor trained in a conventional western approach would glean information by asking questions of the patient, and come to a diagnosis in a different way. There would seem to be much to learn from diverse approaches.

One of the most difficult tasks, however, is that of the "sick" role that becomes much more clearly defined and acted out. To motivate an individual who has become the focus of the family because of illness frequently requires slotting into that approach and working from there.

INDIVIDUAL VERSUS COLLECTIVE IDENTITY—NUCLEAR AND EXTENDED FAMILY SYSTEMS

The Individual Within the Community

Western views also usually differ quite significantly from the traditional African view with regard to personal identity and the relative importance assigned to individual versus group needs. Western society encourages the development of a strong personal identity, whereas the traditional African perspective prizes a group identity. In the same way that there is an integration of body and spirit within a person, so too is there an integration of the individual within the community. As the westernized children develop, they learn to introspect, to be aware of their own needs, and to strive for "personal happiness." In contrast, the Africanized children learn to submerge their own desires in favor of the needs of the community—adaptive functioning is to "turn outwards," to be aware of and participate in the welfare of the society, and to negate personal desires. It must however always be borne in mind that cultural values are also impacted on by the prevailing ecological climate, such as poverty and apartheid.

This difference between western and African cultures was supported by Bentley (1983). He compared Scottish (western) and Swazi (African) individuals, and found significant differences in the frequency of responses that mentioned matters relating to marriage and family responsibilities. Bentley's results were congruent with Mehta, Rohila, Sundberg, and Taylor's (1972) findings on Americans, and this, he asserted, reflects a "Western society that emphasizes individuality rather than concern for family responsibilities which can be considered more characteristic of societies in which the extended family is extant" (Bentley, 1983, p. 228).

The differential effects that individually based and collectively based societies exert on the behavior of their members are pervasive and far-reaching. For example, westernized offspring tend to be nurtured by a nuclear family, or even a single parent, whereas in a traditional Zulu family, parental responsibility is diffused because the whole community takes responsibility for the upbringing of the child—hence the adage: "it takes a village to raise a child."

Traditional African society also consists of nuclear family units, but these units live within a close-knit community or clan, often sharing the same surname. The group takes precedence over the individual, because the individual is perceived to be unable to exist apart from the group (Thorpe, 1991). People within each community regard themselves as brothers, sisters, cousins, and so forth without necessarily being biologically related.

This familial structure confounds clinicians in various ways, namely:

1. Difficulties arise when trying to ascertain the primary parent/caretaker of a child, particularly when trying to establish stability of parenting.
2. The attempt to establish potential genetic patterns as a basis for behavioral dysfunction is not always possible because of the difficulties involved in determining who is in fact biologically related to whom.

Self-Awareness

The degree to which individuals accurately assess their strengths and weaknesses in relation to the rest of their society is considered an important prognosticator for rehabilitative success. Stuss (1999) pointed to the integrity of frontal lobe functioning as vital for an accurate evaluation of the self. However, a major problem stemming from individuals with different conceptions of their role within the society relates to the technique of introspection. The evaluation of responses and treatments based on introspection is an integral requirement when a behavioral assessment is made. However, the ability to focus on the "self," to explore inner feelings and needs would be highly developed in a society emphasizing "personal happiness," but not so in a society concerned with "group happiness." The community—socialized person learns to submerge personal feelings and personal needs in favor of group needs, and so develops skills for interpreting social cues and group requirements. Thus the question "how are you?" tended to elicit minimal response from our Zulu-speaking subjects, but not from their English first-language peers. Furthermore, when a traditional African parent is asked the age of their child, they may respond with the year of the child's birth, rather than the actual age, and if asked for the day and month, the parent may reply—"when the flowers grow," or "when there was the big rain." This reflects the significance of the social and environmental conditions at a particular time, rather than absolute age, which may not carry the same importance for the community. Answers such as these have been considered "ignorant"!

DATA ANALYSIS

Populations in Transition: A Rapid Rural–Urban Drift

In this section, the assumptions inherent in psychometric data are examined, and the importance of collecting qualitative data for cross-cultural neuropsychology is emphasized.

In 1936 the Marxist Party's Central Committee on pedagogical perversions banned all forms of psychometric testing on the grounds that it was antithetical to Marxist–Lenninist ideology (Cole & Maltzman, 1969). Cole and Maltzman (1969, p. 5) described this as "the single most important event in the development of Soviet Psychology during that era."

In South Africa, the issue is being revisited. On May 24, 1998, our most widely read newspaper, the Sunday *Times*, published the results of meetings that have decided to scrap many IQ tests and "Eurocentric" psychometric tests. It was stated, "Some intelligence tests are about to be scrapped because they 'favour whites.'" The move followed a meeting the previous week of top psychologists in Pretoria called in by the Government's advisory statutory council, the Human Sciences Research Council, which is responsible for standardizing IQ tests used at schools, hospitals, clinics, and in industries across South Africa. Psychologists have also raised major concerns recently about "Eurocentric" IQ tests used to stream all pupils in schools. Too often, test scores are not balanced against a pupil's cultural background. In the year 2000, revealing children's IQ test scores was banned, and further legislation for "culture fair" assessments are being tabled.

I believe that there is a parallel thread running between these two events: Both events occur at a time of social change, at a time of turbulence when the existing social order was, and still is, being restructured. It follows, therefore, that the existing tests are seen as preventing the process of change—and so we need to ask ourselves, in our pursuit of the "scientific" study of behaviour—why?

The Nature–Nurture Issue and Psychometric Versus Qualitative Information

Although the motives of the psychologists and politicians that led to such a dramatic rejection of our psychometric wisdom is arguable, one cannot deny its significance nor that embedded within each philosophical approach lies the riddle of the nature–nurture influences. However, in the same way that nature versus nurture is now accepted as a nonissue, so too, given the complexity of human behavior and its evanescent character psychometric versus qualitative is surely a nonissue—they are not mutually exclusive.

It is a truism that during development our intellectual activity becomes inextricably linked to our cultural, historical, and institutional settings. It is these that are not unraveled by psychometric tests alone. When there is a restructuring of society, existing tests must be adapted to encompass the changes. Tests that do not allow for different cultures, and for movement viz from rural to urban, from illiterate to literate, must be developed.

As neuropsychologists, our task is to develop assessment procedures that will reliably and validly allow us to identify intact and impaired cognitive, social, and emotional processes as a result of brain trauma (or any other form of environmental disturbance). As stated previously, children are born into a particular ecological system and learn socially to understand, interpret, and interact with the world according to their own historical and sociocultural environment. The influence of education is also integral in developing responses.

Psychometric Tests

Psychometric tests provide the norms for a particular society, and from this, we can determine to what extent the person deviates from the norm in relation to that particular group, and therefore the degree to which they must deviate in order to validly suggest that there is brain dysfunction.

In order to derive a norm for an intact population, the sample must represent a microcosm of a particular society. Thus the sample must be large, about 1,000; and it must be relatively homogenous in terms of culture, socioeconomic status, education, age, and even in some cases, gender.

Luria (1976) found that tests developed and validated in one culture, repeatedly produced experimental failures and invalidated studies of other cultures. Tasks, therefore, have to be developed that subjects of the particular culture in question will find meaningful. These tasks must be meaningful both in terms of culture, and in terms of environmental experience. For example, it would not be meaningful to ask a traditional African person their exact date of birth (although many may know, due to the influence of westernization), or the current date, for that matter. Failure to produce such responses would be seen as disorientation from a western perspective, but this may not necessarily be the case. In addition, environmental experience must be taken into account—it would be futile to ask a child living in a rural area with few resources, to complete a jigsaw puzzle, or to add 5 + 10. Thus, norms that have been derived from one culture cannot readily be translated into another.

CONCLUDING COMMENTS

Neuropsychologists need to understand which mental functions remain intact and which are disturbed as a result of a particular brain trauma. In order to develop techniques to probe mental function and behavior, the LNI has been adapted (with kind permission of Anne-Lise Christensen), for English-speaking South Africans (Tollman), Afrikaans speaking South Africans (Craig, Du Preez, Tollman, & Watts, 1983), Zulu first-language South Africans, English-speaking children between the ages of 8 and 14 years (Watts, 1989), as well as Zulu first-language children of 8 years of age (Tollman & Msomi, 1999). For each of these, when tasks/questions were adapted to the relevant culture, no differences were found in any community. By using the concepts of double dissociation and an hypothetical deductive process (i.e., test–retest), syndromes have been reliably pinpointed.

It is not surprising that the South African people, who consist of such a colorful mosaic of different groups and cultures, have difficulty in understanding one another. Nevertheless, our brains have the capacity to learn, and through the development of communicatory skills, we can share ideas. Thus, each of the many cultures in South Africa represents a "collective mind" that is developing a structure for coping with the world. It would seem that if we could all work together, a unique South African culture could be developed ... it is my wish that the rest of the world too could develop a "collective mind" to erase the intolerance and unrest that plagues our communal culture.

ACKNOWLEDGMENTS

Thanks to Nina Shapiro, editorial assistant, for her invaluable comments, guidance, and support, and to the Beare Foundation for their generous financial support.

REFERENCES

Bentley, A. M. (1983). Personal and global futurity in Scottish and Swazi students. *Journal of Social Psychology, 121,* 223"229.
Christensen, A. L. (1962). Luria's neuropsychological investigation: Text and manual. Pictorial perception and educational adaptation in Africa. *Psychological Africana, 9,* 226–239.
Christensen, A. L. (1980). Luria's neuropsychological investigation: Text and manual (3rd ed., reproset). Copenhagen: Munksgaard.
Cole, M., & Maltzman, I. (Eds). (1969). *A handbook of contemporary Soviet psychology.* New York: Basic Books.
Craig, A., Du Preez, J., Tollman, S. G., & Watts, A. D. (1983). *Die Afrikaanse vertaling van die Suid Afrikaanse Weergawe van Luria se Neurosielkundige Ondersoek, met toestemming van Anne-Lise Christensen.* Department of Psychology, University of Natal, Durban.
Kruger, J. S., Lubbe, G. J. A., & Steyn, H. C. (1996). *The human search for meaning: A multireligious introduction to the religions of humankind.* Pretoria: Via Afrika.
Lezak, M. D. (1995). *Neuropsychological Assessment* (3rd ed.). New York: Oxford University Press.
Lugg, H. C. (1975). *Life under a Zulu Shield.* Pietermaritzburg: Shuter & Shooter.
Luria, A. R. (1976). *Cognitive development: Its cultural and social foundation.* Cambridge, MA: Harvard University Press.
Mehta, P. H., Rohila, P., Sundberg, N., & Taylor, L. (1972). Future time perspectives of adolescents in India and the United States. *Journal of Cross-cultural Psychology, 3,* 293–302.
Stuss, D. T. (1999). *Functions of the frontal lobes: A 10 year update.* Workshop INS 25th Annual Conference, Boston.
Sunday Times. (1998, May 24).
Sunday Tribune. (2000, December 3).
Thorpe, S. A. (1991). *African traditional religions.* Pretoria: University of South Africa.
Tollman, S. G. (1987). Physiological psychology. In G. A. Tyson (Ed.), *Introduction to psychology: a South African perspective* (pp. 25–58). Johannesburg: Westro Educational Books.
Tollman, S. G. (1999). *Systematizing the process of rehabilitation after head injury: Workshop handout.* INS 22nd Mid-Year International Conference, Durban, South Africa.
Tollman, S. G., & Msomi, P. (1999). *Manual to Luria's neuropsychological investigation for 8 year old Zulu speaking children adapted and translated into Zulu.* Durban: University of Natal Press.
Tollman, S. G., & Msengana, N. B. (1990). Neuropsychological assessment: Problems in evaluating the higher mental functioning of Zulu-speaking people using traditional western techniques. *South African Journal of Psychology, 20*(1), 20–24.
Turnbull, O. H., & Bagus, R. (1991). The translation of the Luria neuropsychological investigation into Zulu: Its relationship to the work of A. R. Luria and L.S. Vygotsky. *South African Journal of Psychology, 21*(2), 6–66.
Vygotsky, L. S. (1978). *Mind in society.* Cambridge, MA.: Harvard University Press.
Watts, A. D. (1989). *The modification of Luria's neuropschological investigation for use with white, English speaking South African children aged eight to fourteen years.* Unpublished doctoral dissertation, University of Natal, Durban.

Author Index

A

Adams, W., 5, 10, *18*
Airhihenbuwa, C. O., 321, 322, *337*
Albee, G. W., 66, *88*
Anastasi, A., 27, *41*, 120, *121*
Anderson, B., 20 *128*
Antell, S., 155, *159*
Aram, D. M., 204, *210*
Arango, J. C., 15, 18
Ardila, A., 18, 21, *23*, 24, 27, 29, 30, *41*, *48*, 80, 89, *98*, 151, *168*, 200, 201, 211, 215, *223*, 241, 242, 246, *247*, 254, 342, 361, *367*
Arean, P., 56. *59*
Azocar, F., 56, *59*

B

Barnett, W. S., 151, 164, *168*
Barsimantov, J., 150, 164, *169*
Bates, 257
Baydar, N., *xxvii*
Beckwith, L., 21, *48*
Beers, T. M., 131, 132, 138, *147*, 150, 166, *168*
Behr, A., 146, *147*
Beller, A. H., 133, *147*

Berger, M. C., *xxvii*, 104, *125*
Berlin, L. J., 21, *48*
Bernstein, J., 103, *126*
Bianchi, S. M., *xxvii*
Bishop, J., 102, *126*
Black, D. A., *xxvii*, 104, *125*
Blank, H., 36, 36n, *50*, 146, *147*, 204, 221, *223*
Blank, R. M., 101, 102, 103, 104, *126*, *127*
Blank, S., 82, 97, *99*
Blau, D. M., *xxvii*, 82, 97, 104, 105, 109, *126*, *133*, *147*, 150, 164, *168*, 252
Blau, F. D., *xxvii*
Blome, J., 226, *247*
Bloom, D., 79, 83, *97*
Bos, J. M., 83, *97*, *100*, 256
Brayfield, A., 133, *147*
Broberg, A., 81, *98*
Brock, T., 83, *97*
Brooks, J. L., 256, *259*
Brooks-Gunn, J., *xxvii*, 150, *169*
Brown-Lyons, M., 150, *168*
Burchinal, M. R., *xxviii*, 151, 165, 166, *168*, 256, 263, 265, *266*
Burton, L. M., 152, *170*
Byers, C., 21, *50*

C

Campbell, F. A., 263, *266*
Cancian, M., 30, *49*
Capizzano, J., *xxvii*, 80, *98*, 151, *168*, 211, *223*, 254
Card, D., 84, *99*, 101, 103, *126*
Carol, B., 80, *99*
Carrol, B., *xxvii*
Casey, J, 257
Caspary, G. L., 80, *98*
Casper, L., 82, *98*
Casper, L. M., 133, *147*
Cassidy, J., 21, *48*
Cave, G., 81, *100*, 253, 255, *259*
Chang, Y., 82, 87, 95, *98*, *99*
Chaplin, D. D., 82, *98*, 133, *147*
Chapman, J., 103, *126*
Chase-Lansdale, P. L., *xxvii*, 79, 80, *98*, 123, *126*, 151, 152, 164, *170*, 256, *259*
Cherlin, A. J., 152, *170*
Chjerlin, A. J., 256, *259*
Choong, Y., 34, *49*
Chu, D., 215, *223*
Clark-Dauffman, E., 257, *259*
Cleveland, G. H., 133, *147*
Clifford, R. M., *xxviii*, 155, *169*, 256, 263, *266*
Coley, R. L., 79, 80, *98*, 151, 164, *170*, 256, *259*
Collins, A. M., 34, 36, *49*, 81, *98*, 131, *147*, 200, 213, *223*
Connelly, R., *xxvii*, 104, 133, *147*
Coonerty, C., 34, *49*
Corcoran, M., 245, *247*
Cox, A. G., 21, *49*, 130, 132, *148*, 150, 164, 166, *170*
Crosby, D. A., 87, 95, *98*, *259*, 265, *266*
Cryer, D., 151, 155, 165, *168*, *169*, 265, *266*
Culkin, M. L., *xxviii*, 256, 263, *266*

D

Danziger, S. K., 226, 245, *247*
Darlington, R., 263, *266*
Davis, E. E., 34, 36, *49*, 213, *223*
Dearing, E., *xxvii*, 256, 265, *266*
Desai, S., *xxvii*
Divine, P. L., 130, *147*
Dodge, W., 257
Dowsett, C., *98*
Duncan, G. J., 79, 83, 97, *99*, 150, 166, *169*, 257, *259*, 265, *266*

Dunn, L., 81, *99*

E

Earle, A., 21, *49*
Edin, K., 82, *100*, 227, *247*
Eggers-Pierola, C., 150, *169*
Ehrle, J., 89, *98*
Eldred, C., 233, *248*
Elixhauser, A., 21, *49*
Emig, C. A., 256, *259*
Emlen, A. C., 40, *49*, 82, *98*, 155, *169*
English, K., 226, *247*
Engstrom, D., 78, *98*
Ensminger, M., 226, *247*
Eshleman, S., 234, *247*
Ewen, D., 204, *223*

F

Fenichel, E., 21, *49*
Ficano, C. K. C., 103, *126*
Figlio, D. N., 102, 104, *126*
Fleck, M. B., 21, *49*
Folk, K. F., 133, *147*
Fronstin, P., 82, *98*, 133, *147*
Fuller, B., *xxvii*, 34, *49*, 80, *98*, *99*, 150, 159, 165, *169*

G

Galanpoulis, A., 252, *259*
Galinsky, E., 159, *169*, 265, *266*
Gallagher, L. J., *49*, 107n, *126*
Gallagher, M., *49*, 107n, *126*
Garfinkel, I., *xxviii*, 226, 245, *248*
Gasman-Pines, A., 87, *98*
Gauthier, C. A., 80, *98*
Geis, S., 96, *99*
Gelbach, J., 104, *126*
Gennetian, L. A., *xxviii*, 82, 84, 87, 95, *98*, *99*, 256, 257, *259*
Georges, A., 34, 36, *49*, 130n, *147*, 213, *223*
Giannarelli, L., 150, 164, *169*
Gibson, C., 166, *169*, 265, *266*
Glantz, F. B., 81, *98*, 131, *147*, 200, *223*
Glazewski, B., 21, *49*
Gordon, R., 123, *126*
Granger, R., 97, 265, *266*
Greenberg, M., *xxviii*, 30, *49*, 78, 79, *98*, *99*, *100*, 104, *127*, 151, *170*, 200, 222, *223*, 224, 242, *248*
Green Book, 107n

AUTHOR INDEX

Greene, W. H., 241, *247*
Griesinger, H., *xxviii*, 54n, 56, 70, *73*
Griffin, A., 21, *49*
Grossberg, A., *xxvii*
Guerra, N., 21, *50*

H

Hagy, A. P., 104, *126*, 133, *147*, 150, 164, *168*
Hair, E. D., 257, *259*
Han, W., 226, 245. *248*
Harknett, K., 84, *99*
Harms, T., 155, *169*
Harris, K. M., *126*
Heckman, _, 104
Heeb, R., 104, *126*
Heflin, C., 245, *247*
Heintze, T., *xxvii*, 104, *127*, 150, *169*, 200, *223*, 245, *248*
Helburn, S. W., 151, *169*
Henderson, C. R., 45, *49*
Hendra, R., 83, *97*
Henly, J. R., 226, 235, *247*
Heymann, J., 21, *49*
Hiatt, S., 45, *49*
Hofferth, S. L., 82, *98*, 133, *147*, 150, *169*
Holcomb, P., 211, *223*
Holloway, S. D., 150, 165, *169*
Hotz, V. J., 102, 104, 106n, *126*
Howes, C., *xxviii*, 21, *49*, 81, *98*, *99*, 151, 152, 159, *169*, *170*, 252, 255, 256, *259*, 263, 265, *266*
Hsu, H., 81, *99*
Hsueh, J., 151, *170*
Hughes, M., 234, *247*
Hurst, A., 96, *100*
Huston, A., 82, 83, 87, 95, 96, *97*, *98*, *99*, 251, 256, 257, 265, *266*
Huston, A. C., *259*
Huston, R. Q., 78, *98*
Hutchins, J., 242, *248*
Hwang, C. P., 81, *98*
Hyatt, D. E., 133, *147*

I

Ivnik, R. J., 48, 55, *60*

J

Johansen, A. S., 150, *169*

Joseph, J. G., 235, *248*

K

Kagan, S. L., *xxvii*, *xxviii*, 80, *98*, *99*, 159, *169*, 256, 263, *266*
Kalil, A., 226, 245, *247*
Kalmanson, B., 21, *49*
Kass, B., 21, *49*
Kemple, J. J., 83, *97*
Kendler, K. S., 234, *247*
Kerachasky, S., 131, *148*
Kessler, R. C., 234, 235, *247*, *248*
Kilburn, M. R., 104, 106n, *126*
Killingsworth, M., 112, *126*
Kimmel, J., 133, *147*
Kipnis, F., 34, *49*
Kirby, G., *49*, 201n, *223*
Kisker, E. E., *xxviii*, 21, *49*, 131, *148*, 152, 159, *170*, 255, *259*
Knox, V. W., *xxviii*, 82, 97, *99*, 257, *259*
Kontos, S., 81, *99*, 159, *169*, 265, *266*
Koralek, R., 211, 215, *223*
Koren, P. E., 40, *49*, 82, *98*
Korfmacher, J., 45, *49*
Kosinski, M., 234, *248*
Kreader, J. L., 34, 36, *49*, 81, *98*, 131, *147*, 200, 213, *223*
Kuhlthau, K., 226, *247*
Kurka, R., 201n, *223*

L

Laird, 257
Lally, J. R., 21, *49*
Lamb, M. E., 78, 81, *98*, *99*, 150, 151, 164, *169*, 253, *259*, 262, *263*, 265, *266*
Lane, J., 215, *223*
Layzer, J. I., 81, *98*, 131, *147*, 150, *168*, 200, *223*, 264
Lazar, I., 263, *266*
Lee, L.-F., 137, *147*
Lehrer, E., 133, *147*
Leibowitz, A., 133, *147*, 150, *169*
Lein, L., 227, *247*
Lemke, R. J., *xxvii*, 72
Lennon, M. C., 226, *247*
Leos-Urbel, J., 227, 229, *248*
Levine, J., 245, *247*
LeVine, R. A., 150, *169*
Levin-Epstein, J., 78, *98*
Lieberman, J. B., 102, 104, *127*

Lieberman, M., 227, 235, *248*
Li-Grining, C. P., 79, 80, *98*
Loeb, S., *xxvii*, 80, *99*
Lohman, B. J., 256, *259*
Lombardi, J., 242, *248*
London, A., 82, 96, 97, *99*, *100*, 257, *259*
Long, S. G., 201n, *223*
Loprest, P., 29, *50*, 130, *147*, 226, *247*
Lowe, E. D., 82, 83, 87, 96, 97, *99*
Lowe, T., 95, *98*
Lu, H.-H., 130n, *147*
Luckey, D. W., 45, *49*
Lyons, S., 226, *247*

M

Maddala, G. S., 137, *147*
Magnuson, K., 265, *266*
Manolatos, T., 246, *247*
Mariner, C. L., 81, *100*, 253, 255, *259*
Martinson, K., 215, *223*
Mason, K., 226, *247*
Maynard, R., 131, *148*
Mazelis, J., 82, *100*
McCartney, K., *xxvii*, 252, 256, *259*, 265, *266*
McCormick, M. C., 21, *49*
McCune, L., 21, *49*
McGonagle, K. A., 234, *247*
McGroder, S. M., 81, *100*, 253, 255, 256, *259*
McLoyd, V. C., 83, 97, *259*, 265, *266*
McMahon, P., 227, 229, *248*
Melton, L., 83, *97*
Menaghan, E., 227, 235, *248*
Meyer, B. D., 102, 104, *126*
Meyers, M. K., *xxvii*, 104, *127*, 150, *169*, 200, 213, *223*, 226, 245, *247*, *248*
Mezey, J., 78, *99*, 222, *223*, 242, 246, *248*
Michael, R. T., *xxvii*
Michalopoulos, C., *xxviii*, 79, 83, 84, 95, 97, *98*, *99*, 133, *148*
Miller-Johnson, S., 263, *266*
Mistry, R., 265, *266*
Moffitt, R. A., 105n, *127*, 152, *170*, 256, *259*
Moore, K. A., 256, *259*
Morris, P. A., *xxviii*, 83, 97, 256, *259*
Mullan, J., 227, 235, *248*
Mullin, C., 102, 104, *126*
Myers, M., 34, 36, *49*

N

Nada, E., 102, 104, *127*
Nelson, C. B., 234, *247*
Nelson, L., 166, *168*
Newman, K., 226, *248*
Ng, R. K., 45, *49*

O

O'Brien, K., 235, *248*
O'Brien, R., 45, *49*
O'Connell, M., 133, *147*
Olds, D. L., 45, *49*
Olson, J. A., 34, 36, *49*, 213, *223*
Olson, K., 226, *248*
Ooms, T. J., 78, *98*
Ostrosky, F., 24, 25, 31, 33, 39, *42*, *49*, 130, 132, 133, *148*, 150, 164, 166, *170*

P

Papillo, 256
Parrott, S., 246, *248*
Pavetti, L., 226, *248*
Pearlin, L., 227, 235, *248*
Peck, L. R., 34, 36, *49*, 213, *223*
Peisner-Feinberg, E. S., *xxviii*, 256, 263, *266*
Perese, K., *49*, 107n, *126*
Peters, H. E., *xxvii*, 104, *125*
Pettit, L. M., 45, *49*
Pontón, M. O., 10, *20*, 46, 48, 54, *60*, 79, *98*, *99*, *100*, 104, *127*, 151, *170*, 200, 222, *223*, 224, 242, *248*, 268, 269, 271, *280*, *281*
Posner, J. K., 257, *259*
Powell, L. M., 133, *148*
Presser, H. B., 21, *49*, 130, 132, 133, *148*, 150, 164, 166, *170*
Puffer, L., *49*
Pungello, E. P., 263, *266*

Q

Queralt, M., *xxvii*, *xxviii*, 54n, 56, 70, 72, *73*
Quint, J. C., 83, *100*

R

Raikes, H., 21, *49*, 78, *100*

AUTHOR INDEX

Ramanan, J., *xxviii*, 257
Rambaud, M. F., 150, *169*
Ramey, C., 263, *266*
Rangarajan, A., 215, *223*
Raphael, J., 226, *248*
Redd, Z. A., 256, *259*
Ribar, D. C., *xxviii*, 104
Ripke, M. N., 257, *259*
Robertson, A., 150, *168*
Robins, P. K., *xxvii*, *xxviii*, 82, 84, *98*, *99*, 101, 103, 104, *126*, 133, *147*, *148*
Robinson, J., 45, *49*
Roff, J., 256, *259*
Rohacek, M., 34, 37, *48*, 200, *223*, 241, 242, 246, *247*
Romich, J., 265, *266*
Rosen, D., 226, 235, 245, *247*, *248*
Rosenbaum, D. T., 102, 104, *126*
Rosman, E. A., 151, *170*
Ross, C., 37, *49*

S

Sandfort, J., 34, *48*, 200, 201n, *223*
Savner, S., 30, *49*
Schexnayder, D., 34, 36, *49*, 213, *223*
Schochet, P., 215, *223*
Schoeni, R. F., 102, 103, 104, *127*
Scholz, J. K., 102, 104, *126*
Schreiber, S., *49*, 107n, *126*
Schroeder, D., 34, 36, *49*, 213, *223*
Schulman, K., 36, 36n, *50*, 146, *147*, 204, 221, *223*
Schultze, K. H., 40, *49*, 82, *98*
Schumacher, R., *xxviii*, 78, 79, *98*, *99*, *100*, 104, *127*, 151, *170*, 200, *222*, *223*, *224*, 242, *248*
Scott, E. K., 82, 96, 97, *99*, *100*
Scrivener, S., 83, *97*
Seefeldt, K., 245, *247*
Seefeldt, K. S., 227, 229, *248*
Segal, M., 21, *49*
Shapiro, M. D., 132n, *148*
Sheff, K. L., 45, *49*
Shinn, M., 159, *169*, 265, *266*
Shonkoff, J. P., 21, *50*
Siefert, K., 245, *247*
Sillari, J., 21, *49*
Simpson, L., 21, *49*
Smith, K., *xxviii*, 82, *100*, 103, 124, *127*
Snow, K. K., 234, *248*

Snyder, K., 34, 36, *48*, 200, 201n, 211, *223*, 227, 229, *248*
Sonenstein, F., *xxvii*, 80, *98*, 151, *168*, 254
Spiegelman, R. G., 133, *148*
Staines, G. L., 132, *148*
Sternberg, K. J., 150, *169*
Straus, M. A., 235, *248*
Szanton, E., 21, *49*

T

Taylor, B. A., *xxvii*, 256, 265, *266*
Tekin, E., 104, 105, 109, *126*, 130n, *148*
Thompson, J., 21, *49*
Tolman, R. M., 226, 235, 245, *247*, *248*
Tout, K., 89, *98*, 256, *259*
Turetsky, V., 78, *98*
Tvedt, K., 130, *147*

U

Urrutia, C. P.,
Uswatte, G.,
Uzzell, B., 108, *367*

V

Vandell, D. L., *xxviii*, 68, *73*, 253, 257, *259*
Vargas, W. G., 257, *259*
Ventura, A., 265, *266*
Verma, N., 83, *97*
Voran, M., *xxviii*, 21, *49*, 152, 159, *170*, 255, *259*
Votruba-Drzal, E., 151, 164, *170*, 256, *259*

W

Wagmiller, R. L., Jr., 130n, *147*
Waite, L. J., 133, *147*, 150, *169*
Wald, E. R., 21, *50*
Waldfogel, J., 226, 245, *248*
Waldman, D. M., *xxvii*, 104, *125*
Walker, J., *xxviii*
Walter, J., 83, *97*
Ware, J. E., 234, *248*
Waters, S., 201n, *223*
Watson, K., *49*, 107n, *126*
Weber, R., 34, 36, *49*, 213, *223*
Weisner, T. S., 82, 83, 96, 97, *99*, *259*
Weissbourd, B., 21, *49*

Werner, A., 81, *98*, 131, *147*, 200, *223*
Wessels, H., 81, *98*
Whitebook, M., *xxviii*, 21, *49*, 151, 152, 159, *170*, 252, 255, *259*
Wilkinson, G., 235, *248*
Wilson, W. J., 152, *170*
Winston, P., 152, *170*
Wissoker, D. A., 82, *98*, 133, *147*
Witsberger, C., 133, *147*
Witt, R., *xxvii*, *xxviii*, 54n, 70, 72, 73
Wittchen, H. U., 234, *247*
Witte, A. D., *xxvii*, *xxviii*, 54n, 56, 70, 72, 73
Wolf, D. A., *xxvii*, 104, *127*, 150, *169*, 200, *223*, 245, *248*
Wolfe, B., 68, *73*, 253
Wortman, C. B., 235, *248*

Y

Yazejian, N., *xxviii*, 256, 263, *266*
Yoshikawa, H., 81, *100*, 151, 164, *170*, 253, *259*

Z

Zaslow, M. J., 81, *100*, 233, *248*, 253, 255, 256, 257, *259*
Zedlewski, S. R., 29, *50*, 226, *248*
Zhao, S., 234, *247*
Ziliak, J. P., 102, 104, *126*

Subject Index

A

Absolutism, 2
Acculturation, 4–5
Alexia and agraphia, 255–257
Ancestral influences in a society
    African customs of burial, 374–375
    behavioral pathology of differing religions and cultures, 375–376
APIL-B, *see also* TRAM-1, TRAM-2
    constructs measured, 238–240
    material, 236–238
    statistical properties, 244
    usage without bias and validity, 231
    validity, 244–245
Asian Indian ethnicity, gender, and age match
    interlanguage issues, 312
    language of testing, 312
    pragmatics, 309–311
    report of results, 313
    source of information, 311
    stimuli and task selection, 311–312
    use of translators, 312–313
Asian Indian interview and evaluation, 308–309
Asian Indian therapy or treatment of medical condition
    age differences, 314–315
    first psession expectations, 313–314
    gift giving, 315
    religious issues, 315
    role of family, 314–315
    topics and tasks selection, 315
Assimilation, 57
Attachment theory, behaviors derived from, 4–5

B

The Bell Curve, 63, 65, 67, 68, 86, 99, 245
Bias in IQ testing
    broadening the canvas, 68
    inflating scores, 67–68
Black–white test score gap
    African American (AAE), 131–137
    testing older African Americans, 137–140
Brain damage and illiteracy, 189–190

C

Cognition and culture, 51–54
Cognitive reserve and outcome measures, 216–218
Cognitive test performance

389

conventions of communication, 26–27
education, 30–34
factors influencing, 120–121, 128–140
familiarity, 29–30
language, 30
modes of knowing, 26
values and meaning, 26–29
Community-based rehabilitation
   advantages and challenges, 366
   politics of implementing the natural recovery model, 364–366
Constructivist theories of development
   Piaget's, 146–148
   Vygotsky, 148–151
Cross–cultural assessments
   assessment for neurorehabilitation, 13–14
   cross–cultural neurorehabilitation, 12–13
   cultural concepts in assessment, 11–12
   cultural concepts in rehabilitation, 14–18
   language factors during assessment, 8–11
   quantitative assessment, 97–100
Cross-cultural neuropsychological data collection
   IQ tests, 378–379
   Marxist-Leninist ideology, 378
   nature-nurture influence, 379
   psychometric tests, 379–380
   psychometric tests versus qualitative information, 379
Cross-cultural quantitative assessment, 97–100
Cross-cultural reality and multiculturalism
   culture, acculturation, and assimilation, 4–7
   ethnicity, 7–8
Cultural and cognition, 94–95
Cultural values
   background authority, 28
   best performance, 28
   cultural values, 27
   internal or subjective issues, 28–29
   isolated environment, 28
   one-to-one relationship, 27
   patterns of abilities, 27
   special type of communication, 28
   speed, 28
   use of specific testing elements and testing strategies, 29
Cultural contrasts relevant to neuropsychological rehabilitation
   cultural contexts, 344–346
Culturally variable concepts, 100–102
Culture, definition of, ix–x, 4, 24
Cultural diversity, ix, 1, 2, 6, 8, 45, 97, 304

E

Education and age-related cognitive decline during normal aging, 219–222
Education in the context of brain-behavior relationships
   dementia, 208–210
   hemispheric competence for language and other functions, 203–205
   language, 205–208
   target populations for studying, 202–203
Emotions and attitudes
   ancestral influences, 374–376
   cultural differences in emotional presentations and meaning, 373–374
   data analysis, 378–380
   nuclear and extended systems, 376–378
   social and emotional influences, 372–373
English-Afrikaans IQ Differences
   continued but diminishing gap, 85–86
   difference of six scale points, 84–85
Environmentalism triumphant, nativism resurgent, 64–66
Epistemological foundation
   phenomology, 103–104
   systems theory, 104–105
Ethnicity, 7–8
Executive function in Hispanics
   an evolving construct, 165–172
   studies, 172–176

F

Facilitation of recovery
   activity analysis, 353–354

SUBJECT INDEX

contextual assessment, 352–353
environmental analysis, 354–356
family and community training (natural helpers), 356–359
goals, 352
incorporating cognitive and emotional strategies, 359–360
training generalization, 359
zone of recovery, 350–352

H

Heredity an and the social construction of hope, 66
Hispanic patient assessment process
  patient's preferred language, 269–271
  pediatric assessment, 273–277
  use of measures, 271–273
Hispanic patient evaluated
  assessment process, 268–277
  culture, 268
  language, 266–268
HIV/AIDS, 330–336
Holistic, qualitative approach, 102–103

I

Idiographic (individual-based) epistemological sources, 46–49
Illiteracy disadvantage debate, 191–194
Immigration issues within Asian Indian community
  education, 305
  model minority myth, 305–306
  vocation, 305
India historical and geographical background
  belief system, 306
  communication styles, 307–308
  gender differences, 306
  immigration issues, 305–306
  multiculturalism, 304
  multilingualism, 304
  notions of guilt and shame, 307
  role of family, 306
  role of women, 307
Information processing paradigm, 73
Irrelevancy of the angular gyrus hypothesis, 254–255

L

Language

classification systems, 118–119
language disturbances in different languages, 119–120
phoneme discrimination, 116–117
universals in language, 117–118
Linking psychometrics and information processing
  componential subtheory, 80–83
  contextual subtheory, 74
  experiential subtheory, 74–77
  Wechsler intelligence scales, 77–80

M

Marxist-Leninist ideology, 378
Measures,
  modification of, 54–57
Memory, 115–116
Minority group testing
  anger, 37
  cultural solitude, 36
  culture, 35
  decreased self-esteem, 36
  depression, 37
  feelings of failure and/or success, 37
  frustration, 36
  homesickness, 37
  isolation, 36
  language, 35
  nationality, 35
  normality, 35
  paranoia, 36
  reference group, 36
  social image, 36
Modifying measures for cross-cultural use, 54–57

N

Natural recovery model
  community based rehabilitation, 363–366
  conventional neurorehabilitation, 348
  cosmopolitan rehabilitation, 347–348
  definition of, 346–347
  direct neuropsychological rehabilitation services, 361–363
  facilitation of recovery, 349–360
  overprotection, 360–361
Neuropsychological assessment, 95–97
Neuropsychological evaluation of the developing child, 154–158

Neuropsychological problems in development
  cerebral palsy, 151–152
  learning disabilities, 153–154
  traumatic brain injury, 152–153
Neuropsychological test performance in illiterates
  language, 185–187
  memory, 187–188
  praxic and motor abilities, 188–189
  visuospatial and visuoconstructive abilities, 187
Neuropsychology as an epistemic task, 46–57
Nomothetic (law-based) epistemological sources, 47
Normal versus abnormal test performance, 50–51
Norms in different national and cultural groups
  culture, 38–41
  language, 38
Nuclear and extended family systems
  African versus Western view, 376–377
  self awareness, 377–378

P

Patterns of abilities, 27
Perceptual abilities
  perceptual constancy, 112
  sensory discrimination, 111–112
  visual illusions, 112–113
PET scan studies on reading process in Japanese language, 258–261
Piaget's theory of development, 146–148
Practice effects, 71–72
Problems of bias
  pernicious consequences of *inflating* IQ scores, 67–68
Psychometric and information-processing paradigms
  information processing paradigm, 73
  psychometric paradigm, 69–70
  education, 70–71
Psychometric paradigm, 69–70

R

Relativism, 3

S

Science and neuropsychology, 45–46
South African case studies
  Africanization of Westerners, 72–73
  brain injuries, 322–326
  education and urbanization, 70–71
  English-Afrikaans IQ differences, 83–88
  HIV/AIDS, 330–336
  IQ scores, 68–69
  evaluation of the developing child, 154–158
  practice effects, 71–72
  stroke, 326–330
  TRAM-2, 242–243
  unbundling social and emotional influences, , 372–373
Spanish speakers' clinical neuropsychology,
  acculturation, 285–286
  culture defined, 284–285
  demographics, 286
  heterogeneity, 285
Spatial abilities
  cultural differences in visuospatial abilities, 114–115
  reference systems, 113–114
Statistical properties of visuospatial genotype testing
  APIL-B, 244–245
  TRAM-1, 241–242
  TRAM-2, 242–243
Stroke in rural South Africa
  perceptions of stroke, 329–330
  summary of age and sex patterns, 327–329

T

TRAM-1, *see also* APIL-B
  material, 233–234
  statistical properties, 241–242
TRAM-2, *see also* APIL-B
  concept formation test, 235
  material, 234–235
  memory and understanding test, 236
  statistical properties, 242–243
  SymTran test, 235
  usage without bias and validity, 231

Translating neuropsychological concepts in tests into Spanish
case of measuring intelligence, 287–289
clinical neuropsychology in Spain evaluation, 289–292
instruments, 292–298
rehabilitation, 298–299
samples of neuropsychological tests available in Spanish, 287

U

Universalism, 3
Use of measures, 49–51

V

Visuospatial arena, 229–231
Visuospatial genotype testing
applications to visuospatial assessment tools, 247–249
APIL-B, 236–240
TRAM-1, 231–234
TRAM-2, 234–236
Vygotsky's theory of development, 148–151

W

Wechsler intelligence scales, 77–80